PREPECTORAL TECHNIQUES IN RECONSTRUCTIVE BREAST SURGERY

Allen Gabriel, MD, FACS
Clinical Professor of Plastic Surgery
Loma Linda University Medical Center
Loma Linda, California
and
Private Practice
Vancouver, Washington

G. Patrick Maxwell, MD
Clinical Professor of Surgery
Department of Plastic Surgery
Loma Linda University Medical Center
Loma Linda, California

Maurice Y. Nahabedian, MD, FACS
Professor of Plastic Surgery
Virginia Commonwealth University—Inova Branch
National Center for Plastic Surgery
McLean, Virginia

Steven R. Sigalove, MD, FACS
Department of Plastic Surgery
Northwestern Medicine Central DuPage Hospital
Winfield, Illinois

Wolters Kluwer

Philadelphia • Baltimore • New York • London
Buenos Aires • Hong Kong • Sydney • Tokyo

Executive Editor: Brian Brown
Development Editor: Ashley Fischer
Editorial Coordinator: John Larkin
Production Coordinator: Sadie Buckallew
Design Coordinator: Holly McLaughlin
Manufacturing Coordinator: Beth Welsh
Prepress Vendor: S4Carlisle Publishing Services

9 8 7 6 5 4 3 2 1

Printed in China

Library of Congress Cataloging-in-Publication Data

Names: Gabriel, Allen, editor. | Nahabedian, Maurice Y., editor.
Title: Prepectoral techniques in reconstructive breast surgery / [edited by] Allen Gabriel, Maurice Nahabedian.
Description: First edition. | Philadelphia : Wolters Kluwer Health, [2019] | Includes bibliographical references and index.
Identifiers: LCCN 2018039785 | ISBN 9781496388278
Subjects: | MESH: Breast Implantation—methods | Mammaplasty—methods | Pectoralis Muscles—surgery | Breast Implants | Acellular Dermis | Mastectomy
Classification: LCC RD539.8 | NLM WP 910 | DDC 618.1/90592—dc23 LC record available at https://lccn.loc.gov/2018039785

Care has been taken to confirm the accuracy of the information presented and to describe generally accepted practices. However, the authors, editors, and publisher are not responsible for errors or omissions or for any consequences from application of the information in this book and make no warranty, expressed or implied, with respect to the currency, completeness, or accuracy of the contents of the publication. Application of this information in a particular situation remains the professional responsibility of the practitioner; the clinical treatments described and recommended may not be considered absolute and universal recommendations.

The authors, editors, and publisher have exerted every effort to ensure that drug selection and dosage set forth in this text are in accordance with the current recommendations and practice at the time of publication. However, in view of ongoing research, changes in government regulations, and the constant flow of information relating to drug therapy and drug reactions, the reader is urged to check the package insert for each drug for any change in indications and dosage and for added warnings and precautions. This is particularly important when the recommended agent is a new or infrequently employed drug.

Some drugs and medical devices presented in this publication have Food and Drug Administration (FDA) clearance for limited use in restricted research settings. It is the responsibility of the health care provider to ascertain the FDA status of each drug or device planned for use in his or her clinical practice.

shop.lww.com

CCS1018

CONTRIBUTORS

John G. Apostolides, MD, FACS
Chief
Defy Plastic and Reconstructive Surgery
Scripps La Jolla Hospitals
San Diego, California

C. Coleman Brown, MD, FACS
Chief
Department of Plastic Surgery
Sibley Memorial Hospital, Johns Hopkins Medicine
Washington, District of Columbia

Gregory Christopherson, PhD
Associate Director
Research and Development
LifeCell (an Allergan Affiliate)
Bridgewater, New Jersey

Rafi Fredman, MD
Plastic Surgery Resident
Division of Plastic and Reconstructive Surgery
University of North Carolina
Chapel Hill, North Carolina

Allen Gabriel, MD, FACS
Clinical Professor of Plastic Surgery
Loma Linda University Medical Center
Loma Linda, California
and
Private Practice
Vancouver, Washington

Scot Bradley Glasberg, MD
Department of Plastic Surgery
Lenox Hill Hospital/Manhattan Eye, Ear, and Throat Hospital
Northwell Health System
Hofstra School of Medicine
New York, New York

John R. Harper, PhD
Chief Technology Officer
Research and Technology
KCI, an Acelity Company
San Antonio, Texas

John Hijawi, MD, FACS
Director of Breast Reconstruction Program
Division of Plastic Surgery
Intermountain Healthcare
Salt Lake City, Utah

Steven R. Jacobson, MD
Jacobson Plastic Surgery
Rochester, Minnesota

Glyn Jones, MD
Professor of Surgery
Department of Surgery
University of Illinois College of Medicine
Peoria, Illinois

Victor King, MD
Department of Plastic Surgery
Rhode Island Hospital
Providence, Rhode Island

G. Patrick Maxwell, MD
Clinical Professor of Surgery
Department of Plastic Surgery
Loma Linda University Medical Center
Loma Linda, California

Maurice Y. Nahabedian, MD, FACS
Professor of Plastic Surgery
Virginia Commonwealth University—Inova Branch
National Center for Plastic Surgery
McLean, Virginia

Michelle C. Roughton, MD
Assistant Professor
Department of Surgery
Division of Plastic and Reconstructive Surgery
University of North Carolina
Chapel Hill, North Carolina

Arthur H. Salibian, MD
Clinical Professor
Aesthetic and Plastic Surgery Institute
University of California
Irvine Medical Center
Orange, California

Hani Sbitany, MD
Division of Plastic and Reconstructive Surgery
Department of Surgery
University of California, San Francisco
San Francisco, California

Noemi M. Sigalove, MD, FACS
Comprehensive Breast Center of Arizona
Scottsdale, Arizona

Steven R. Sigalove, MD, FACS
Department of Plastic Surgery
Northwestern Medicine Central DuPage Hospital
Winfield, Illinois

Toni Storm-Dickerson, MD
Co-director
Compass Oncology Breast Specialists
Medical Director—Surgical Services
Kearney Breast Center, PeaceHealth
Vancouver, Washington

Aran Yoo, MD
Surgery Resident
Department of Plastic Surgery
Louisiana State University
New Orleans, Louisiana

PREFACE

The world of prosthetic breast reconstruction has passed many milestones since its inception in the 1960s. The introduction of the breast implant, in 1962, has opened the door to a myriad of innovations and advancements that have helped women around the world in the setting of cosmetic and reconstructive surgery. Prosthetic devices have evolved into a variety of shapes, sizes, textures, and filler materials and are available as tissue expanders and permanent implants. Breast reconstruction techniques have advanced based on our ability to predictably provide one- or two-stage reconstruction following skin or nipple-sparing mastectomy. The use of acellular dermal matrices and autologous fat grafting has refined our technique such that surgical outcomes now mimic those of breast augmentation. Despite these advancements, it is the nature of plastic surgeons to innovate and continuously strive to pursue perfection in order to better meet the needs of our patients.

One of the controversies and discussion points with prosthetic breast reconstruction has centered on where the ideal location of the implant should be. Early on, devices were placed in the subcutaneous space because the pectoralis major muscle was frequently removed with the more radical mastectomy techniques of the time. Complication and reconstructive failure rates were high because the mastectomies were aggressive and extensive.[1] With the advent of the modified radical mastectomy, the pectoralis major muscle was preserved, and prosthetic devices could now be placed under the muscle with fewer complications and reconstructive failure compared to subcutaneous. However, issues related to implant displacement, animation deformity, and muscle spasm were frequent occurrences and determined to be sequelae of subpectoral device placement.[2] For decades, this was a source of patient dissatisfaction without a real solution.

Over the years, as breast and plastic surgeons began to "team-up," greater attention has been directed toward optimizing mastectomy skin flaps in order to preserve the subcutaneous fat and maintain perfusion. Acellular dermal matrix use was demonstrated to be effective as a means of maintaining the position of the breast implant on the chest wall and to reduce the incidence of capsular contracture.[3] Autologous fat grafting has been shown to be safe and effective in correcting contour abnormalities and improving skin quality.[4] Thus, the concept of the "Bioengineered Breast" was born and has revolutionized the performance of prosthetic breast reconstruction.[5] As this concept has propagated, the evolution to prepectoral reconstruction has again revolutionized the world of prosthetic breast reconstruction.[6-8] By leaving the pectoralis major muscle completely undisturbed, the incidence of muscle spasm, animation deformity, and implant displacement has been reduced. Thus, prepectoral breast reconstruction represents the latest advancement in prosthetic breast reconstruction and is the focus of this book.

This book represents the first of its kind and is focused on the technical nuances, strategies, and options associated with prepectoral breast reconstruction. The contributors to this text are all surgeons with extensive experience with this technique and represent the thought leaders with the various techniques. It begins with the chapter from Pat Maxwell, MD, who has arguably been the most influential plastic surgeon in promoting the use and techniques of prosthetic breast reconstruction. He and Dr. Gabriel chronicle the history of prosthetic breast reconstruction from its origin in the 1960s to the present. There are chapters from leading breast surgeons such as Toni Storm-Dickerson and Noemi Sigalove, who are experts in nipple-sparing mastectomy and the guiding principles for performing an oncologically sound mastectomy. Steve Jacobsen and Steve Sigalove are two pioneers with this technique and have performed hundreds of prepectoral reconstructions. Their chapters will focus on specific techniques and maneuvers that will optimize outcomes. The role of proper patient selection, direct to implant, staged prepectoral and conversion from subpectoral to prepectoral reconstruction will be reviewed by notable surgeons, including Glyn Jones, Maurice Nahabedian, Hani Sbitany, John Hijawi, Cole Brown, Michelle Roughton, and John Apostolides.

In conclusion, we hope that this book on prepectoral prosthetic breast reconstruction will provide a start-to-finish review of the salient aspects of this procedure in order to make it predictable, reproducible, and safe. It represents an up-to-date and state-of-the-art approach to breast reconstruction, which we believe represents the next paradigm shift. As plastic surgeons, we now practice our craft in an era of maximal preservation of natural form and function in order to enhance aesthetics and to reduce morbidity. Preservation of the pectoralis major muscle and prepectoral placement of prosthetic devices should be the overriding goal of all breast and plastic surgeons alike.

Maurice Y. Nahabedian

Allen Gabriel

REFERENCES

1. Schlenker JD, Bueno RA, Ricketson G, Lynch JB. Loss of silicone implants after subcutaneous mastectomy and reconstruction. *Plast Reconstr Surg*. 1978;62:853-861.
2. Becker, H, Fregosi N. The impact of animation deformity on quality of life in post-mastectomy reconstruction patients. *Aesth Surg J*. 2017;37(5):531-536.
3. Salzberg CA, Ashikari AY, Berry C, Hunsicker LM. Acellular dermal matrix-assisted direct-to-implant breast reconstruction and capsular contracture: a 13-year experience. *Plast Reconstr Surg*. 2016;138(2):329-337.
4. Spear SL, Coles CN, Leung BK, Gitlin M, Parekh M, Macarios D. The safety, effectiveness, and efficiency of autologous fat grafting in breast surgery. *Plast Reconstr Surg Glob Open*. 2016;4:e827.
5. Maxwell GP, Gabriel A. Bioengineered breast: concept, technique, and preliminary results. *Plast Reconstr Surg*. 2016;137:415-421.
6. Sigalove S, Maxwell GP, Sigalove NM, et al. Prepectoral implant-based breast reconstruction: rationale, indications, and results. *Plast Reconstr Surg*. 2017;139(2):287-294.
7. Woo A, Harless C, Jacobson SR. Revisiting an old place: single surgeon experience on post-mastectomy subcutaneous implant-based breast reconstruction. *Breast J*. 2017;23(5):545-553.
8. Nahabedian MY, Cocilovo C. Two-stage prosthetic breast reconstruction: a comparison between prepectoral and partial subpectoral techniques. *Plast Reconstr Surg*. 2017;140:22S-30S.

ACKNOWLEDGMENTS

I would like to thank and acknowledge several individuals who were instrumental in the preparation and publication of our book, *Prepectoral Techniques in Reconstructive Breast Surgery*. First and foremost, I would like to thank Allen Gabriel, whose enthusiasm and contributions to this project have inspired all of us. I would also like to thank all of the contributors whose combined efforts have resulted in a truly outstanding book. These are all busy surgeons and scientists who are exceptionally talented and key opinion leaders in prepectoral breast reconstruction. A huge thank-you goes to my friend and mentor, Scott Spear, MD, who suddenly and unexpectedly passed on in March 2017. He was a thought-leader and the source of inspiration to many as he continuously challenged us to innovate and advance the specialty of plastic surgery. I am sincerely grateful to the staff at Wolters Kluwer for their hard work, energy, and commitment to this book and for believing that we could create this remarkable book. Finally, I would like to thank my wife Anissa and my two daughters, Danielle and Sophia, for standing by my side throughout my career and providing support, patience, and understanding. Thank-you to all as this project represents a culmination of all of our hard work and effort in preparing what I believe to be a state-of-the-art book on prepectoral breast reconstruction.

Maurice Y. Nahabedian

I would like to acknowledge all who supported and contributed toward the preparation and publication of our book, *Prepectoral Techniques in Reconstructive Breast Surgery*. First and foremost, I thank all of my coeditors, Maurice Nahabedian, Steven Sigalove, and Pat Maxwell, for their support, guidance, and contributions. Also, this book would not have been possible without all the dedicated and talented contributors, who took time out of their busy schedules to prepare their outstanding chapters. I would also like to thank my mentor, Pat Maxwell, who has supported me through the years and introduced me to a prepectoral approach, in 2008. This idea would not have become so popular without his vision on how breast surgery should be performed in the future. The staff at Wolters Kluwer worked tirelessly, and we appreciate the energy and commitment they invested in this book and their belief that we could create this remarkable book. I also want to acknowledge my parents, sister, and extended family, who have all made sacrifices and supported me in my goals of becoming a physician and surgeon. Finally, I thank my wife Cassie, who has always stood by me and has provided me with patience through the preparation of this book. Thank-you to all as this project introduces a new era in breast reconstructive surgery and crowns our hard work and effort in preparing what I believe to be a state-of-the-art book on prepectoral breast reconstruction.

Allen Gabriel

CONTENTS

CHAPTER 1

THE EVOLUTION OF PROSTHETIC BREAST RECONSTRUCTION: FROM SUBPECTORAL TO PREPECTORAL UTILIZING THE BIOENGINEERED CONCEPT

Allen Gabriel and G. Patrick Maxwell

KEY POINTS

- Regenerative scaffolds of acellular matrices and regenerative cells of physiologically processed fat have changed the face of breast enhancement and breast reconstruction.
- Animation deformities caused by muscle contraction, chest tightness, pain, and muscle spasm are other significant concerns in dual-plane reconstructions.
- The evolution of breast reconstruction has been possible only with close collaboration of breast surgeons delivering viable flaps and the availability of form-stable implants, ADMs, and high-quality processed fat for creation of bioengineered breasts.
- Principles of breast surgery and the utilization of form-stable implants and regenerative constructs and cells are applied to all aspects of breast surgeries, such as in primary augmentations and reconstructions as well as in secondary revisionary augmentation and reconstructions.

INTRODUCTION

Implant-based breast reconstruction is the most frequently performed reconstructive technique following breast ablative surgery.[1] For the past 15 years, this technique has been performed primarily with subpectoral implant placement via the dual-plane approach. The coverage and support provided by the pectoralis major muscle has not only minimized implant-related complications but has also mitigated the risk of capsular contracture and produced a more natural-looking breast. However, a concern with this approach is the risk of functional impairment of the pectoralis muscle and animation deformities, both of which are a direct consequence of muscle elevation.[2,3] Changing the implant site to a prepectoral placement may help resolve some of these concerns. Application of the bioengineered breast concept—utilizing a combination of form-stable and/or higher fill implants, regenerative dermal matrices, and fat grafting— can produce predictable results with both the prepectoral and the dual-plane approach.[4]

The authors introduced the term "bioengineered breast" in 2009, defining it as an enhanced breast form consisting of a combination of form-stable or higher fill breast implant, regenerative scaffold, and regenerative cells (**Figure 1.1**).[1] Use of regenerative scaffolds of acellular matrices and regenerative cells of physiologically processed fat has changed the face of breast enhancement and breast reconstruction. No longer is the implant alone the sole factor in replacing or enhancing the female breast form, but now, the soft-tissue cover overlying the implant is further enhanced. Enhancing the soft-tissue cover not only supplements volume and shape but further alters how the recipient's host tissue responds to the foreign body implant. This powerful combination of constructs better allows us to achieve the ultimate goal of breast

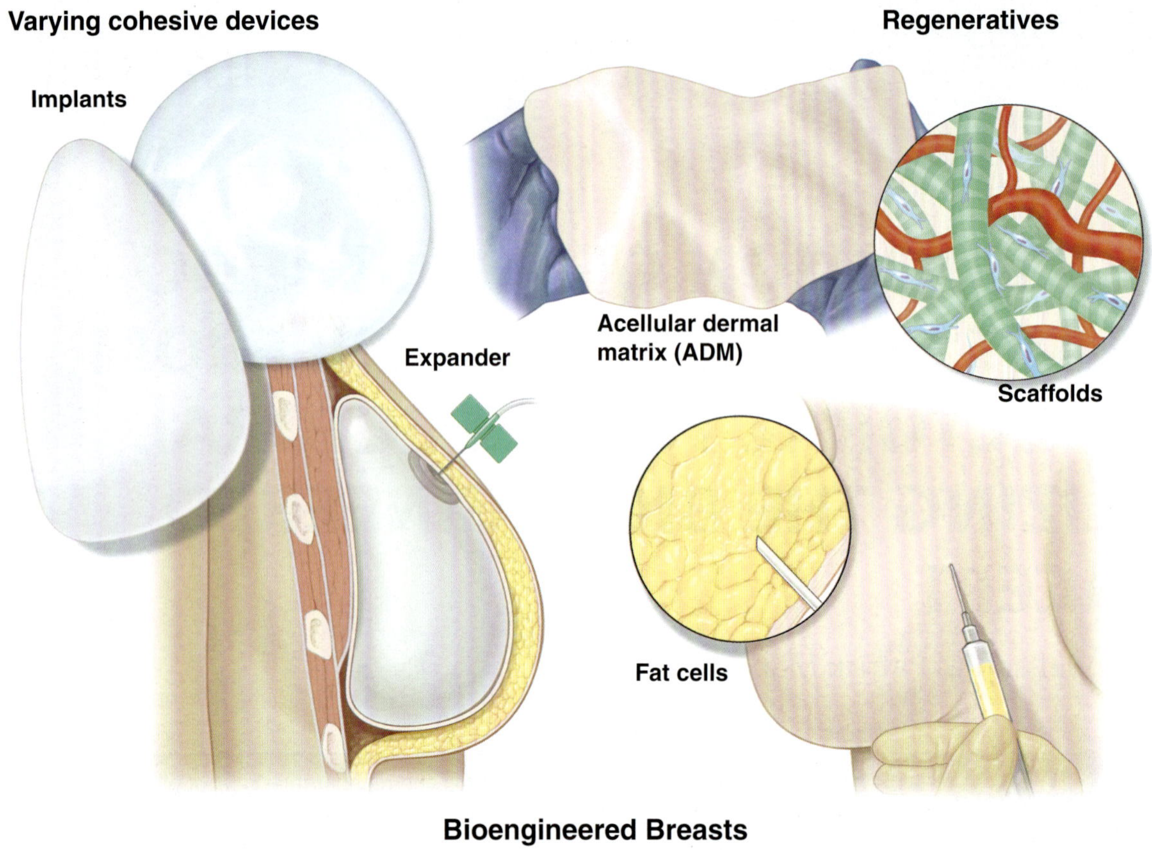

Figure 1.1 The advances in the availability of more cohesive and higher fill implants, and scaffolds, (acellular dermal matrices) and regenerative cells, (processed fat with good quality), have revolutionized modern day breast reconstruction utilizing this bioengineered concept to "Aesthetic Breast Reconstruction."

reconstruction—to recreate a breast that looks and feels like the natural breast (**Figure 1.2**). The bioengineered breast can be created by the use of an acellular matrix with an expander or implant in a first-stage reconstruction procedure and fat grafting in a second-stage procedure, or combining all three elements in a reconstructive or aesthetic revision. This concept combined with prepectoral reconstruction makes the reconstruction and results more aesthetically pleasing.

HISTORY OF SUBPECTORAL PLACEMENT

Silicone breast implants, introduced in the early 1960s, marked the beginning of the modern era of implant-based breast reconstruction. The first breast reconstructions, performed in the early 1960s with the introduction of the silicone implant, involved placement of the implant in a subcutaneous pocket, beneath the mastectomy skin but over the pectoralis major muscle. This subcutaneous approach was simple and quick and preserved the integrity of the pectoralis muscle, but it was associated with a number of complications. Implant malposition (bottoming out), visibility, and palpability; rippling/wrinkling; implant exposure subsequent to skin breakdown; and capsular contracture were some of the most commonly reported complications.[5] With the realization that these complications arose from insufficient soft-tissue coverage, the breast reconstruction technique evolved to moving the implant from the subcutaneous to the submuscular position.

In submuscular placement, the implant is placed under the pectoralis major muscle without releasing the inferior origin of the muscle. Full-muscle coverage of the implant is achieved by recruitment of muscle flaps (serratus anterior and rectus abdominis sheath) for lateral and inferior coverage of the implant. Full-muscle coverage eliminated the soft-tissue coverage limitations of the subcutaneous approach, but it resulted in unnatural-looking breasts. The inferior restrictions imposed by the submuscular pocket prevents lower pole expansion that results in poor breast projection, ptosis, and definition of the breast shape.[6] In addition, recruitment of muscle flaps introduced donor site morbidity.

To address the inferior restriction of full-muscle coverage, the partial muscle coverage or dual-plane technique was introduced. In partial muscle coverage, the implant is covered partially superiorly by the pectoralis major and partially inferiorly by only the mastectomy flap.[5,7,8] The inferior subcutaneous coverage not only allows for lower pole expansion but also eliminates the need for

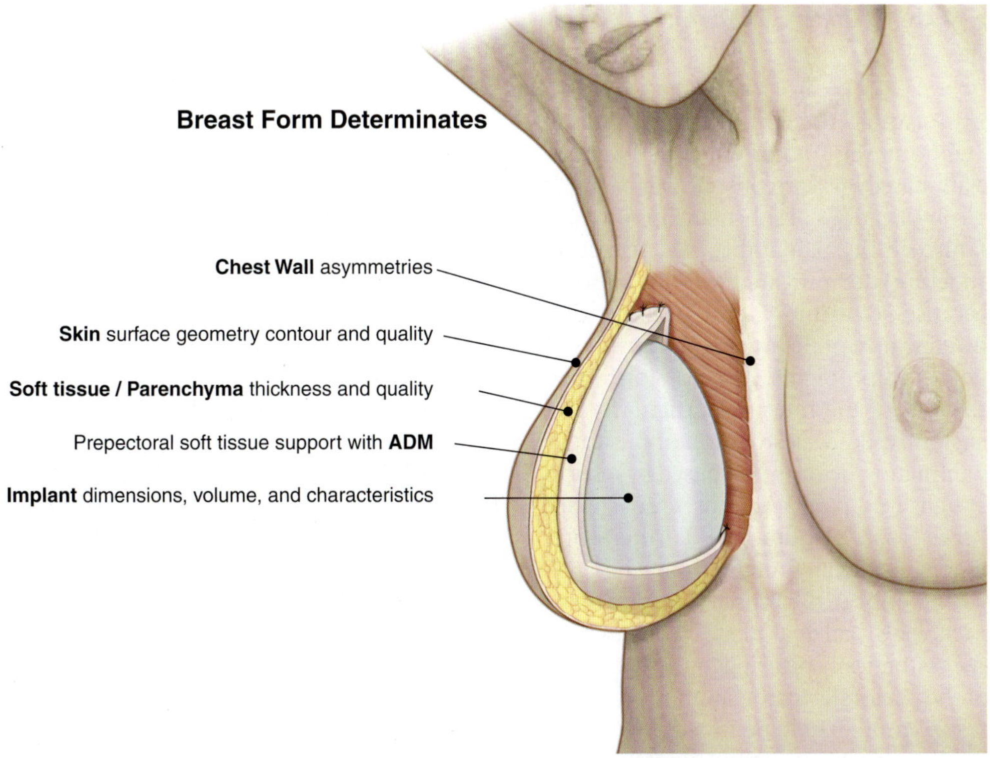

Figure 1.2 All layers of the breast form should be addressed planning the reconstruction.

flap recruitment for lower pole coverage. Partial muscle coverage, however, introduced a new problem. Without its inferior attachment, the pectoralis major is free to migrate superiorly, which causes "window shading". Moreover, subcutaneous coverage at the lower pole reintroduced the problems seen with subcutaneous implant placement.

To address the problem of lower pole coverage, acellular dermal matrices (ADMs) were introduced in breast reconstruction in 2006. In this widely utilized modification of the partial muscle coverage technique, ADM sutured at the lower pole provides the additional support needed at the inferior pole.[9-12] With lower pole ADM placement, complications associated with subcutaneous coverage are minimized without restricting lower pole expansion.[13] Although this technique resolves some of the concerns of partial muscle coverage (without ADM), the pectoralis major muscle remains elevated, and window shading remains a problem. Window shading can, however, be minimized by stabilizing the muscle and altering the degree of release of the muscle origins. The evolution of breast reconstruction has been possible only with close collaboration of breast surgeons delivering viable flaps and the availability of form-stable implants, ADMs, and high-quality processed fat for creation of bioengineered breasts (**Figure 1.3**).

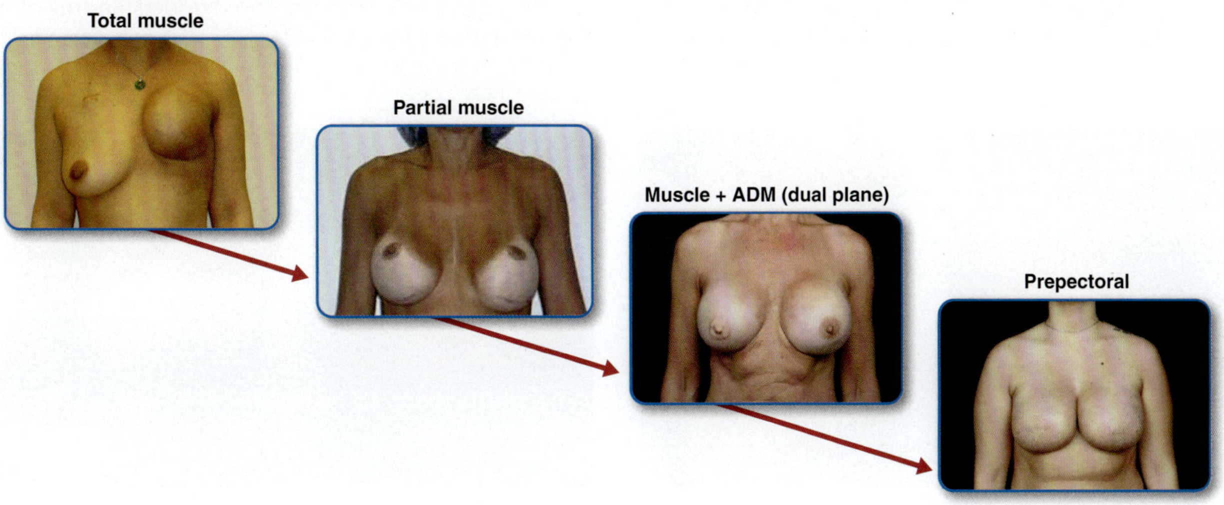

Figure 1.3 Evolution of device based breast reconstruction.

RATIONALE FOR PREPECTORAL PLACEMENT

Subpectoral prosthesis placement with partial muscle coverage, with or without ADM, is currently the standard technique for implant-based breast reconstruction. Many of the disadvantages/complications of subcutaneous implant placement (implant visibility, palpability, and exposure; and capsular contracture) are mitigated with the subpectoral technique because of the thicker coverage provided by the muscle. The elevation of the muscle, however, has introduced its own set of problems. A major concern is functional impairment of the muscle, particularly the adduction, anteversion, and inward rotation of the upper limb. In addition, animation deformities caused by muscle contraction, chest tightness, pain, and muscle spasm are other significant concerns[2,3] (**Figure 1.4**). Furthermore, subpectoral placement creates an unnatural state because the natural breast is anterior to the muscle. Despite these concerns, patients who have had dual-plane reconstruction with ADM can have aesthetically pleasing results; but with any contraction of the pectoralis major, animation deformity on the chest can immediately be noted.[14] We have utilized fat grafting as a means of establishing a natural gliding surface between the thin mastectomy flap and the pectoralis–ADM interface, which decreases the pain and the visual deformities associated with the scarred mastectomy flap being pulled by the pectoralis major.[4] This ameliorates but does not eliminate animation deformity, and some degree of animation remains.

As a further means to alleviate muscle-related issues, we resorted to moving the implant from the subpectoral back to the prepectoral (subcutaneous) position in certain revision cases. We then utilized our bioengineered breast concept to overcome the limitations of subcutaneous placement and improve the aesthetic outcome.[4] Using form-stable and/or higher fill implants, we reinforced the entire breast pocket with ADM to mimic muscle coverage and performed fat grafting to enhance the thickness and the gliding ability of the subcutaneous pocket. This has produced consistent outcomes with resolution of animation deformity and implant-related complications in appropriately selected patients.

We have been using the prepectoral approach in our revision cases since 2008 and have refined the technique further. Initially, we placed the ADM anteriorly over the implant, but given the complexity of placement of the ADM and its suturing, we attempted to find a more efficient solution to simplify ADM utilization. To this end, various off-label constructs of prosthesis and ADM were configured for placement into the prepectoral space. We continue to utilize both of these techniques for ADM placement in our practices, and more details of these constructs are included in another chapter.

Given the simplicity of the prepectoral concept and the good outcomes in revision cases, we then adopted the concept into our primary reconstructions and have performed prepectoral implant placements in select primary reconstructions as a means to proactively address complications associated with subpectoral placement as well as to simplify the reconstructive process.

Patient selection is discussed in Chapter 9 because it is imperative to approach patient selection from a multidisciplinary standpoint, involving the surgical team (reconstructive and oncologic) as well as medical oncology and, most definitely, radiation oncology in any case where adjuvant radiotherapy is anticipated.

DISCUSSION

Prepectoral implant placement is not a novel concept, because the first subcutaneous breast reconstructions were essentially prepectoral. However, prepectoral reconstructions performed in the 1960s were limited by the extent of mastectomy, reconstructive technique, technology, and perhaps also by the lower expectations of breast aesthetics. Over the past several decades, great strides have been made in implant designs and reconstructive and soft-tissue augmentation techniques. Mastectomies are now less aggressive, with improved understanding of skin flap limitations; hence, the damage to the skin flap and its

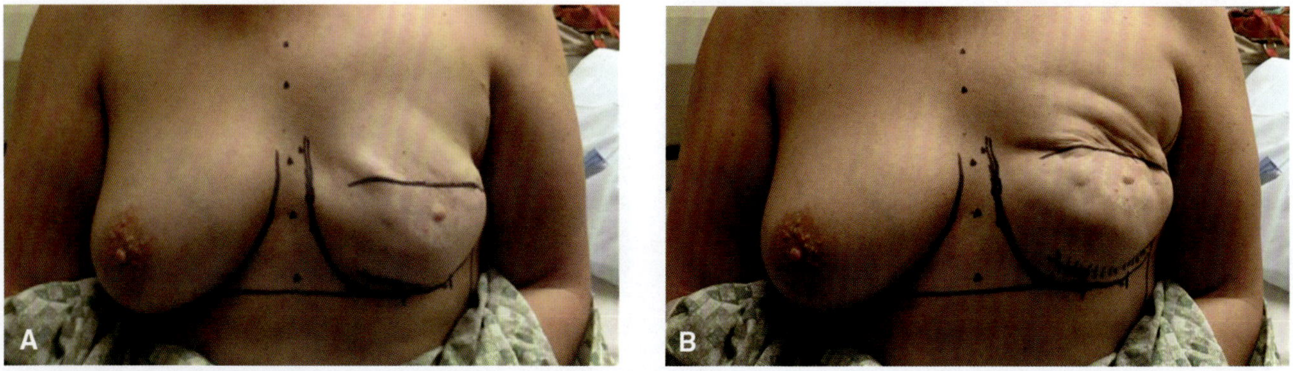

Figure 1.4 Patient with animation deformity years after mastectomy and dual plane reconstruction with silicone implants.

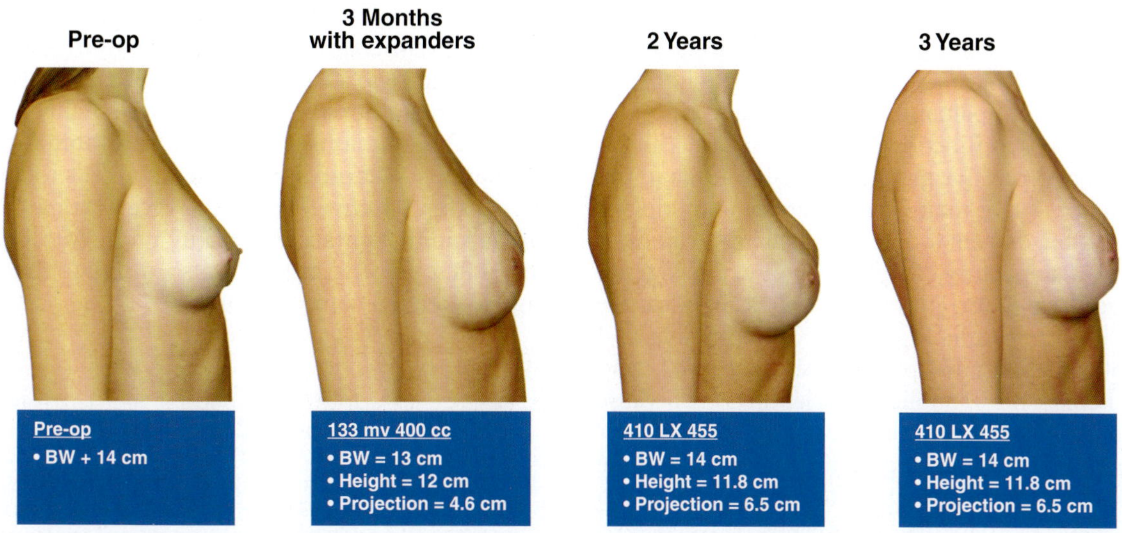

Figure 1.5 Patient following bilateral nipple sparing mastectomy and immediate 2 stage reconstruction utilizing the bioengineered approach. All layers were addressed and results remain stable at 3 years post op.

vasculature is minimized. The availability of devices that assess tissue perfusion has further allowed assessment of perfusion and viability of the skin flap that help guide decisions on the suitability of the prepectoral approach for a particular patient. The availability of ADMs that can be utilized as a layer of vascularized regenerative tissue between the implant and mastectomy flap is a prerequisite for prepectoral placement. Improvement in fat grafting techniques have made fat grafting a routine procedure in breast surgery, thereby allowing the utilization of adipose tissue to support and augment the soft-tissue volume between the implant and the mastectomy flap. Finally, improvement in implant designs have resulted in highly cohesive, form-stable, and higher fill implants that are associated with less rippling. It is the combination of all these factors that have made the prepectoral approach feasible, more than half a decade after early attempts failed.

Our preliminary results suggest that the prepectoral approach can lead to predictable outcomes and aesthetically stable reconstructions at least in the short term[1] (**Figure 1.5**). Integral to the success of this approach is our bioengineered breast concept of enhancing soft-tissue

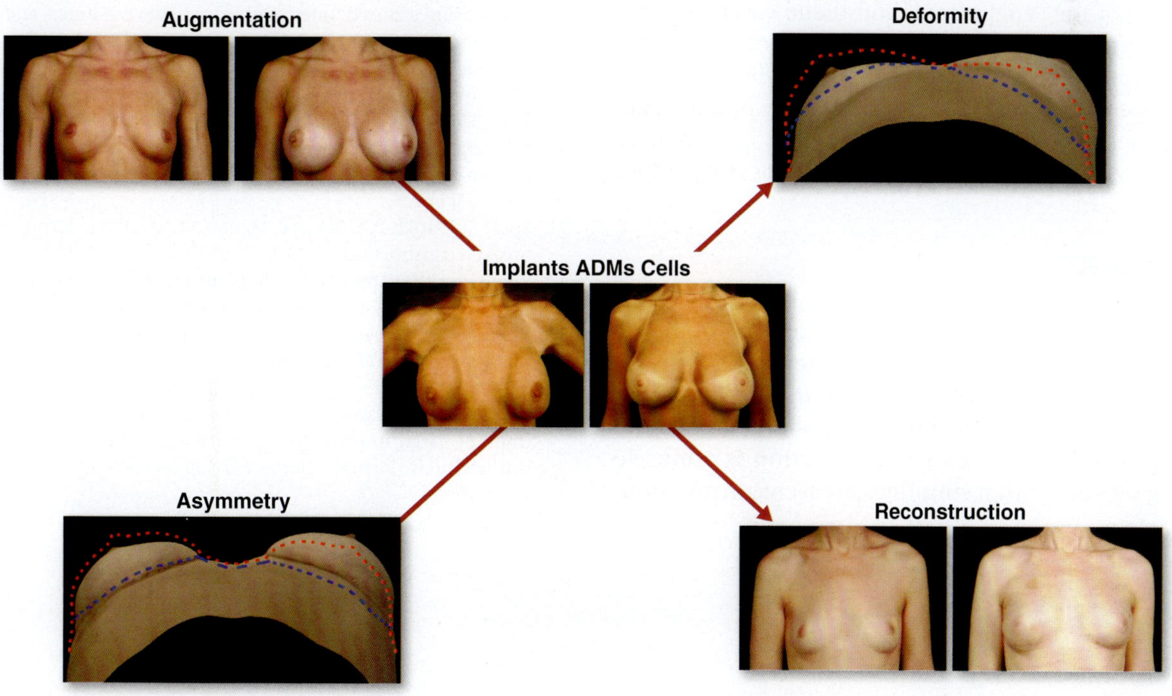

Figure 1.6 The principles described utilizing the bioengineered concept (implants, ADMs, and cells) are interchangeable between, augmentations, revisions and reconstructions. ADM, acellular dermal matrix.

coverage using a combination of regenerative scaffold (ADM) and regenerative cells in conjunction with form-stable implants. Volume enhancement is critical for aesthetics, such as masking implant palpability, visibility, and rippling/wrinkling, as well as functionality of the breast. Thicker flaps are more protective given that small trauma to the breast will not lead to major complications and implant loss. In addition, diligent follow-up of patients to monitor for signs of postoperative complications and their aggressive management is also critical for a successful outcome.

In addition to producing aesthetically pleasing and predictable outcomes, the prepectoral procedure is also attractive because of its simplicity. It is less invasive because it obviates the need to elevate the pectoralis major muscle. With muscle sparing, surgical time is shortened, the requirement for intravenous pain control or a pain pump is diminished, and patients can typically be discharged after one night of hospital stay. For patients, it is a less traumatic procedure with less pain and a faster recovery. In the future, patients may be able to be discharged home on the same day after prepectoral reconstruction.

The immediate prepectoral procedure, however, is not suitable for all patients; refer to Chapter 10 for detailed patient selection criteria. Prepectoral placement can be performed in single- or two-stage procedures.

The breast reconstructive process is continuously evolving, given the increasing expectations of both patients and surgeons for stable aesthetic outcomes with minimal complications and a fast recovery. Whether prepectoral implant placement using the bioengineered breast concept would fulfill these expectations remains to be seen. Evaluation of longer term outcomes will be necessary to ensure the adequacy of the "engineered" soft-tissue coverage. Principles of breast surgery and the utilization of form-stable implants and regenerative constructs and cells are applied to all aspects of breast surgeries, such as in primary augmentations and reconstructions as well as in secondary revisionary augmentation and reconstructions (**Figure 1.6**).

SUMMARY

Bioengineered breasts represent an evolution of the reconstructive process that aims to augment the soft-tissue envelope of reconstructed breasts to produce breasts that not only look but also feel like natural breasts. Prepectoral implant-based breast reconstruction is a muscle sparing procedure that simplifies breast reconstruction. By placing the implant prepectorally, the attendant problems associated with pectoralis muscle elevation are avoided. The success of this approach rests on the bioengineered breast concept, wherein highly cohesive, form-stable implants are utilized in combination with regenerative scaffold and regenerative cells to augment the soft-tissue envelope of the reconstructed breast. Tissue supplementation not only improves the overall aesthetic outcome but may also mitigate the risk of implant-related complications.

KEY REFERENCES

1. Sigalove S, Maxwell GP, Sigalove NM, et al. Prepectoral implant-based breast reconstruction: rationale, indications, and preliminary results. *Plast Reconstr Surg*. 2017;139(2):287-294.
2. de Haan A, Toor A, Hage JJ, Veeger HE, Woerdeman LA. Function of the pectoralis major muscle after combined skin-sparing mastectomy and immediate reconstruction by subpectoral implantation of a prosthesis. *Ann Plast Surg*. 2007;59(6):605-610.
3. Spear SL, Schwartz J, Dayan JH, Clemens MW. Outcome assessment of breast distortion following submuscular breast augmentation. *Aesthetic Plast Surg*. 2009;33(1):44-48.
4. Maxwell GP, Gabriel A. Bioengineered breast: concept, technique, and preliminary results. *Plast Reconstr Surg*. 2016;137(2):415-421.
5. Hammond DC, Capraro PA, Ozolins EB, Arnold JF. Use of a skin-sparing reduction pattern to create a combination skin-muscle flap pocket in immediate breast reconstruction. *Plast Reconstr Surg*. 2002;110(1):206-211.
6. Glasberg SB, Light D. AlloDerm and Strattice in breast reconstruction: a comparison and techniques for optimizing outcomes. *Plast Reconstr Surg*. 2012;129(6):1223-1233.
7. Serra-Renom JM, Fontdevila J, Monner J, Benito J. Mammary reconstruction using tissue expander and partial detachment of the pectoralis major muscle to expand the lower breast quadrants. *Ann Plast Surg*. 2004;53(4):317-321.
8. Spear SL, Pelletiere CV. Immediate breast reconstruction in two stages using textured, integrated-valve tissue expanders and breast implants. *Plast Reconstr Surg*. 2004;113(7):2098-2103.
9. Breuing KH, Warren SM. Immediate bilateral breast reconstruction with implants and inferolateral AlloDerm slings. *Ann Plast Surg*. 2005;55(3):232-239.
10. Salzberg CA. Nonexpansive immediate breast reconstruction using human acellular tissue matrix graft (AlloDerm). *Ann Plast Surg*. 2006;57(1):1-5.
11. Spear SL, Parikh PM, Reisin E, Menon NG. Acellular dermis-assisted breast reconstruction. *Aesthetic Plast Surg*. 2008;32(3):418-425.
12. Zienowicz RJ, Karacaoglu E. Implant-based breast reconstruction with allograft. *Plast Reconstr Surg*. 2007;120(2):373-381.
13. Breuing KH, Colwell AS. Inferolateral AlloDerm hammock for implant coverage in breast reconstruction. *Ann Plast Surg*. 2007;59(3):250-255.
14. Vardanian AJ, Clayton JL, Roostaeian J, et al. Comparison of implant-based immediate breast reconstruction with and without acellular dermal matrix. *Plast Reconstr Surg*. 2011;128(5):403e-410e.

CHAPTER 2

THE SCIENCE OF ACELLULAR DERMAL MATRIX INCORPORATION

Gregory Christopherson and John R. Harper

KEY POINTS

- Surgical usage and understanding of ADMs has evolved over the past 25 years.
- ADM incorporation can be divided into four key phases: cohesion (ADM recognition and initial adherence), engraftment (initial graft "take"), integration (stronger bonding of native and grafted ADM tissues), and remodeling (long-term compositional alteration of the ADM in response to surrounding biochemical and mechanical cues).
- ADM incorporation is dependent on many of the same factors as is native wound healing (surrounding tissue oxygenation/vascularity, ablation of dead space, bioburden reduction, etc.); and ADMs should be treated with care, similar to that given to any tissue flap and/or sterile medical device.

THE INTRODUCTION OF ACELLULAR DERMAL MATRICES

The reconstructive ladder provides guidance to surgeons when addressing a broad spectrum of reconstructive challenges. Although there have been many versions of the ladder over the years, the principles of choosing the most appropriate reconstructive approach suited to the complexity of the patient and to the goal have remained the same. In the past decade, technology and innovation have provided surgeons with alternatives that reduce the complexity of the reconstruction, as well as reducing the morbidity to the patient, while often improving the quality of the outcome. Janis, et al.[1] have described the impact of key innovations on the ladder, and one of the notable contributions to the "New Reconstructive Ladder" has been acellular dermal matrices (ADMs). Originally, in the early 1990s, ADMs were developed with the intention of serving as an "off-the-shelf" source of dermal scaffold in split-thickness skin grafting procedures in debrided, full-thickness burn wounds. By placing the ADM in a debrided wound bed with an overlying thin, epithelial graft, surgeons could obtain an acceptable result while minimizing the thickness of the donor site and associated morbidity to the patient.[2] From grafting of debrided burn wounds to treating lower extremity chronic wounds, such as diabetic foot ulcers, ADMs have been shown to allow surgeons to place more dermal tissue thickness in wound beds in patients who are poor candidates for thick skin grafts. Once plastic surgeons observed how effectively patients incorporated the dermal matrix, other applications of this technology were contemplated that provided similar reductions in patient morbidity, such as facial contouring, oral surgery, sports medicine, wound care, complex abdominal wall reconstruction, and breast reconstruction. In each of these examples, ADMs have been shown to provide the surgeon with an additional tool for the reconstructive tool box that either supplements or replaces the patient's own tissues in a variety of operations.

EVOLUTION OF ACELLULAR DERMAL MATRIX UNDERSTANDING AND SURGICAL USAGE

A major component of mesenchymal tissue, such as the dermis, is an extracellular matrix (ECM) made up primarily of fibrillar collagen, but also contains specialized structural components that help direct the behavior of the cells within the tissue. To produce a tissue substrate that is packaged and available to surgeons in the operating room for use as a tissue substitute in reconstructive surgery, the cells must be removed without damaging the ECM, and the material must be preserved to prevent degradation upon storage. Furthermore, it is important to sterilize the material in a manner that does not alter the ADM integrity, because this may trigger an adverse reaction in the patient. It is important that surgeons understand the way patients respond to ADMs before considering their use as an adjunct in device-assisted breast reconstruction.[3]

To better describe the acceptance of ADMs by patients and the ingrowth of their own cells and tissues into the scaffold, studies were conducted in relevant preclinical models of skin grafting, abdominal wall reconstruction,[4] and breast reconstruction.[5] Seminal experiments stemmed from a guinea pig abdominal wall reconstruction model that studied material fibrogenesis, or a tendency to stimulate adhesion formation of ADMs compared to a synthetic hernia mesh that is known to elicit significant adhesion formation. The authors found that the synthetic mesh control caused significant adhesions to form against the mesh, whereas ADMs were surprisingly adhesion free.[6] But beyond that, ADMs appeared to protect the synthetic mesh from adhesion formation when interposed between the mesh and the animal's visceral tissues. In another related example, it was observed that certain ADMs seemed to have a protective effect on the foreign body response to synthetic materials. This was shown by implanting silicone sheet in rodents with or without an ADM wrap and comparing the ADM-protected response to the silicone sheet implants alone. Although denuded silicone generated the expected encapsulation response, those wrapped with ADM were surrounded by a layer of tissue that was clearly superiorly distinguishable from the scar-like capsule surrounding the control. This work suggested that by placing the ADM between a breast implant or tissue expander and the patient's tissue, an encapsulation response might be minimized if not completely prevented. In a primate model of breast reconstruction that involved placing miniature breast implants in the subcutaneous plane, it was shown that when ADM was wrapped around the implant, there appeared to be a protective effect against capsule formation when compared to bare implants. The incorporation of the ADM into the primate tissues when placed between the implant and the animal's native tissues was like that seen in scores of explants taken at the tissue expander to permanent implant exchange during the second stage of breast reconstruction in humans.

Concurrently with increased scientific understanding, ADMs were used in continuously more innovative surgical applications since their inception. Nearly two decades ago, surgeons began deriving an approach of using ADM to reinforce or stabilize the pectoralis major in a dual-plane, implant-based breast reconstruction.[7] This approach helped revolutionize breast reconstruction, greatly reducing serious complications associated with breast implant–based techniques, while also providing new avenues of surgical intervention and control. Involvement of the pectoral muscle in conjunction with an ADM prevented lateral or inferior migration of the tissue expander and the permanent implant, while also nearly eliminating capsular contracture and providing a stable, cosmetically enriching outcome for patients. By incorporating ADM into the dual-plane reconstruction, both surgeons and patients have responded favorably to the postoperative cosmetic result, helping eliminate a large portion of the stigma of surviving breast cancer. In addition to providing tissue support in the primary reconstruction, ADMs were shown to be useful in revision procedures, such as repositioning of the implants in the event of bottoming-out or other forms of implant malposition. As presented in great detail throughout other chapters of this book, ADMs allowed for continued surgical innovation beyond a dual-plane approach, and in conjunction with other technologic advances (cohesive implants, perfusion assessment systems), have ushered in further reconstructive options, with potentially even greater advantages to the patient. As ADMs become an even more integral aspect of breast reconstruction—providing nearly complete mechanical support of the soft-tissue envelope and complete anterior (and potentially posterior) contact/coverage of the breast implant—it becomes even more critical for surgeons to conceptually understand the mechanisms by which ADMs interact with the patient, and change over time. The goal of this chapter is to provide that context at a level appropriate to a surgeon's perspective; those interested in greater mechanistic detail are encouraged to read the key citations provided within the bibliography. When reviewing ADM literature, it is important to keep in mind that the inability to effectively study human ADMs in any nonprimate preclinical model limits the current level of scientific rigor: the host response of lower phylogenetic mammals is triggered by the human characteristics of the ADM, greatly altering the cellular cascade, confounding the ability to effectively analyze advanced elements of incorporation. Although there is a great deal left to understand regarding ADM incorporation and the underlying mechanisms of action, the key characteristics are in relatively clear focus at a high level.

PHASES OF ACELLULAR DERMAL MATRIX INCORPORATION

Despite the variability that still exists with ADM usage—and the occasional uncertainty in surgical outcomes—key aspects of ADM incorporation have been clearly defined, both clinically and preclinically. ADM incorporation mirrors the phasic nature of traditional wound healing, with key characteristics that define early, middle, and late stages. It can be generally bucketed into intervals but actually behaves as more of a continuum, belying a delicate temporal balance of cellular infiltration and matrix turnover, which is likely highly dependent on the biochemical and mechanical cues of the local microenvironment (which includes patient factors) as well as the nature of the ADM itself. When applied with tight apposition to native tissue in a well-perfused surgical plane, ADMs will fuse to their surroundings in a short time (cohesion), fully coalescing with the native tissue as a largely intact acellular tissue graft (engraftment). That bond with the surrounding wound bed is secure, but weak initially, relying on a provisional protein matrix. As healing proceeds, the ADM–tissue interface integrates more heavily, with the nascent matrix maturing into a collagen-rich structure with increased vascularity throughout the entire graft (integration). Over the course of months and years, a properly integrated ADM will slowly respond to a cascade of cellular and mechanical induction to continuously turn over new collagen matrix (remodeling), retaining elements of the original ADM graft but *incorporating* more patient tissue over time (**Figure 2.1**). The timing of the different phases can be patient and treatment specific, influenced by a multitude of factors, both known (radiation, comorbidities) and unknown (patient genetics, ADM/donor quality).

Cohesion

Much like traditional wound healing, there is an equilibrium state achieved early on that initiates subsequent phases. With any physical injury, hemostasis propagates the wound-healing cascade. ADMs are unique in that hemostasis still occurs (there is obviously still sharp dissection in surgery), but inclusion of a mature ECM likely alters the healing paradigm going forward. The initial phase has not been clearly described to this point in literature, but in this view probably involves two overriding factors: the host immune response will immediately recognize the implanted ADM and respond with a cellular cavalcade (positive or negative) specifically tailored to the ADM; in addition, assuming properly perfused and apposing native tissue–ADM placement, early adherence of two tissue planes with nearly identical structural composition will

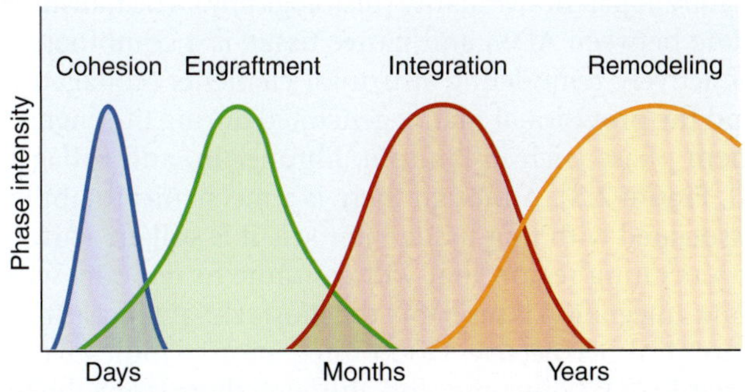

Figure 2.1 Phases of acellular dermal matrix (ADM) incorporation. Similar to wound healing, ADM incorporation is a complex spatial and temporal continuum that is easily divided and understood as discrete stages, each with unique characteristics. Overall, ADMs transition from latent acellular structural constructs into responsive incorporated tissues within the patient.

occur, commonly known as cohesion. From a practical standpoint, there are not likely the same definitive cellular mechanisms in ADM incorporation as in hemostasis to so clearly delineate cohesion from engraftment (they are at best currently undefined, scientifically); but it is helpful to identify how critical the initial ADM placement is to a successful surgical outcome. Cohesion is a vital step within 0 to 3 days to properly jumpstart subsequent phases of ADM incorporation, despite being largely poorly understood mechanistically at this point in time.

Engraftment

The engraftment phase has the most in common with traditional wound healing, overlapping heavily with inflammation mechanisms, and is likely most critical for successful incorporation long term. Engraftment can be thought of as the stage where the ADM is accepted by the patient as an intact (albeit acellular) tissue graft, mostly unchanged from its starting form, aside from early-stage integration at the ADM periphery. From a mechanistic view, leukocytes present in the area remove cellular debris remaining from surgical trauma, as well as enzymatically debride any compromised tissues and police the area for bacterial infiltration. Inclusion of an ADM for this phase of wound healing is influential in two major ways: the existence of an intact ECM prevents the need for a provisional wound matrix and somehow influences macrophage behavior to be more constructive toward remodeling long term. To the first point, it is unclear whether a decellularized scaffold occludes platelet clotting and autolysis (of proinflammatory modulators) or operates through an alternative mechanism, but providing an intact tissue scaffold clearly alters tissue deposition during the inflammatory and granulation phases of wound healing. Fibronectin, laminin, and collagen III are still deposited in large quantities, but as more of a layered interface between the native tissue and the ADM, as opposed to filling large tissue deficits. Perhaps as a result of this more localized and controlled deposition, there appears to be a pronounced shift in the macrophage activity from a proinflammatory state to a reconstructive phenotype. This is most clearly seen in preclinical experimentation and is enormously reliant on the characteristics of the implanted ADM.[8] Any damage or alteration caused by processing or donor variability may manifest as diseased tissue, resulting in markedly increased inflammatory infiltrate that is of a more traditional (negative) immune response. In the event chronic inflammation is avoided, enzymatic and proteolytic activity proceeds in a logical manner, and within the course of days to weeks a protein- and proteoglycan-rich bonded layer attaches the ADM to the adjacent native tissue. A key difference between ADMs and living tissue grafts is the source of vascularization: early inosculation occurs in tissue grafting when both sides of the tissue interface can provide sufficient blood vessels to seek and combine as a response to hypoxic conditions. With an ADM, there is no living bundle of capillaries or microvessels, and true neovascularization must occur in lieu of revascularization—the two terms are often used synonymously, but neovascularization is a much more difficult condition, highly dependent on the ability of cells to infiltrate the graft. In the event that inflammation does not override cell migration and vessel induction, healthy neovascularization occurs at the periphery of the graft (not to be confused with chronic blood vessel formation, which is counterproductive to vessel generation throughout the ADM), initiating an "edges to center" transport that allows further maturation of the ADM–tissue interface to occur. This new vessel formation appears in the form of centripetal budding from vascularized tissues into the periphery of the ADM, continuing inward and maturing over time (**Figure 2.2**). It should be noted that

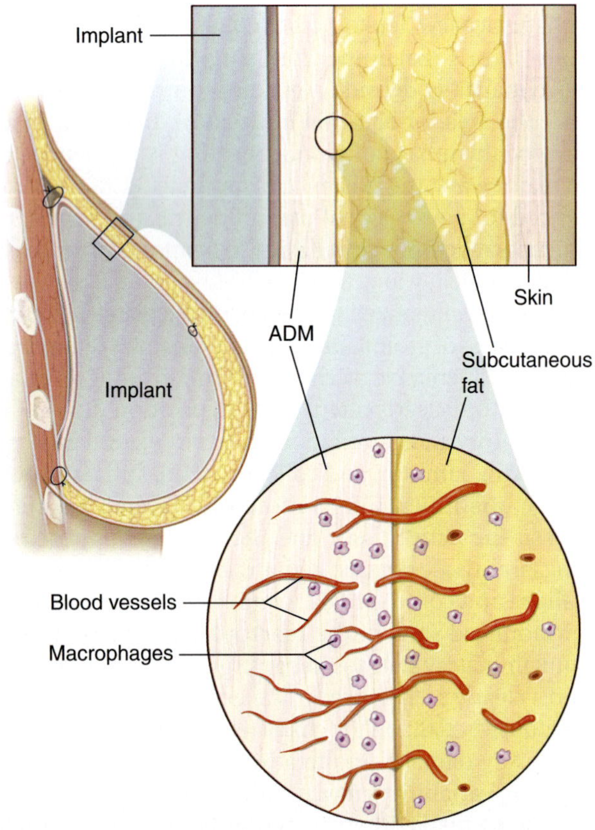

Figure 2.2 Engraftment. The critical early stage of acellular dermal matrix (ADM) incorporation, engraftment is dependent on a combination of ADM quality and surgical application, and is likely complete at 14 to 21 days from implantation, depending on patient factors. A delicate balance of acute inflammation and provisional scaffold deposition creates a physical coupling of the ADM to the surrounding tissue plane. Immune cells enzymatically remove residual ADM damage, whereas reconstructive cells (fibroblasts, endothelial cells, and mesenchymal stem cells) migrate into the periphery of the ADM and start the process of neovascularization and early physical integration of the ADM.

inflammation and vascularization are closely linked, but controlled recellularization of healthy infiltrate (fibroblasts, endothelial cells, and mesenchymal stem cells) relies on the biointegrity of the ADM. Any damage that exists in the ADM likely slows the process of engraftment and following stages of incorporation, as cellular mechanisms work to remove "diseased" tissue, and the immune response conflicts with regenerative cascades. If inflammatory infiltrate proceeds to a chronic state, as a result of either a hostile surgical environment or altered ADM or both, it is possible that engraftment will be prevented, and later aspects of ADM incorporation will be compromised as well, if not bypassed entirely.

Integration

Integration can be thought of as a maturation of the engraftment phase, where the foundational strength, vascularity, and cellularity of the ADM are established to allow for long-term reconstruction in later phases. Integration is the stage when the ADM transitions from an intact graft that completely resembles its starting state to an intermediary tissue that now belongs to the patient and is responding to the surrounding environment. This is also the most common phase referred to by surgeons during any second-stage surgery, where there is obvious physical marriage between the ADM and overlying soft tissue but a clear visual delineation of where the graft starts and ends compared to the native tissue. The engraftment phase is a story of cellular mechanisms, whereas the integration phase is much more grossly observed (particularly late-stage integration), with large punctated blood vessels and a clear (if small) transition zone of newly created connective tissue linking the ADM and soft-tissue envelope. The integration ("integrating") phase generally can be described as lasting between a few weeks and several months. Hallmarks of this phase would be the virtual elimination of any inflammation, with dispersion of fibroblasts throughout the ADM, and readily apparent vascularity (histologically). The transition zone between ADM and native tissue is a combination of actively remodeling structural elements (collagen I) and the provisional matrix generated during the engraftment phase (rich in laminin, fibronectin, and collagen III; **Figure 2.3**). Although there is a mechanical stability associated with that tissue interface, it is still an actively regenerating region that will continue to remodel with time. Integration is probably **the** most relevant phase from a surgical perspective. Good integration is indicative of a stable ADM outcome; and although there is absolutely the capacity of that to change over time (discussed in the next section), a robust connection between the ADM and surrounding native tissue that is devoid of scar is a sign of reliable ADM behavior going forward. Warning signs of ADM behavior at this stage of incorporation manifest in more readily observable ways (erythema, edema, lack of

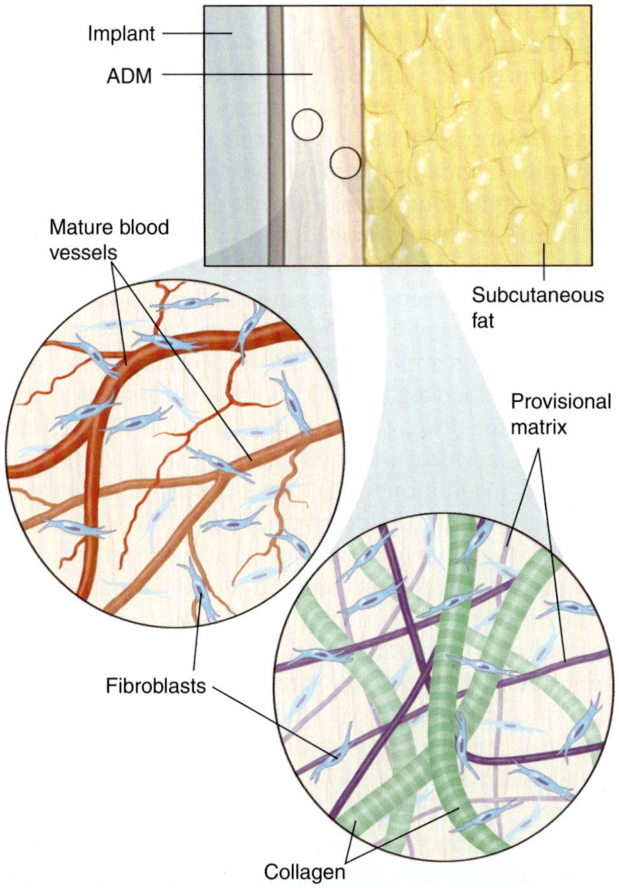

Figure 2.3 **Integration.** As engraftment proceeds, cellular elements and vasculature permeate the entirety of the acellular dermal matrix (ADM). When fully integrated, inflammation subsides, and the host response begins to transition into a reconstructive phase. The ADM is still readily apparent grossly and histologically, but the graft has been accepted by the patient, and the provisional ADM–tissue interface has matured into a mechanically strong and well-perfused transitional connective tissue.

vascularity, or connective tissue strength). Drawing back to the integrity of ADMs, there appears to be evidence now that different types of alteration to the matrix can present at later stages (perhaps even after successful engraftment). This, unfortunately, speaks to the large gaps of working knowledge that scientists and clinicians need to reconcile moving forward.

Remodeling

Remodeling (or regeneration) is perhaps the most debated aspect of incorporation.[9] There is strong preclinical evidence to suggest that—especially in demanding mechanical applications such as abdominal wall or tendon/ligament applications—ADMs readily remodel to the applied traction forces over time, to create connective tissue able to withstand the demands of that tissue space. Despite starting out as a "dead" (or at least dormant) tissue construct, the body can bring them alive and utilize them as a natural component of the patient's own soft tissue over time. By the time a remodeling phase is reached (as early as 2 months, but typically a few months later, and then potentially extending through the lifetime of the patient), fibroblasts (and other connective tissue cell types) are dispersed throughout the graft, with a healthy neovascularized infrastructure to feed and transport them throughout the tissue (**Figure 2.4**). Fibroblasts are known to be a mechanosensing cell type that will reorient collagen bundles under allowable conditions. This type of physical restructuring of the tissue has been clearly shown in primate models and has been corroborated with human samples. Human ADMs generally have unique histologically identifiable aspects that can be identified from clinical biopsies (especially elastin), providing indelible evidence that—at least in some conditions—ADMs can transition from off-the-shelf implantable goods to a living, reactive tissue. Similar to wound healing, elements that influence collagen production will likely impact the kinetics of remodeling—diabetes, smoking, genetic deficiencies,

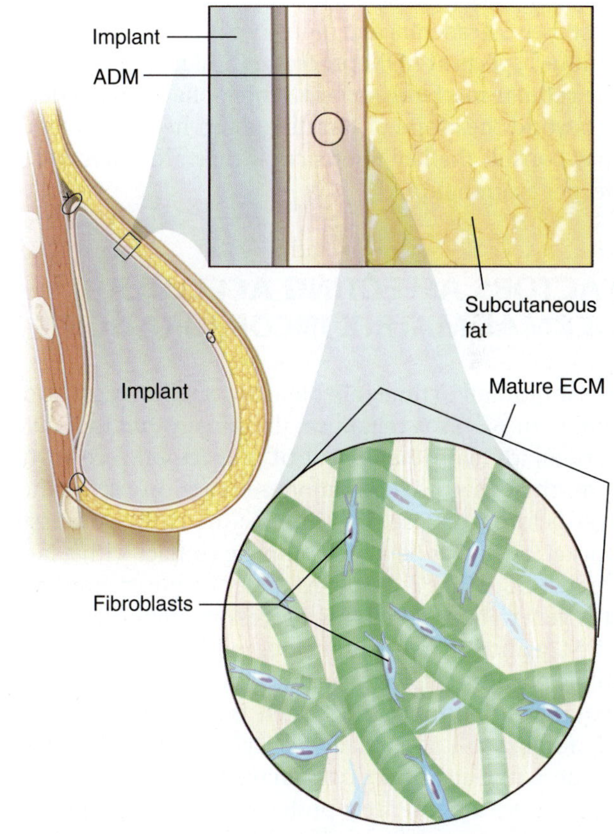

Figure 2.4 **Remodeling.** The acellular dermal matrix (ADM) has reached a stable equilibrium with the patient constantly in a state of natural turnover. There is full cellular infiltration and robust vascularization throughout the ADM. The collagen structural elements are actively—but slowly—reorganizing in response to biochemical and biomechanical stimuli. The remodeling phase can be described as lasting years or potentially even the lifetime of the patient. For all intents and purposes, the ADM is a viable grafted tissue within the patient, and will more completely incorporate over time.

and so on. Patient elements likely impact earlier phases as well, making it difficult to optimize patient outcomes with so many virtual unknowns at the time of surgery. Like any other surgery, this is a case where surgeon judgment is crucial, and despite not knowing the exact impact of comorbidities on ADM incorporation, we can infer some aspects to better inform those decisions, as discussed in the next section.

As stated earlier, the phases of ADM incorporation are more of a continuum than discrete intervals, with kinetics heavily dependent on patient and surgical factors, as well as the integrity of the ADM itself. Generally speaking, a well-processed ADM is treated by the body as a dormant tissue plane and accepts an acute inflammatory infiltrate to strip away any residual ECM damage. Connective tissue cell infiltration proceeds simultaneously with vascular budding, generating a juvenile protein-rich interface with surrounding tissue that can mature into robust collagen integration over time. A complex series of interactions lead to acceptance of the graft into a native tissue state that reacts to the surrounding microenvironment to remodel over time and continuously incorporates into true functional host tissue. Academia and industry continuously examine unique aspects of ADM processing and how they impact the cellular mechanisms of all three phases. Such detail is beyond the scope of our discussion here, but readers may consult the key references if they are interested in deeper examination.

FACTORS AFFECTING ACELLULAR DERMAL MATRIX INCORPORATION

It is important to remember that any surgical reconstruction with ADMs is reliant on the surgery *and* the ADM. Particularly with the advent of prepectoral reconstruction, there is potentially more reliance on ADMs than ever before (it is used to reinforce the entire soft-tissue pocket, as well as being in complete contact with a large foreign body like a tissue expander or breast implant). It is generally accepted that processing methods impact ADM quality. There are numerous publications that point to the preclinical effects generated by various proprietary manufacturing approaches. There is a delicate balance of identifying solutions that effectively decellularize dense tissue without impacting remaining matrix integrity. Companies are intensely protective of their proprietary approaches to solving this problem, and the literature is mixed on how processing differences may manifest clinically.[10] Regardless of processing methods, for human tissues, donor variability is an overarching challenge. Genetics and lifestyle greatly impact skin quality, as well as potentially other factors such as age, diet, sun exposure, cosmetics and narcotics use (chemical exposure), and a host of other variables. Even with rigorous screening and medical records analysis, it is currently cost prohibitive to stratify donor quality. Likely because of this, every manufacturer will have difficulty producing universally excellent goods, and any caustic elements apparent in processing will have an even more deleterious effect given the spread of incoming tissue quality. Despite that difficulty, it remains that variations in ADM quality likely impact surgical outcomes. If aspects of the ECM (primarily collagen) are compromised during solution processing and/or sterilization—these altered elements are readily apparent during sensitive in vitro and in vivo testing—the immune system will respond by enzymatically removing the damaged components. This inflammatory cascade is believed to increase complication rates, acting as a likely nidus for the propagation of side effects such as seroma, infection, necrosis, red breast, and capsular contracture. As stated, in addition to ADM quality, surgical application of the grafts critically determines patient outcomes. For reference here, aspects that particularly impact the application of ADMs are the focus: any acellular matrix needs a baseline level of perfusion to allow the early cellular mechanisms of engraftment to proceed, and these aspects are examined in detail in later chapters. In addition to multiple brands of ADMs available on the market, there is a constant evolution of different forms within each brand, the most recent of which are intentionally patterned perforations/fenestrations. There are interesting questions around the benefit of removing ECM construct (which many surgeons have done by hand for quite some time) to allow fluid transduction and soft-tissue ingrowth, but there is, unfortunately, a dearth of data to support any conclusions, especially as meshing patterns become more aggressive—although fenestrations allow for easier ADM expansion, they are also problematic as areas of scar tissue formation (especially for ADMs that may be compromised during processing, leading to more inflammation). In fact, increasing fenestrations run counter to the principles (mechanical and immunoprotective) that support ADM choice in the first place. As industry continues to respond to technical demands from the surgical community, more product choices will present to the market, making downstream clinical decisions even more challenging. All anyone can urge is to make data-driven decisions.

HUMAN VERSUS XENOGENEIC ACELLULAR DERMAL MATRICES

Discussion provided in this chapter is intended principally for the understanding of human-derived ADMs. Public knowledge of the differences of human and xenogeneic ADMs is limited, making it difficult to universally apply aspects of ADM incorporation across species. Regardless of the different regulatory pathways of human versus animal sources (human ADMs are generally a cell/tissue pathway regulation in the United States; xeno-ADMs are a medical device, with different restrictions or requirements), some literature seems to indicate that in sensitive surgical applications such as breast reconstruction (extensive tissue trauma and soft-tissue undermining, potential oncologic concerns, compromised perfusion, presence of a large foreign body, etc.) xenogeneic differences are more impactful, leading to increased difficulty in successful reconstructions. It is possible that the majority of xenogeneic ADMs (generally porcine derived, but bovine sources are also popular) are more prone to undergo a resorb-and-replace mechanism than are human ADMs, but harshly processed human ADMs can occasionally display resorption as well. Inflammatory enzymatic degradation appears to be the main culprit for resorption, which may be more readily triggered by the presence of nonhuman antigenic material that remains following the processing of animal tissues. Despite this current limitation, there is significant excitement around xenogeneic tissues moving forward, because of their much more consistent "donor" profile. As genomic and proteomic profiling continues to mature, expect xenogeneic tissues processed with more thorough and/or targeted solutions that can strip away nonconserved proteins to catch up with human sources as a viable surgical option, although the regulatory environment is much more complicated. In addition, more "human-like" xeno-ADMs will allow for more thorough scientific examination, because they can be effectively studied in small animal models, benefiting the clinical community with an increased understanding of how to most successfully apply and monitor the tissues during use.

SUMMARY

The invention (reappropriation?) of ADMs has afforded surgeons the option to radically alter how they treat patients, especially in the realm of breast reconstruction. The process of ADM incorporation shares many elements of traditional wound healing: a critical starting phase triggers a host immune response while immediately starting the early adherence process (cohesion); inflammation and protein deposition work in tandem to generate a provisional matrix connection between the ADM and the patient, creating a tissue-inductive environment where the graft is weakly adhered, but largely unchanged from its initial state (engraftment); that interface matures and strengthens over time (integration), evolving to a collagen-rich transition zone as fibroblasts and blood vessels infiltrate the entirety of the graft, elements specific to the patient that vivify the ADM; the neovascularization and neocellularization across the ADM allow for long-term responsiveness to the surrounding biochemical and mechanical cues transduced from the microenvironment (remodeling), inducing the ADM to slowly reorganize and continuously incorporate over the years.

KEY REFERENCES

1. Janis JE, Kwon RK, Attinger CE. The new reconstructive ladder: modifications to the traditional model. *Plast Reconstr Surg*. 2011;127(suppl 1): 205S-212S.
2. Sheridan RL, Choucair RL. Acellular allogenic dermis does not hinder initial engraftment in burn wound resurfacing and reconstruction. *J Burn Care Rehabil*. 1997;18(6):496-499.
3. Harper JR, McQuillan DJ. A novel regenerative tissue matrix (RTM) technology for connective tissue reconstruction. *Wounds*. 2007;19(6):163-168.
4. Xu H, Wan H, Sandor M, et al. Host response to human acellular dermal matrix transplantation in a primate model of abdominal wall repair [published online ahead of print July 1, 2008]. *Tissue Eng. Part A*. 2008;14(2).
5. Stump A, Holton LH III, Connor J, Harper JR, Slezak S, Silverman RP. The use of acellular dermal matrix to prevent capsule formation around implants in a primate model. *Plast Reconst Surg*. 2009;124:82-91.
6. Butler CE, Prieto VG. Reduction of adhesions with composite AlloDerm/polypropylene mesh implants for abdominal wall reconstruction. *Plast Reconstr Surg*. 2004;114:464.
7. Jones GE, Harper JR. Technologic advances in breast surgery, acellular dermal matrix preparation, pp. 229-236; Skin flap perfusion with ICG, pp. 237-250, In: Jones GE. *Bostwick's Plastic and Reconstructive Breast Surgery*. 3rd ed. St. Louis, MO: Quality Medical Publishing, Inc.; 2010.
8. Sandor M, Leamy P, Assan P, et al. Relevant in vitro predictors of human acellular dermal matrix-associated inflammation and capsule formation in a nonhuman primate subcutaneous tissue expander model. *Eplasty*. 2017;17:e1.
9. Novitsky YW, Rosen MJ. The biology of biologics: basic science and clinical concepts. *Plast Reconst Surg*. 2012;130(suppl 2):9S.
10. Kim JYS, Mlodinow AS. What's new in acellular dermal matrix and soft-tissue support for prosthetic breast reconstruction. *Plast Reconstr Surg*. 2017;140:30S.

CHAPTER 3

GUIDING PRINCIPLES OF ONCOLOGIC APPROPRIATE MASTECTOMIES: NIPPLE-SPARING MASTECTOMY VERSUS SKIN-SPARING MASTECTOMY VERSUS MASTECTOMY WITHOUT RECONSTRUCTION

Toni Storm-Dickerson and Noemi M. Sigalove

KEY POINTS

- Why it is safe to retain the nipple in nipple-sparing mastectomy performed for breast cancer
- Oncologic selection criteria and safety of prepectoral reconstruction following mastectomy performed for breast cancer

INTRODUCTION

Breast cancer is the most common type of cancer and accounts for nearly 14.6% of all newly diagnosed cancers in the United States.[1] One in four people will be diagnosed with cancer in their lifetime, and for women one-half of these will be breast cancer.[1] There were an estimated 252 710 new cases of breast cancer in 2017.[2] Estimated deaths from breast cancer in 2017 were 40 610, representing 1 in 37 women diagnosed with breast cancer, and 6.8% of all cancer-related deaths.[3] Further, breast cancer survival after breast conservative surgery (BCS) or mastectomy (with or without reconstruction) is based on stage at diagnosis with an overall 5-year relative survival rate (2006-2012) of 89.7%.[4-7] Most studies[4] agree there is similar 5-year survival with breast-conserving therapy (BCT) and mastectomy, although some studies suggest a survival benefit in mastectomy at 20 years and greater.[8] Regardless of the surgical approach, the oncologic principles of complete tumor removal, appropriate lymph node assessment, and patient selection remain constant. Although we are beginning to understand that tumor biology is a major predictor of tumor behavior guiding treatment recommendations as reflected in the new AJCC (American Joint Committee on Cancer) 2018 staging guidelines, these complexities of cancer biology are covered elsewhere, and we focus on the oncologic safety of the various mastectomy techniques and patient selection.

There are two basic approaches to the surgical treatment of breast cancer—BCS and mastectomy. BCS is the preservation of the breast and combines lumpectomy, lymph node assessment, and complete removal of a breast tumor, generally, with breast radiation (XRT), allowing for survival benefit similar to that of mastectomy. Mastectomy is the removal of the entire breast gland with variation in degree of skin preservation based on plan for reconstruction.[2] Without addressing the axilla, there are three basic types of mastectomy: (1) mastectomy with or without reconstruction (maximal removal of the overlying breast skin); (2) skin-sparing mastectomy (SSM), preservation of the skin envelope less the nipple–areolar complex and usually includes reconstruction; and (3) nipple-sparing mastectomy (NSM), preservation of the entire skin envelope, and reconstruction.[2]

Although today, BCS is the treatment of choice for most (59% of early-stage vs. 13% of advanced stage) women with early-stage I/II breast cancer, mastectomies have retained a role in multicentric, locally advanced stage III/IV (59% of advanced stage vs. 36% of late-stage) disease, tumors not visualized on imaging or deleterious gene carriers.[2] However, this has been true only in the past 30 to 40 years. Halstead's radical mastectomy,[9] involving removal of the entire breast with surrounding tissue, lymph nodes, and the pectoral muscles, was the standard of care from the 1880s until the 1980s, when Dr. Bernard Fischer first suggested trials to evaluate the validity of radical mastectomy. NSABP-04 (National Surgical Adjuvant Breast and Bowel Project),[10] published in 1980, showed equivalent survival with radical mastectomy compared to simple mastectomy, and the NSABP-06 trial, published in 1985, showed equivalent survival for BCS (lumpectomy and radiation) as for mastectomy.[11,12] These studies were pivotal in changing our surgical approach to breast cancer. It was then not until the early 1990s that BCS was considered a universal standard of care.

Since 2005, there has been an increasing preference for mastectomies in the United States, especially among patients with early-stage breast cancer.[11,12] Between 2002 and 2012, rates of contralateral prophylactic mastectomies (CPMs) in the United States have more than doubled (from 3.9% to 12.7%),[13] despite evidence that CPM does not increase overall survival (OS) in most cases and is not routinely recommended by the National Comprehensive Cancer Network (NCCN) for most women.[14] This trend is likely fueled by a combination of events, including improved reconstructive options, increased patient awareness, and choice. In spite of improved survival, attributable in large part to better systemic therapies, improved early diagnosis,[15] and improved BCT cosmetic outcomes with oncoplastic techniques, we continue to see a trend toward more aggressive breast surgery.[16]

ONCOLOGIC SAFETY OF NIPPLE- AND SKIN-SPARING MASTECTOMIES

Over the past 50 years, there have been increasing data on the oncologic safety of both NSMs and SSMs, starting with Barbara Freeman performing 1500 subcutaneous mastectomies for patients with painful fibrocystic breast disease and finding a 0.4% incidence of breast cancer in 10-year follow-up,[17] and followed by the work of Hinton who published his data in 1984 showing no difference in different disease-free survival (DFS) and OS in patients with stage I and II breast cancer undergoing subcutaneous mastectomies.[18] There have also been several large population studies, evaluating the safety of prophylactic mastectomies[19-21] in patients considered to be high risk secondary to family history, showing significant decrease in the incidence of both recurrent and contralateral breast cancers. Agarwal et al[22] used SEER (Surveillance, Epidemiology, and End Results) data to compare the DFS and OS following NSM and modified radical mastectomy/NSM and found no significant differences between the procedures. Although their data supported the oncologic safety of NSM, they acknowledged possible selection bias (lower tumor grade, negative nodes, no lymphovascular invasion, etc), and suggested careful patient selection, as reflected in the NCCN guidelines.[23]

Newer data supports preservation of the uninvolved nipple regardless of tumor size. Several studies have shown that, although locoregional recurrence is clearly elevated in locally advanced disease, preservation of the uninvolved nipple does not increase the risk of local recurrence. Further, when locoregional recurrence does occur, it is not at the nipple.[24] Smith et al[25] published their data in September 2017, showing that in 2182 patients with stage 0 to III breast cancer, who underwent NSM at Massachusetts General Hospital between 2007 and 2016, at a mean follow-up of 51 months, they saw 2.7% distant recurrence, with two deaths, and no recurrences at the nipple.

Li Mingzhu et al used SEER data to look at cancer-specific survival (CSS) and OS in 2440 patients undergoing NSM between 1998 and 2013 with a median age of 50, including Tis, T1-3 (79.6% T2-3), and N0-3. Of the NSM cases, 26%, 20%, and 13.8% were T2-3, N1-3, and estrogen receptor negative. In patients diagnosed between 1998 and 2010 ($N = 763$), median follow-up was 69 months with 5- and 10-year CSS, 96.9% and 94.9%, respectively, and the OS; 94.1% and 88.0%, respectively. Ethnicity, T-stage and N-stage were independently associated with CSS, and age and T-stage were factors independently associated with OS.[26] They showed a 10-year OS of 72% for N2-3 patients after NSM. This was significantly better than the reported outcomes following traditional mastectomy in patients with a similar tumor burden per National Cancer Database 8-year OS was 66.6% and 53.5%, respectively, following complete mastectomy in N2-3 patients with and without radiation therapy (RT), respectively.[27]

Therefore, these data repeatedly show that nipple preservation in NSM is safe in patients with breast cancer and that disease extent is a general predictor of increased risk for locoregional and distant recurrence rather than for nipple recurrence in patients without pathologic evidence of nipple involvement. These data include extensive evaluation of patients with Tis and T1-3, and N1-3 disease with follow-up beyond 10 years.

ONCOLOGIC SAFETY AND SELECTION CRITERIA FOR PREPECTORAL RECONSTRUCTION FOLLOWING MASTECTOMY

Prepectoral implant placement is not a novel concept, because the first subcutaneous breast reconstructions were, in fact, prepectoral. Reconstructions performed in the 1960s, however, were limited by aggressive mastectomy dissection, paucity of reconstructive techniques, and lack of innovative

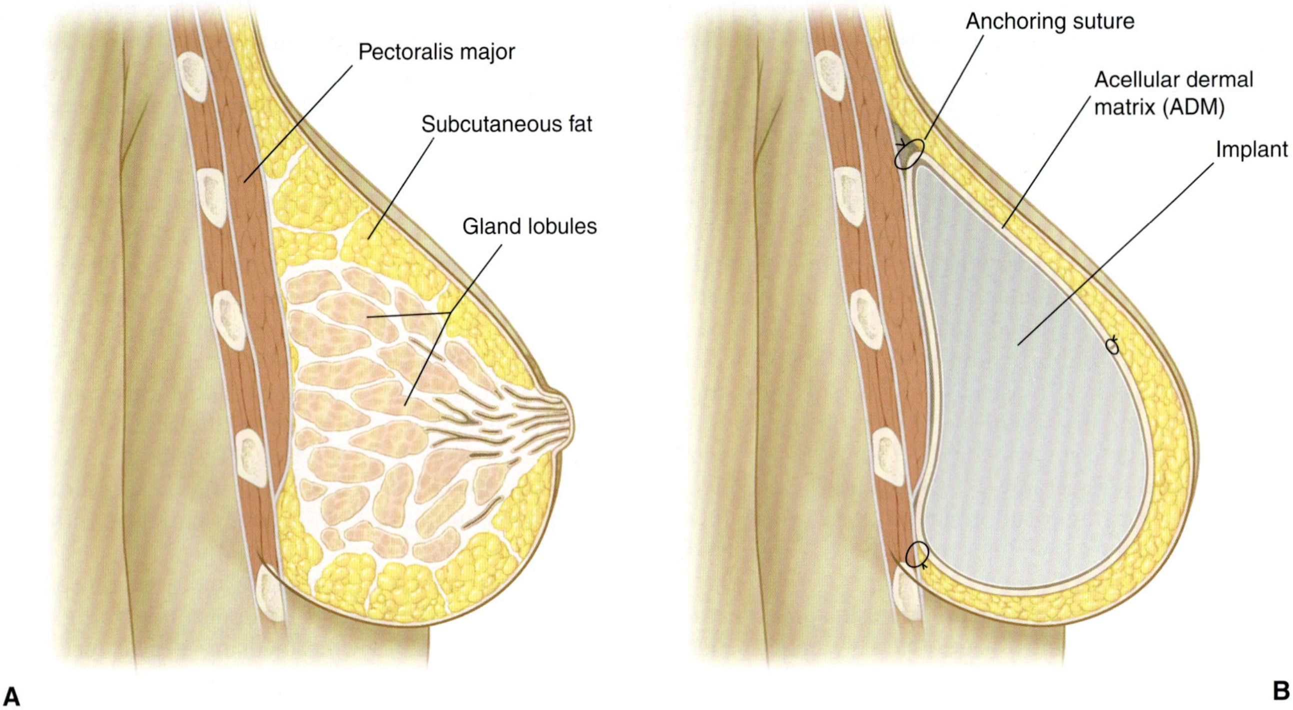

Figure 3.1 Position of the native breast as compared to the prepectoral implant. A, Native breast. B, Postmastectomy breast with prepectoral implant.

technology. Patient acceptance of marginal aesthetic outcomes may also have contributed to the slower change in surgical technique. Over the past several decades, tremendous strides have been made in oncologic care, implant design, and reconstructive as well as soft-tissue augmentation techniques. Mastectomies are more precise, fueled by the recognition that breast cancer is a disease defined by biology rather than by anatomy alone. Understanding the importance of skin flap perfusion and vascular integrity in the success of reconstruction has led to changes in surgical technique that aim to minimize flap necrosis. The availability of tissue perfusion assessment devices has also allowed objective determination of perfusion and skin flap viability. The use of these devices helps the reconstructive surgeon determine whether a patient is suitable for immediate reconstruction. Critically important to these quantum shifts has also been the use of acellular dermal matrices. These materials serve as a layer of vascularized regenerative tissue between the implant and the mastectomy flap, allowing for stabilization of the reconstructed breast.

The main patient benefits of the prepectoral approach include elimination of animation deformity and comfort derived from leaving the pectoralis muscle undisturbed. Leaving the muscle in its native position allows for a procedure that is less invasive and better tolerated by patients than its subpectoral counterpart.[28,29] Postoperative complications with the prepectoral approach have been shown to be comparable in type and incidence to those reported with partial muscle coverage.[30-33] A less traumatic procedure leads to minimal pain with decreased need for narcotics, faster recovery, elimination of animation deformity, improved long-term comfort, as well as a more natural appearing breast.[28,29,32,33] These advantages arise from the fact that the reconstructed breast takes the place of the excised one without any additional disruption to natural anatomy (**Figure 3.1**).

It is important to note that the prepectoral procedure is not suitable for all patients. Selection criteria for prepectoral reconstruction combine variables that are unique to each individual with parameters that are felt to be oncologically safe. General exclusion criteria include ischemic, poorly vascularized skin flaps after mastectomy; patients with a history of preoperative breast irradiation or uncontrolled diabetes (hemoglobin A_{1c} >7.5%); patients who are active smokers, immunocompromised, or morbidly obese (body mass index >40); and patients who lack fat donor sites (**Table 3.1**).[32]

TABLE 3.1 GENERAL EXCLUSION CRITERIA

1. Ischemic, poorly vascularized skin flaps after mastectomy
2. Patients with a history of preoperative breast irradiation
3. Uncontrolled diabetes (hemoglobin A_{1c} >7.5%)
4. Patients who are active smokers
5. Immunocompromised
6. Morbidly obese (BMI >40)
7. Patients who lack fat donor sites

These are general exclusion criteria, and they should be used on a case-by-case basis in conjunction with multidisciplinary team comfort with surgical approach and reconstruction. Abbreviation: BMI, body mass index.

TABLE 3.2 ONCOLOGIC EXCLUSION CRITERIA

Oncologic Indications for Prepectoral Reconstruction	Oncologic Contraindications for Prepectoral Reconstruction
1. Use the same oncologic parameters as for any skin-sparing or nipple-sparing mastectomy 2. Multidisciplinary approach essential to ensure that each discipline is willing to embrace and safely adapt to the new technique	1. *Large tumors (>5 cm)* 2. Late cancer stage 3. *Deep tumors* 4. Chest wall involvement 5. Grossly positive axillary involvement 6. High risk of recurrence (based on multidisciplinary approach)

Any patient qualifying for chemotherapy should be considered for delivery in the neoadjuvant setting to potentially downstage the patient and sterilize the axilla, avoiding additional morbidity and increasing a patient's surgical options.

In addition, we have identified a number of oncologic contraindications for the prepectoral reconstructive approach (**Table 3.2**). Patients with late-stage breast cancer, posterior tumors near to or involving the pectoralis major muscle, and patients at high risk for recurrence are felt to be poor candidates for prepectoral placement. It is important to note that the oncologic safety of this procedure has not yet been documented. As with subpectoral reconstruction, extreme caution should be exercised for large tumors and for clinically positive lymph nodes. An attempt can be made to downstage the tumor using neoadjuvant chemotherapy, whereby prepectoral reconstruction is deemed safe after a favorable clinical and radiographic response. Although a history of RT negatively impacts prepectoral reconstruction, the converse is not the case. RT can and should be used for all prepectoral reconstruction patients who have an oncologic indication for postmastectomy radiation. Issues worthy of discussion are the timing of implant placement and possible benefit from using additional muscle coverage such as a latissimus flap. In our experience, to date, complications associated with adjuvant radiation are not significantly different than those seen with dual-plain reconstruction. Although complications of skin necrosis can occur, the more common complications tend to be skin tightening and stiffness with associated reduction in size.

Since the prepectoral approach has been performed consistently for fewer than 5 years, oncologic guidelines will continue to undergo evolution as with any new technique. We feel that it is prudent to err on the side of caution until data from randomized, prospective clinical trials and results of oncologic outcomes become available.

Patient selection should be approached from a multidisciplinary standpoint and should involve the entire care team. Reconstructive and oncologic surgeons, medical oncologists, and radiation oncologists should understand and be comfortable with the implementation of the prepectoral technique. As long as oncologic safety criteria are upheld, prepectoral implant-based reconstruction can be used for both SSMs and NSMs.

KEY REFERENCES

1. Howlader N, Noone AM, Krapcho M, et al, eds. SEER Cancer Statistics Review (CSR), 1975-2014. Bethesda, MD: National Cancer Institute. http://seer.cancer.gov/csr/1975_2014/, based on November 2016 SEER data submission, posted to the SEER web site, April 2017.
2. American Cancer Society. *Cancer Treatment & Survivorship Facts & Figures 2016-2017*. Atlanta, GA: American Cancer Society; 2016.
3. American Cancer Society. Surgery for breast cancer. 2016. https://www.cancer.org/cancer/breast-cancer/treatment/surgery-for-breast-cancer.html
4. McCready D, Holloway C, Shelley W, et al. Surgical management of early stage invasive breast cancer: a practice guideline. *Can J Surg*. 2005;48(3):185-194.
5. van Dongen JA, Voogd AC, Fentiman IS, et al. Long-term results of a randomized trial comparing breast-conserving therapy with mastectomy: European Organization for Research and Treatment of Cancer 10801 trial. *J Natl Cancer Inst*. 2000;92:1143-1150. doi:10.1093/jnci/92.14.1143.
6. Fisher B, Anderson S, Bryant J, et al. Twenty-year follow-up of a randomized trial comparing total mastectomy, lumpectomy, and lumpectomy plus irradiation for the treatment of invasive breast cancer. *N Engl J Med*. 2002;347:1233-1241.
7. Veronesi U, Cascinelli N, Mariani L, et al. Twenty-year follow-up of a randomized study comparing breast-conserving surgery with radical mastectomy for early breast cancer. *N Engl J Med*. 2002;347:1227-1232. doi:10.1056/NEJMoa020989.
8. Cao JQ, Olson RA, Tyldesley SK. Comparison of recurrence and survival rates after breast-conserving therapy and mastectomy in young women with breast cancer. *Curr Oncol*. 2013;20(6):e593-e601.
9. Halsted WS. I. The results of operations for the cure of cancer of the breast performed at the Johns Hopkins hospital from June, 1889, to January, 1894. *Ann Surg*. 1894;20:497-555.
10. Fisher B, Montague E, Redmond C, et al. Findings from the NSABP protocol no. B-04: Comparison of radical mastectomy with alternative treatments for primary breast cancer. I. Radiation compliance and its relation to treatment outcome. *Cancer*. 1980;46:1-13.
11. Fisher B, Bauer M, Margolese R, et al. Five-year results of a randomized clinical trial comparing total mastectomy and segmental mastectomy with or without radiation in the treatment of breast cancer. *N Engl J Med*. 1985;312:665-673.
12. Wickerham DL, Anderson SA, Fisher B, Margolese R, Mamounas T, Wolmark N. NSABP protocol B-06: a randomized clinical trial comparing total mastectomy with lumpectomy with or without irradiation in the treatment of breast cancer—Results after 15 years of follow-up. *Eur J Cancer*. 1998;34(suppl 5):S38.
13. Arora NK, Gustafson DH, Hawkins RP, et al. Impact of surgery and chemotherapy on the quality of life of younger women with breast carcinoma: a prospective study. *Cancer*. 2001;92(5):1288-1298.
14. National Comprehensive Cancer Network. Updated NCCN guidelines for breast cancer discourages prophylactic mastectomy in women other than those at high risk. 2009. http://www.nccn.org/about/news/newsinfo.aspx?NewsID=226. Accessed December 7, 2016.
15. Plevritis SK, Munoz D, Kurian AW, et al. Association of screening and treatment with breast cancer mortality by molecular subtype in us women, 2000-2012. *JAMA*. 2018;319(2):154-164.
16. Taylor KL, Lamdan RM, Siegel JE, Shelby R, Hrywna M, Moran-Klimi K. Treatment regimen, sexual attractiveness concerns and

psychological adjustment among African American breast cancer patients. *Psychooncology*. 2002;11(6):505-517.

17. Freeman BS. Subcutaneous mastectomy for benign breast lesions with immediate or delayed prosthetic placement. *Plast Reconstr Surg*. 1962;30:676-682.
18. Hinton CP, Doyle PJ, Blamey RW, Davies CJ, Holliday HW, Elston CW. Subcutaneous mastectomy for primary operable breast cancer. *Br J Surg*. 1984;71:469-472.
19. Hartmann LC, Sellers TA, Schaid DJ, et al. Efficacy of bilateral prophylactic mastectomy in BRCA1 and BRCA2 gene mutation carriers. *J Natl Cancer Inst*. 2001;93(21):1633-1637.
20. Hartmann LC, Schaid DJ Woods JE, et al. Efficacy of bilateral prophylactic mastectomy in women with a family history of breast cancer. *N Engl J Med*. 1999;340:77-84.
21. Rebbeck TR, Friebel T, Lynch HT, et al. Bilateral prophylactic mastectomy reduces breast cancer risk in BRCA1 and BRCA2 mutation carriers: the PROSE Study Group. *J Clin Oncol*. 2004;22(6):1055-1062.
22. Agarwal S, Agarwal S, Neumayer L, Agarwal JP. Therapeutic nipple-sparing mastectomy: trends based on a National Cancer Database. *Am J Surg*. 2013;208:93-98.
23. NCCN.org. Clinical Practice Guidelines in Oncology-Breast Cancer. Version I. 2016:1-184.
24. Burdge EC, Yuen J, Hardee M, et al. Nipple skin-sparing mastectomy is feasible for advanced disease. *Ann Surg Oncol*. 2013;20(10): 3294-3302.
25. Smith B, Tang R, Rai U, et al. Oncologic safety of nipple-sparing mastectomy in women with breast cancer. *J Am Coll Surg*. 2017;225(3): 361-365.
26. Li M, Chen K, Liu F, Su F, Li S, Zhu L. Nipple-sparing mastectomy in breast cancer patients and long-term survival outcomes: an analysis of the SEER database. *PLoS ONE*. 2017;12(8):e0183448. doi:10.1371/journal. pone.0183448.
27. Chen K, Liu J, Zhu L, Su F, Song E, Jacobs LK. Comparative effectiveness study of breast-conserving surgery and mastectomy in the general population: a NCDB analysis. *Oncotarget*. 2015;6:40127-40140. doi:10.18632/oncotarget.5394.
28. Gabriel A, Sigalove S, Sigalove NM, et al. Can surgical technique impact length of stay and post-operative outcomes in breast reconstruction? Abstract: The American Society of Breast Surgeons 18th Annual Meeting. 2017; Las Vegas, NV.
29. Gabriel A, Sigalove S, Sigalove NM, et al. Does surgical technique impact post-operative outcomes of breast reconstruction? Abstract. International Society for Pharmacoeconomics and Outcomes Research 22nd Annual International Meeting. 2017; Boston, MA
30. Cordeiro PG, McCarthy CM. A single surgeon's 12-year experience with tissue expander/implant breast reconstruction: part I. A prospective analysis of early complications. *Plast Reconstr Surg*. 2006;118:825-831.
31. Kim JY, Davila AA, Persing S, et al. A meta-analysis of human acellular dermis and submuscular tissue expander breast reconstruction. *Plast Reconstr Surg*. 2012;129:28-41.
32. Sigalove S, Maxwell PG, Sigalove NM, et al. Prepectoral implant-based breast reconstruction: rationale, indications and preliminary results. *Plast Reconstr Surg*. 2017;139(2):287-294.
33. Maxwell GP, Storm-Dickerson T, Whitworth P, Rubano C, Gabriel A. Advances in nipple-sparing mastectomy: Oncological safety and incision selection. *Aesthet Surg J*. 2011;31:310-319.

CHAPTER **4**

THE MASTECTOMY AND INCISION PLACEMENT

Toni Storm-Dickerson and Noemi M. Sigalove

KEY POINTS

- Surgical consideration when performing an ontologically appropriate nipple-sparing mastectomy
- Appropriateness of intraoperative nipple assessment
- The blood supply and anatomy of the breast
- Sensory innervation to the breast and nipple
- Strategies to minimize tissue ischemia from lymph node dye injection
- Understanding breast anatomy and perfusion to plan incision placement, and maximize mastectomy flap viability

INTRODUCTION

The potential that malignant tumor cells remain in the preserved nipple–areolar complex (NAC) is the major concern regarding the oncologic safety of nipple-sparing mastectomy (NSM). Although NSM has been repeatedly proved to be safe, the extent to which the nipple is surgically cored at the time of mastectomy and the value of intraoperative frozen core assessment remain somewhat controversial.

Rusby et al[1] looked at 48 specimens from 7 nonirradiated and 5 irradiated nipples and found that preservation of a 2-mm peripheral rim of tissue removes 96% of the nipple ducts while preserving 50% of the blood supply. Preservation of a 3-mm peripheral rim of tissue removes 87% of the ducts and preserves 66% of the blood supply. Therefore, overdissection of the nipple does not improve survival or decrease local recurrence, but does increase nipple ischemia and can result in unnecessary nipple loss.

The role of intraoperative frozen section of the NAC, however, remains controversial. Eisenberg et al[2] looked at the nipple pathology from 325 patients with NSM and frozen section, evaluating for occult disease and found a sensitivity and specificity of 64% and 99%, respectively. Alperovich et al[3] looked at 501 patients undergoing NSM between 2006 and 2013 (216 therapeutic, 285 prophylactic). Of the 480 with subareolar biopsies/nipple core, 307 had intraoperative frozen assessment with subsequent permanent sections and 173 had permanent evaluation only. Among the 307 intraoperative frozen sections, 12 were positive on permanent, 5 of which had a false negative (FN) on frozen (41% FN, and a 3.9% overall positivity of NAC cores). Of the positive NAC biopsies, 62% were ductal carcinoma in situ. Only 30% of the resected specimens had abnormal residual pathology. The authors concluded that intraoperative frozen assessment was highly specific but only moderately sensitive in detecting NAC disease and, thus, they felt it was worth doing.

Others, such as Suarez-Zamoraal et al[4] found significant interobserver variability. Among 34 NSMs, the frozen section FN and false-positive (FP) rates were 5.9% and 8.8%, respectively. The sensitivity and specificity were 77.8% and 88.0%, respectively. These authors explained the FN as sampling errors and cautery artifacts, and the FP as freezing artifacts and intraductal papillomas. They described subareolar frozen section as a specific test with moderate sensitivity with vast improvement, "almost perfect" when performed by a breast pathologist.

Although there is no true right or wrong answer to intraoperative nipple core assessment, we have found several useful tips. First, discuss your approach thoroughly with your patient and the potential need for delayed nipple removal depending on the final pathology. Perform sharp dissection of the subnipple tissue to minimize cautery artifact. Do not overdissect the nipple. Assess preoperative imaging to evaluate possible nipple involvement. Know your pathologist's expertise (Does your center have a breast pathologist?). Determine on a case-by-case basis the benefit and risk of intraoperative assessment. Lastly, when you do perform a nipple resection, consider nipple sharing from the unaffected nipple. If involvement is localized to the nipple, preserve the areola because this will improve the overall cosmetic outcome.

Even in institutions without frozen section evaluation, the rate of NAC positivity has been identified at 2.7% to 14%.[5] However, recurrence at that nipple remains very uncommon. Amara et al[6] looked at 751 patients and 1176 breasts undergoing NSM with a follow-up of 31.3 months. The NAC had a positive margin or involvement of nipple tissue in 2.7% (32 breasts), 56% were invasive cancer, and 44% had in situ disease. Management included repeat excision (11 cases, 34% of cases), 16% underwent adjuvant radiation only (NAC included as part of the post-mastectomy breast field), without further excision, 25% had complete NAC removal, and 25% had no additional treatment. The authors saw a significant decrease in NAC excision during the study period ($P = 0.003$). The overall local recurrence rate was 6.2%, with no recurrence at the preserved NAC skin, regardless of treatment. Petit et al[7] reported that when combined with intraoperative radiotherapy, patients with a positive NAC margin identified during NSM may not need further treatment after surgery. Taken together, these data further support the oncologic safety of nipple preservation in NSM.

BLOOD SUPPLY AND ANATOMY OF THE BREAST

Understanding the basic anatomy of the breast is key to any breast surgeon, both for cancer management and maximizing patient surgical outcomes. By understanding the anatomy, we can minimize postoperative pain, fat necrosis, and skin and NAC necrosis, while maximizing oncologic outcomes of tumor removal and preservation of retained tissues. What we are coming to understand is that the blood supply to the breast skin and NAC is tremendously variable.[8] The main sources of blood supply to the breast are the internal thoracic (IT), lateral thoracic (LT), anterior intercostal (AI), and thoracoacromial arteries. van Deventer et al, in their cadaver study, found that in 7 of 27 breast dissections, branches from the LT artery did not supply the NAC; and that in 8 breasts, branches from the AI arteries were absent (**Figure 4.1**). However, in all breasts examined, the NAC was fed by one or more branches from the IT artery. Given these complexities and the unpredictability of the blood supply in the setting of mastectomy with reconstruction, we

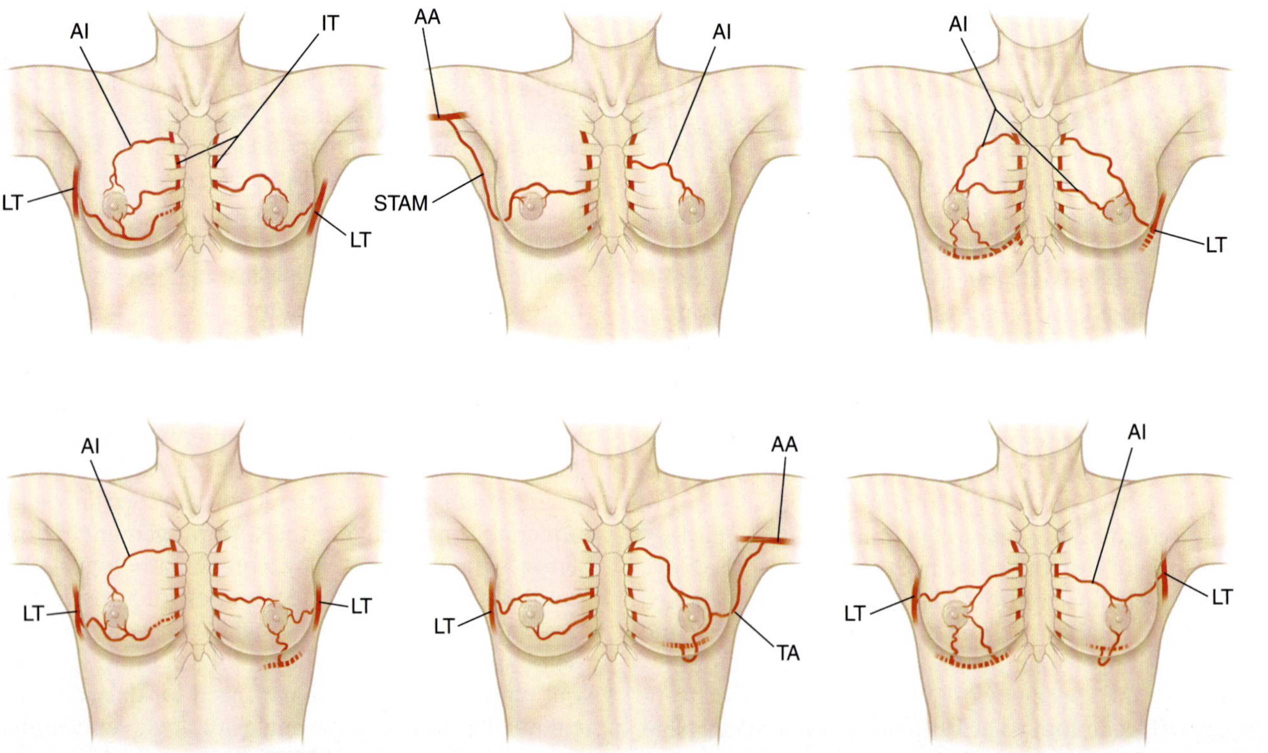

Figure 4.1 Blood supply to the breast–nipple–areolar complex (NAC). Main blood supply: internal thoracic (IT), lateral thoracic (LT), anterior intercostal (AI), thoracoacromial (TA) arteries. van Deventer found 7 of 27 branches from the LT artery did not supply the NAC; and in eight breasts, branches from the AI arteries were absent. In all breasts examined, the NAC was fed by one or more branches from the IT artery.

need to take advantage of any tools that may be available to us, such as preoperative magnetic resonance imaging (MRI) and perioperative perfusion assessment devices. These tools can be used, often at no additional expense having been obtained for other purposes, to assess patients for aberrancies in blood supply/arterial distribution so that we can be more cognizant of what perfusion challenges we may be facing and operate accordingly.

The skin of the nipple rests directly on a thin layer of smooth muscle, areolar muscle fibers which are distributed in two directions: radial (muscle of Meyerholz) and circular (muscle of Sappey) and are responsible for the telotism of the papilla, "mimicking an erection." Sensation carries onto the NAC, as the main blood supply to the NAC and the inner half of the breast. Seitz et al[9] used MRI in to the nipple is thought to derive primarily from the lateral cutaneous branch of T4.[1] The importance of the IT 52 breasts to classify the blood supply to the NAC into five anatomic zones or "NACsomes" (**Figure 4.2**). They further demonstrated that the vast majority of the blood supply is from the medial perforates or a mix of medial and other anatomic zones; medial (type I), lateral (type II), central (type III), inferior (type IV), and superior (type V). As would be expected following much along the lines of the breast proper, the distribution was very heavily medially based; type I, 54%, multizone (type I + II, *N* = 20; type I + III, *N* = 2), 42%, one breast had type II only blood supply, 0.4% and one breast had type III only blood supply, 0.4%. Further, the blood supply was found to be symmetrically distributed between the breasts 96% of the time.

As seen with the NACsomes and the breast blood supply as mentioned,[8,10] in *most cases*, the vast majority of the blood supply comes from a medial distribution. The IT accounts for approximately 60% of the total blood supply to the breast. This makes understanding the planned parameters of dissection before initiation of a mastectomy imperative. Overdissection into the medial/central plains of the breast will result in devastating skin necrosis.

We suggest drawing out the borders of the breast on the patient, before starting the surgery, taking special care to not violate the intercostals originating along the midline (**Figure 4.3**). This is an area that can easily be overdissected, with devastating results because it is responsible for the majority of the blood supply in most patients.

SENSORY INNERVATION TO THE BREAST AND NIPPLE

Although nerves and vessels do run relatively together, the origins of the sensory distribution to the breast are primarily laterally derived from the anterolateral thoracic

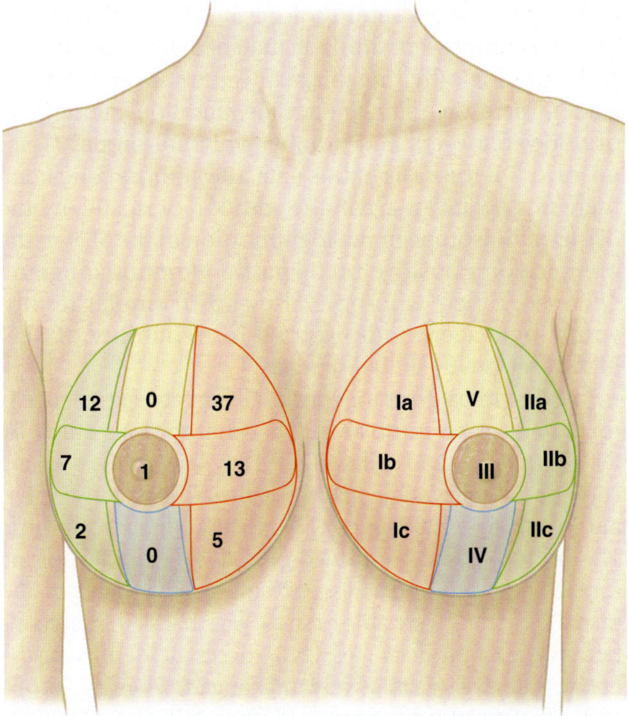

Figure 4.2 NACsomes are the blood supply to the NAC. Type I (medial), type II (lateral), type III (central), type IV (inferior), type V (superior). Type I, 54%. Multizone, 42%, (type I + II, *N* = 20; type I + III, *N* =2). Type II, one breast, 0.4%. Type III, one breast, 0.4%. Generally, blood supply was symmetrically distributed between the breasts 96% of the time.

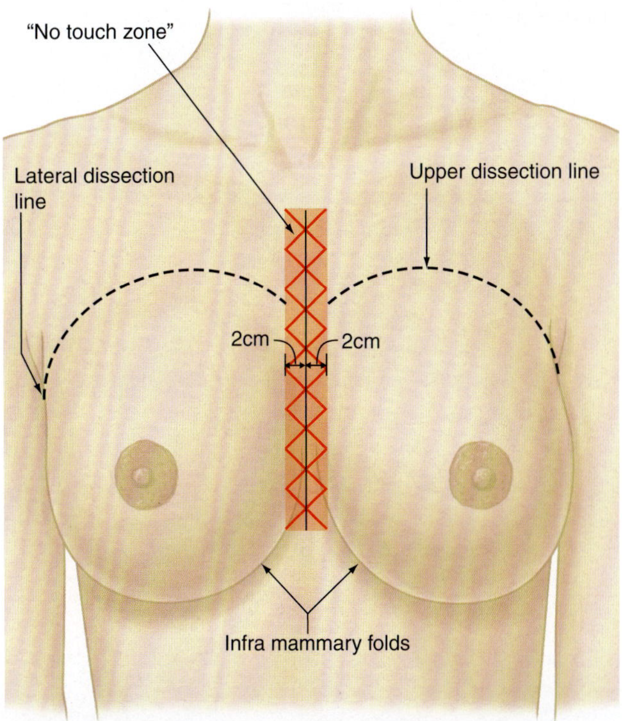

Figure 4.3 Drawing of the breast markings with patient in the supine position. Middle line Xs demarcate the midline "No touch zone" where the majority of the blood supply originate (internal thoracic and anterior intercostal), the dotted lines are the lateral and upper dissection lines to help avoid overdissection.

intercostal, with the majority of the blood supply arising medially from the internal mammary artery (IMA).[11,12] Additional sensory input comes from the anteromedial branches of the thoracic intercostal nerves T3-T5, and the supraclavicular nerves from the cervical plexus also provide innervation to the upper and lateral portions of the breast.[13] Schulz et al demonstrated the primary innervation to the nipple from the lateral branch of the fourth intercostal nerve and also the trajectory of innervation to the nipple and translated these findings into preservation of nipple sensation. They looked at 86 women who underwent Wise pattern reduction mammoplasty and found that by avoiding dissection in the inferolateral quadrant or what they called the "unsafe zone" of the breast, they were able to reliably spare nipple sensation. Although we currently expect loss of nipple sensation with NSM, this may change as we better understand breast anatomy and the extent of dissection needed for optimal oncologic outcomes while preserving tissue integrity. Preservation of the fourth intercostal and nipple sensation may yet be possible with NSM as we continue to learn and to hone our skills. Further, understanding the nerve distribution can impact incision placement choice in BCS and NSM (**Figure 4.4**).

Reproduction of the intercostal nerve innervation to the nipple. The red dashed lines demarcate the inferolateral breast quadrant to be avoided during surgical dissection to minimize nerve injury and loss of nipple sensation. II, III, IV, V = Anterior cutaneous T2-5, Lateral cutaneous T3-5.

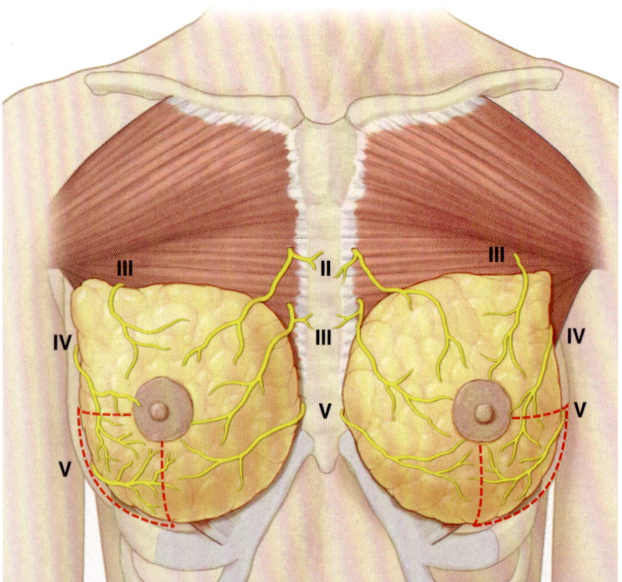

Figure 4.4 Nervous distribution to the breast. The red dashed lines demarcate the inferolateral breast quadrant. II, III, IV, V = Anterior cutaneous T2-5, Lateral cutaneous T3-5.

ROLE OF BLUE DYE FOR SENTINEL LYMPH NODE BIOPSY

Management of the axilla is beyond the scope of this chapter and we practice both society surgical oncology (SSO) best practice guidelines and American Society of Breast Surgeons (ASBrS) consensus statement recommendations on management of the axilla. However, we briefly discuss the use of blue dye and radioisotope for sentinel lymph node biopsy (SLNB) detection in the setting of NSM in particular. SLNB is the gold standard for axillary staging. However, debate remains as to the optimal method of sentinel lymph node (SLN) detection. Determine whether patients are undergoing an SLNB with isosulfan blue dye, methylene blue dye, and radioisotope should be considered before entering the operating room. There are reports in the literature of both isosulfan blue and methylene blue causing cutaneous necrosis[14]; and although the data have shown improved sensitivity and specificity with dual tracer, the number of SLN sampled seems to be more important than the use of dual tracer.[15,16] For this reason, we prefer to forgo the use of blue dye and use only radioisotope for SLNB in patients without a history of neoadjuvant chemotherapy, always assuring a 2 to 3 node harvest.

O'Reilly et al[17] performed a prospective randomized controlled trial comparing the combination of radioisotope and blue dye versus radioisotope alone on 667 clinically node-negative women with positive preoperative lymphoscintigram. Combination dye and isotope was given to 342 patients and radioisotope alone to 325 patients. The two groups were similarly matched demographically and pathologically (mean age, mean tumor size 2.4 cm, grade). There was a similar node identification rate, number of nodes retrieved, and number of lymph nodes (LNs) positive. On the basis of this data, the authors concluded there was no advantage in the addition of isosulfan blue dye to radioisotope in the identification of the SLN in the presence of a positive preoperative lymphoscintigram. There are others who have also shown similar results, with single-agent radioisotope for reliability of SLN identification, in skilled hands.[18,19]

We would caution that, as in all surgery, experience is important as seen illustrated in an ambitious study by Dr. Hirum Cody and colleagues.[20] They showed the learning curve of eight new surgeons during their initial, consecutive, and combined 2000 cases of SLNB at a single institution. The protocol used combined blue dye and radioisotope for SLN mapping and assessed results at increments of 500 cases. What they were able to show was that as the surgeons became more proficient at SLNB, success at identifying the LN by blue dye was relatively unchanged, whereas isotope identification steadily increased from 86% to 94%.

Although we prefer to use only radioisotope in the nontreated patient, in the post neoadjuvant setting we minimize our FN rate to well below 10% by continuing to utilize the dual tracer, confirming removal of the clinically positive node (cN1), and by assuring a three lymph node harvest. Removal of the cN1 node can be done with preoperative or intraoperative localization of the lymph node using ultrasound (US) or by radiographic confirmation that the clipped/biopsied node has been removed. In this way, if the cN1 has sterilized we perform a three-node assessment to minimize FNs,[21] and remove no more nodes. Lastly, although we do use blue dye in the post neoadjuvant setting, we dilute it, be it isosulfan blue or methylene blue, at a 1 to 3 with injectable saline.

We also assess the axilla clinically preoperatively with US and have a full discussion with the patient regarding the risks associated with the blue dye including skin necrosis and tissue and implant loss and with isosulfan blue, rare anaphylaxis. We strongly encourage surgeons to find what is right for them and fully discuss the issues, options, and concerns with their patients.

MASTECTOMY FLAP MAXIMIZATION

The ultimate goal of a mastectomy is to remove the breast tissue to minimize local recurrence while preserving healthy skin to maximize rapid healing of healthy tissues. This goal remains the same regardless of the extent of skin retained or if reconstruction is immediate, delayed, or never to happen. Although our incisions and the extent of skin preserved may vary, the principles remain constant and are based on the complete removal of the breast gland with preservation of the skin and hypodermis.

The more we understand about the role biology plays in cancer, the more we understand bigger is not necessarily better. Mastectomy flap viability is not determined by flap thickness but is rather defined by anatomy.[22-24] The skin is made up of three layers: the epidermis, dermis, and hypodermis. The blood supply lies within the hypodermis (**Figure 4.5**).[9,23-25] The subcutaneous fat, or the fat of the hypodermis, is made up of adipose cells. Numerous studies have shown that adipose cell growth is subject to both hyperplasia (increase in number) and hypertrophy (increase in size).[23-26]

In obese patients, in comparison to thin patients, adipose cells express both hyperplasia and hypertrophy, which leads to an overall increase in the size of their hypodermis. As a consequence, obese patients are more likely to have thicker flaps, whereas nonobese patients tend to have thinner flaps (**Figure 4.6**). The dermal layer remains relatively unchanged.[27,28] As long as the oncologic surgeon observes the anatomic division between the hypodermis and breast glandular tissue, both types of flaps will remain viable and oncologically sound. They will also both ensure maximal removal of the breast gland while preserving blood flow. It is important to understand that there is no survival benefit to taking tissue beyond the breast gland.[29-31]

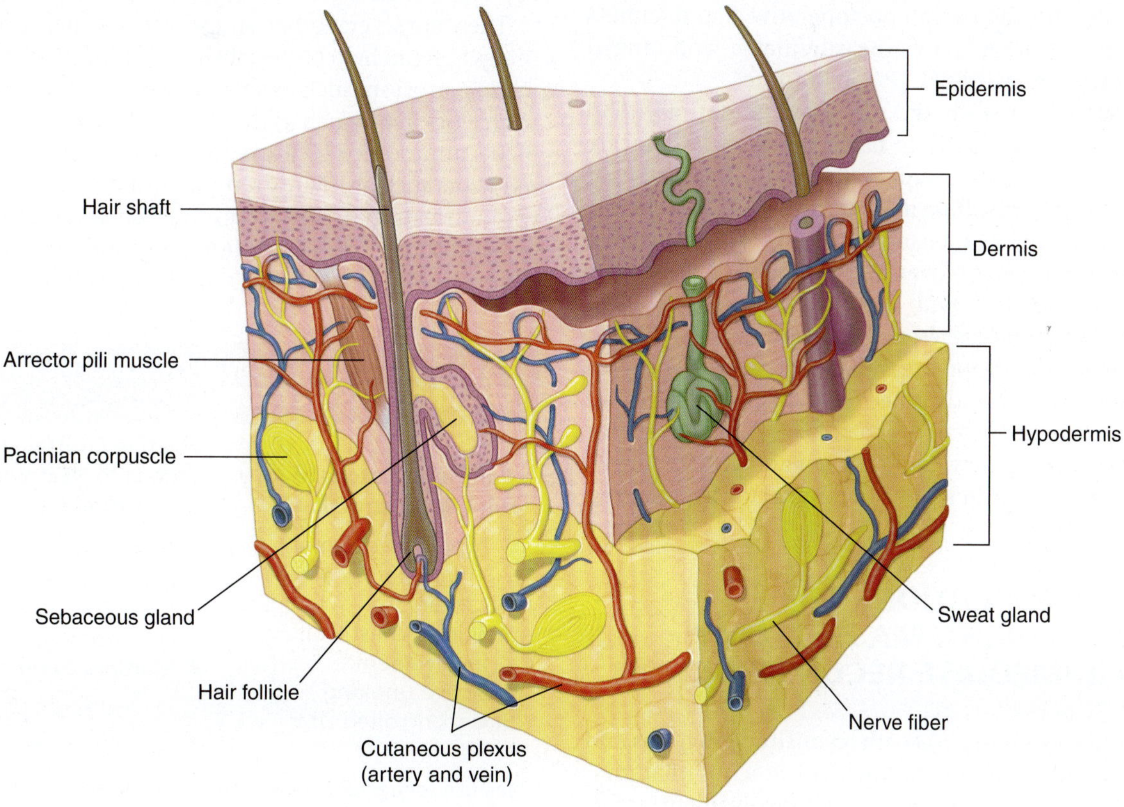

Figure 4.5 Illustration of the layers of the skin. Illustration of the blood supply to the skin running in the hypodermis or bottom layer of the skin just above the breast gland.

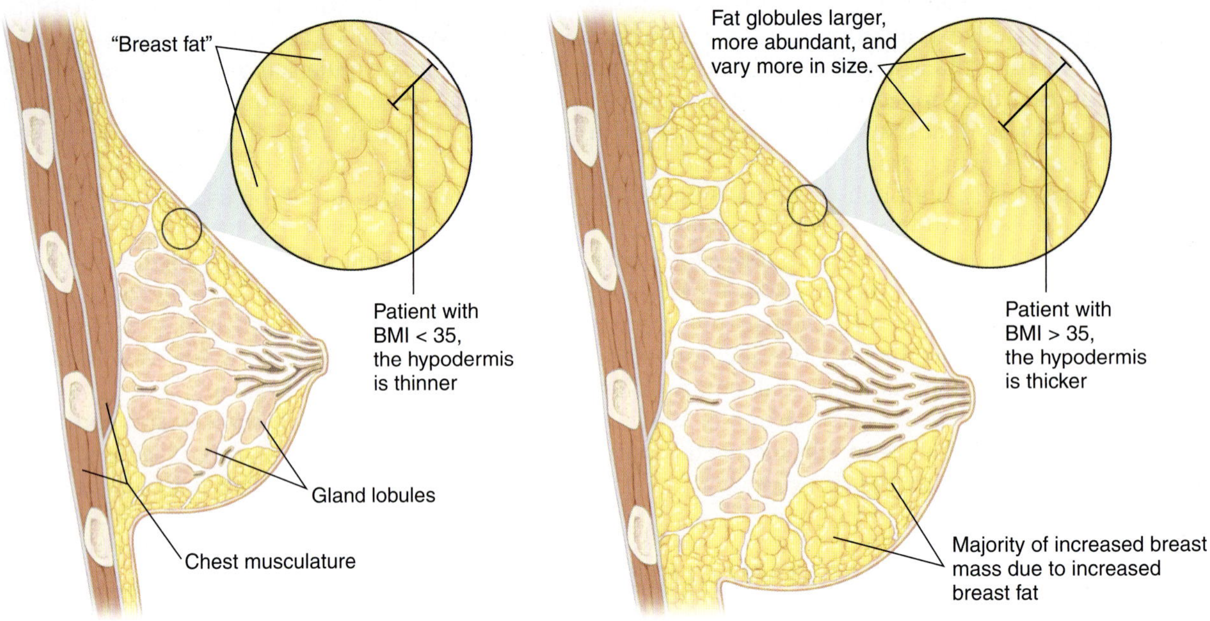

Figure 4.6 Illustration of varied hypodermal thickness. BMI, body mass index.

Frey et al[32] performed MRIs on 420 NSMs, 379 preoperative and 60 postoperative. The average total preoperative skin/subcutaneous tissue "flap" thickness was 11.4 mm and the average total postoperative flap thickness was 8.7 mm. They found that a flap thickness of less than 8 mm was an independent predictor of ischemic complications. By MRI the overall postoperative flap thickness was 68.2% of preoperative measurements, and ranged from 52.0% versus 74.0% ($P < 0.0001$).[32]

Although their study did not correlate BMI and flap measurements uniquely to each patient, it did nicely demonstrate a routine overdissection of the breast flaps at the time of NSM, resulting in significantly higher ischemic complications. In fact, even in the majority of their surviving flaps, the dissection was overaggressive, with flap thickness measured at 8.7 mm with a pre-NSM measurement of 11.4 mm. We would suggest that there is no survival benefit in overdissection of the breast flap, whereas its sequel is significant. Further study is needed to help us understand the ideal extent of dissection; and perhaps with more refinement, may lead to nerve preservation and greater patient satisfaction because these structures run in the hypodermis.

CONTRAINDICATIONS TO NIPPLE-SPARING MASTECTOMY WITH IMMEDIATE RECONSTRUCTION

Contraindications to NSM with reconstruction for us and our plastic surgeons are nipple involvement, inflammatory breast cancer, skin or chest wall involvement, active smoking, and uncontrolled diabetes mellitus (DM)/HbA1c. Relative contraindications are BMI > 40, history of radiation, and multiple comorbidities (**Table 4.1**). An important note is that relative contraindication should be considered contraindication based on you and your plastic surgeon's comfort level and expertise. For instance, we would not hesitate to delay or proceed with a latissimus flap on a patient with high BMI and a history of radiation.

There are several other, simple yet extremely important things that can help protect the mastectomy flaps and maximize perfusion, such as sharp dissection or use of a cool source of energy such as the Photon Blade or the Plasma Blade, tumescence, gentle retraction using nonconducting retractors such as Invuity retractors, sharp dissection, and warm irrigation. Lastly, we strongly encourage the breast surgeon to observe the angiography and watch the perfusion assessment after the mastectomy because this can

TABLE 4.1 CONTRAINDICATIONS TO NIPPLE SPARING MASTECTOMY

Contraindications to NSM with Reconstruction	Relative Contraindications to NSM with Reconstruction[a]
1. Nipple involvement 2. Inflammatory breast cancer 3. Skin or chest wall involvement 4. Active smoking 5. Uncontrolled DM/HbA1c	1. BMI > 40 2. History of radiation (can proceed with muscle coverage) 3. Multiple comorbidities

[a]Relative contraindication should be considered contraindication based on level of comfort and experience.

Abbreviations: BMI, body mass index; DM, diabetes mellitus; NSM, nipple-sparing mastectomy.

be extremely educational for our self-assessment, to see the origins of the blood supply as well as any compromised areas that result from our dissection. This is not a criticism, but an opportunity to improve our techniques and continue to enhance our skills.

INCISION PLACEMENT

To achieve optimal skin flaps and incision placement, the breast surgeon should be cognizant of the exact location of the tumor. Planning and communicating with the plastic surgeon is key. Never hesitate to utilize tumor localization if a nonpalpable malignancy is located at or near a resection edge/margin, that is, very anterior, posterior, superior, and lateral, etc. This can include simple intraoperative US with overlying skin marking, or clips or wire placement per individual surgeon's preference. However, especially in those patients with very peripherally located lesions post neoadjuvant chemotherapy, the ability to confirm complete removal of the tumor foci can be critical. This will help to both assure that the tumor has been removed while limiting potential overdissection of the mastectomy flaps. Also, if you are very concerned that a focal area may need additional resection, you can utilize intraoperative frozen assessment and/or place a small nonabsorbable suture that can be removed in the office once the margin is confirmed benign or, if there is found to be residual disease, used to guide a focused re-excision.

Further, plastic surgeons should plan incision length and location so that it allows for comfortable dissection by the breast surgeon. Suboptimal incision length will increase surgical time, stress and tension on flaps, as well as the potential for errors and ischemia. If isosulfan or methylene blue is used, the site of injection should be located away from incision, not under the nipple and minimized in the case of nipple sparing. Incision placement for the mastectomy is based on these criteria, at the same time ensuring that patient oncologic candidacy aligns with patient preference. We must take into account patient expectations regarding breast appearance, nipple preservation, size, ptosis, and local recurrence risk. Ultimately, surgical decisions are made in concert with the patient, including vigorous patient education while considering the patient's values and preferences with the recommendations of the entire oncologic team.

As breast surgeons, we do not discuss the cosmetic principles guiding reconstructive approach but focus instead on our perspective for incision placement and incision size (**Figure 4.7**). Our personal preference is the inframammary approach, which has proved to be an excellent option for NSM and has been found to be both effective and safe.[33-35] Important issues to consider are surgeon comfort level with the procedure and the ability to properly remove the breast gland while preserving flap viability. At times, elongating the incision or extending in a laterosuperior manner can lead to increased operative efficiency and safety. However, consider the lateral intercostal distribution and potential increased chronic pain with this incision.

We encourage careful patient selection and larger incisions until the operating surgeon masters and feels comfortable with these surgical techniques. With skin-sparing

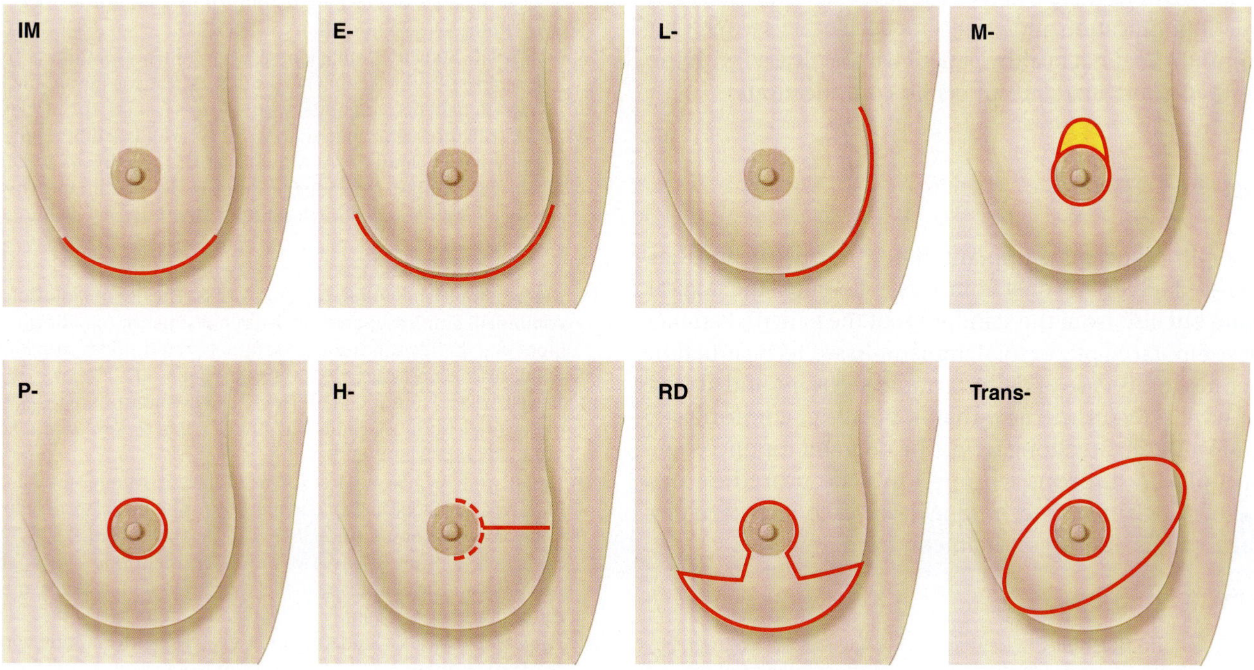

Figure 4.7 Nipple- and skin-sparing mastectomy skin incisions. IMF, inframammary fold incision; E-IMF, extended IMF; L-IMF, lateral IMF; P-NAC, peri-nipple areolar complex, H-Cent, horizontal–pericentral, RDP, reduction pattern.

mastectomy, incision approaches include horizontal central breast, vertical reduction pattern, and periareolar. With the periareolar approach, the incision is made along the areolar border, such that the NAC is removed with the underlying breast gland, and the breast is removed through this circular incision. If necessary, this incision can be extended superiorly in an elliptical manner, allowing for greater visibility, or removal of a larger breast. The periareolar approach allows for maximum skin preservation, providing the reconstructive surgeon the entire skin envelope for use. Reduction of the skin envelope can be achieved by de-epithelialization of the lower pole for overlapping of flaps. We vary our incision approach for skin-sparing mastectomy using the reduction pattern mastectomy or the low horizontal mastectomy. The reduction pattern mastectomy allows for a more natural shape of the breast, with improved anterior projection and less horizontal expanse. The low horizontal mastectomy allows for the entire incision line to be hidden along the inframammary fold with no flap confluence, decreasing risk for skin necrosis.

If available, we recommend the use of skin perfusion assessment devices. Both surgeons should be present to review results. The decision to proceed with prepectoral reconstruction is largely based on adequate flap viability, and the breast surgeon must take ownership of devascularized flaps. Consistently reviewing results also allows the breast surgeon to recognize and avoid future dissection errors. The device should be used as an assessment as well as an educational tool.

Plastic surgeons should also listen to concerns voiced by the breast surgeon regarding their dissection. Single-stage reconstruction should be abandoned when the breast surgeon feels that flaps may become too stressed with inflation. In working together, the best outcome is achieved by communication and respect for each other's work. Our common goal is a healthy patient who is pleased with the aesthetic outcome and suffers no complications.

SUMMARY

Overall, prepectoral implant–based reconstruction has achieved success not only from the standpoint of the surgical team but also from the standpoint of the patient. Patients have embraced prepectoral implant–based reconstruction because of its ease of delivery, rapid recovery, and ability to have a reconstruction that is pleasing, comfortable, and well-tolerated long term. The demand for oncologic and plastic surgeons who perform the procedure has been rising, and the technique deserves to be part of any breast surgical team's armamentarium.

KEY REFERENCES

1. Rusby JE, Brachtel EF, Taghian A, Michaelson JS, Koerner FC, Smith BL. Microscopic anatomy within the nipple: implications for nipple-sparing mastectomy. *Am J Surg*. 2007;194(4):433-437.
2. Eisenberg RE, Chan JS, Swistel AJ, Hoda SA. Pathological evaluation of nipple-sparing mastectomies with emphasis on occult nipple involvement: the Weill-Cornell experience with 325 cases. *Breast J*. 2014;20:15-21.
3. Alperovich M, Choi M, Karp NS, et al. Nipple-sparing mastectomy and sub-areolar biopsy: to freeze or not to freeze? Evaluating the role of sub-areolar intraoperative frozen section. *Breast J*. 2016;22(1):18-23.
4. Suarez-Zamoraa DA, Barrera-Herreraa LE, Palau-Lazaroad MA, et al. Accuracy and interobserver agreement of retroareolar frozen sections in nipple-sparing mastectomies. Ann Diagn Pathol. 2017;29:46-51.
5. Tang R, Coopey SB, Merrill AL, et al. Positive nipple margins in nipple sparing mastectomies: rates, management, and plastic safety. *J Am Coll Surg*. 2016;222(6):1149-1155.
6. Amara D, Peled AW, Wang F, Ewing CA, Alvarado M, Esserman LJ. Tumor involvement of the nipple in total skin-sparing mastectomy: strategies for management. *Ann Surg Oncol*. 2015;22:3803-3808.
7. Petit JY, Veronesi U, Orecchia R, et al. Nipple-sparing mastectomy with nipple areola intraoperative radiotherapy: one thousand and one cases of a five years experience at the European institute of oncology of Milan (EIO). *Breast Cancer Res Treat*. 2009;117:333-338.
8. van Deventer P, Graewe FR. The blood supply of the breast revisited. *Plast Reconstr Surg*. 2016;137(5):1388-1397.
9. Seitz IA, Nixon AT, Friedewald SM, Rimler JC, Schechter LS. "NAC-somes": a new classification system of the blood supply to the nipple areola complex (NAC) based on diagnostic breast MRI exams. *J Plast Reconstr Aesthet Surg*. 2015;68:792-799.
10. Zucca-Matthes G, Urban C, Vallejo A. Anatomy of the nipple and breast ducts. *Gland Surg*. 2016;5(1):32-36.
11. Mathes SJ, Nahai F. *Reconstructive Surgery: Principles, Anatomy, and Technique*. New York, NY: Churchill Livingston; 1997.
12. Pansky B. *Review of Gross Anatomy*. 6th ed. New York, NY: McGraw-Hill; 1996.
13. Schulz S, Zeiderman M, J. Gunn JS, et al. Safe plastic surgery of the breast II: saving nipple sensation. *Eplasty*. 2017;17:e33.
14. Bircan HY, Ozcelik U, Koc B, Kemik O, Demirag A. Cutaneous necrosis as a result of isosulphane blue injection in mammarian sentinel lymph node mapping: report of two cases. *Clin Med Insights: Case Rep*. 2014;7:79-81.
15. Giuliano AE, McCall L, Beitsch P, et al. Locoregional recurrence after sentinel lymph node dissection with or without axillary dissection in patients with sentinel lymph node metastases: the American College of Surgeons Oncology Group Z0011 randomized trial. *Ann Surg*. 2010;252(3):426-433.
16. Boughey JC, Suman VJ, Mittendorf EA, et al; Alliance for Clinical Trials in Oncology. Sentinel lymph node surgery after neoadjuvant chemotherapy in patients with node-positive breast cancer: the ACOSOG Z1071 (Alliance) clinical trial. *JAMA*. 2013;310(14):1455-1461.
17. O'Reilly EA, Prichard RS, Al Azawi D, et al. The value of isosulfan blue dye in addition to isotope scanning in the identification of the sentinel lymph node in breast cancer patients with a positive lymphoscintigraphy: a randomized controlled trial (ISRCTN98849733). *Ann Surg*. 2015;262(2):243-248.
18. Bines S, Kopkash K, Ali A, Fogg L, Wool N. The use of radioisotope combined with isosulfan Blue dye is not superior to radioisotope alone for the identification of sentinel lymph nodes in patients with breast cancer. *Surgery*. 2008;144(4):606-609.
19. Kang T, Yi M, Hunt KK, et al. Does blue dye contribute to success of sentinel node mapping for breast cancer? *Ann Surg Oncol*. 2010;17(suppl 3):280-285.
20. Derossis AM, Fey J, Yeung H, et al. A trend analysis of the relative value of blue dye and isotope localization in 2,000 consecutive cases of sentinel node biopsy for breast cancer. *J Am Coll Surg*. 2001;193(5):473-478.
21. Boileau JF, Poirier B, Basik M, et al. Sentinel node biopsy after neoadjuvant chemotherapy in biopsy-proven node-positive breast cancer: the SN FNAC study. *J Clin Oncol*. 33:258-264.
22. Drolet R, Richard C, Sniderman AD, et al. Hypertrophy and hyperplasia of abdominal adipose tissues in women. *Int J Obes (Lond)*. 2008;32(2):283-291.

23. Freeman BS. Subcutaneous mastectomy for benign breast lesions with immediate or delayed prosthetic placement. *Plast Reconstr Surg*. 1962;30:676-682.
24. Burns DA, Breathnach SM, Cox N, Griffiths CE, eds. *Rook's Textbook of Dermatology*. 7th ed. Malden, MA: Blackwell Science; 2004.
25. Jo J, Gavrilova O, Pack S, et al. Hypertrophy and/or hyperplasia: dynamics of adipose tissue growth. *PLoS Comput Biol*. 2009;5(3):e1000324.
26. Sun K, Kusminski CM, Scherer PE. Adipose tissue remodeling and obesity. *J Clin Invest*. 2011;121(6):2094-2101.
27. Stolier A, Sullivan S, Dellacroce F. Technical considerations in nipple-sparing mastectomy: 82 consecutive cases without necrosis. *Ann Surg Oncol*. 2008;15:1341-1347.
28. Beer GM, Varga Z, Budi S, Seifert B, Meyer VE. Incidence of the superficial fascia and its relevance in skin-sparing mastectomy. *Cancer*. 2002;94:1619-1625.
29. Fisher B, Anderson S, BryantJ et al. Twenty-year follow up of a randomized trial comparing total mastectomy, lumpectomy and lumpectomy plus radiation for the treatment of invasive breast cancer. *N Engl J Med*. 2002;347:1233-1241.
30. Fisher B, Wolmark N, Redmond C, Deutsch M, Fisher ER. Findings from NSABP Protocol No. B-04: comparison of radical mastectomy with alternative treatments. II. The clinical and biologic significance of medial-central breast cancers. *Cancer*. 1981;48: 1863-1872.
31. Fisher B, Bauer M, Margolese R, et al. Five-year results of a randomized clinical trial comparing total mastectomy and segmental mastectomy with or without radiation in the treatment of breast cancer. *N Engl J Med*. 1985;312:665-673.
32. Frey JD, Salibian AA, Choi M, Karp NS. Mastectomy flap thickness and complications in nipple-sparing mastectomy: objective evaluation using magnetic resonance imaging. *Plast Reconstr Surg Glob Open*. 2017;5(8):e1439.
33. Farahat AM, Hashim T, Soliman HO, Manie TM, Soliman OM. Skin sparing mastectomy: technique and suggested methods of reconstruction. *J Egypt Natl Canc Inst*. 2014;26(3):153-159.
34. Rawlani V, Fiuk J, Johnson SA, et al. The effect of incision choice on outcomes of nipple-sparing mastectomy reconstruction. *Can J Plast Surg*. 2011; 19(4):129-133.
35. Colwell AS, Tessler O, Lin AM, et al. Breast reconstruction following nipple-sparing mastectomy: predictors of complications, reconstruction outcomes, and 5-year trends. *Plast Reconstr Surg*. 2014;133: 496-506.

CHAPTER 5

ASSESSING TISSUE VIABILITY

Allen Gabriel, Steven R. Sigalove, Maurice Y. Nahabedian, and G. Patrick Maxwell

KEY POINTS

- Tissue viability can be assessed clinically or by tissue perfusion devices.
- Devices can assess by tissue oxygenation or fluorescence imaging.
- Advantages and disadvantages are described.
- A current list of devices available is summarized.

INTRODUCTION

As mentioned in Chapter 1, the assessment of tissue viability of the skin flaps is an essential component of our bioengineered approach to prepectoral prosthetic breast reconstruction. The most common early postoperative complications after immediate breast reconstruction are flap necrosis, seroma, infection, and capsular contraction.[1,2] Inadequate intraoperative blood supply to the tissue flaps is apparently the main driver of flap necrosis and may be a contributing factor to other complications. Timely and accurate intraoperative identification of insufficient blood supply enables the surgeon to either take remedial measures to improve viability or to debride hypoxic tissue margins, thereby preventing those common early postoperative complications. Furthermore, smoking and uncontrolled diabetes hamper microcirculation to the tissues and should therefore be considered as contraindications to the bioengineered prepectoral method of prosthetic breast reconstruction, as discussed in later chapters of this book. In such higher risk cases (immediate reconstruction following mastectomy), where the surgeon has decided to proceed anyway, meticulous technologic assessment of tissue viability becomes all the more valuable in these patients, to prevent postoperative morbidities associated with inadequate microcirculation in the tissue flaps. So this chapter reviews the various technologies available for assessing tissue viability.

Traditionally, tissue viability has been assessed by direct clinical examination. Direct clinical assessment is based primarily on the tissue color, and sometimes additionally on temperature, turgor, observation of bleeding at the dermal edge, or bleeding reaction to needle pricking. The flaps should have a color and temperature approximating the normal healthy state. If pricked, there should be a normal outflow of bright red blood—neither a lack of bleeding nor a rapid outflow of dark blood. Unfortunately, direct clinical assessment depends substantially on the experience of the assessor. And even with experience, clinical assessment of tissue viability can be challenging in the operating room (OR) because of the conditions under which it is performed. Another limitation of clinical observation is that it cannot be performed continuously. Similarly, whole-body indices of blood circulation (such as blood pressure) can also serve as supplemental warning signs, but they lack specificity to the breast flaps and therefore cannot be relied on as a sufficient indicator of flap tissue viability. There are several types of Doppler probes that can assess blood flow to the tissue, using heat sensors, ultrasound, or laser, to measure temperature, fluid movement, or hemoglobin. The major limitation of all these probes is that they cannot image the entire flap simultaneously and instead require contact with a specific point of the tissue, which implies that the surgeon already knows where exactly the tissue lacks viability. These probes also depend on assessor experience and have not been highly reliable in this application. So they will not be reviewed further here.

For all these reasons, it is preferred to make use of the current imaging devices for locally assessing tissue viability. Sometimes, even though skin flaps appear viable clinically, imaging will reveal areas at risk that may need treatment measures (such as applying topical nitroglycerine) to better maintain viability, or will reveal ischemic margins that need debridement. Viable skin flaps are an essential prerequisite for bioengineered prepectoral prosthetic breast reconstruction, and the current imaging technologies enable us to better maintain truly viable skin flaps.

The devices available today for assessing tissue viability can be categorized into two broad groups: devices that assess blood oxygenation versus devices that assess tissue perfusion. Each of these two broad groups of devices is discussed individually in more detail subsequently. The basic difference between these two broad categories is what they are actually measuring and what information is being provided to the surgeon. In simple terms, devices that assess oxygenation take snapshot measurements of the amount of oxygenated and deoxygenated hemoglobin in the tissue, to then calculate the amount of oxygen that the tissues extract from the blood. By contrast, devices that assess perfusion perform continuous optical measurement of the volume of a fluorescent tracker dye, and thus also a real-time assessment of dynamic blood flow through the tissue. The big picture between the two tissue viability devices are that oxygenation is not real time and does not measure perfusion directly as compared to devices that assess perfusion directly. This can be important when assessing partially failing flaps in the OR.

OXYGENATION ASSESSMENT DEVICES

Bioengineering Background

One "obvious" way to assess the oxygen uptake of tissue is to measure and compare the amount of oxyhemoglobin and deoxyhemoglobin in that tissue region. Near-infrared spectroscopy (NIRS) is a well-established, noninvasive method to do that.[3-5] The basic principle is that the devices shine a spectrum of light onto the tissue and then measure the wavelengths that are reflected back. Because oxyhemoglobin and deoxyhemoglobin absorb different wavelengths of light, the amount of reflected light detected in various wavelengths enables an assessment of the amount of oxyhemoglobin and deoxyhemoglobin in the tissue, and thus a calculation of the amount of oxygen being absorbed by the tissue. Despite the name, NIRS devices typically emit both infrared and near-infrared lightwaves from an emitter. Sensors then measure how much reflected light is received back at various wavelengths. Both infrared and near-infrared light will pass through skin, bone, and other tissues unattenuated. Near-infrared light is absorbed by both oxygenated and deoxygenated blood, whereas infrared light is absorbed only by deoxygenated blood. Thus, the difference in the amount of infrared versus near-infrared reflected light detected by the receiving sensors serves as a way to calculate the amount of oxygen uptake in the tissues.[3-5] NIRS technology is often used for monitoring in surgical and in intensive care unit contexts, whereby only numerical data is provided. Here, we only consider devices that also provide imaging and thus can be used for assessing flap viability.

KD203 (Kent Imaging; Calgary, AB, Canada)

Kent Imaging's KD203 (**Figure 5.1**) is a portable device that uses NIRS to provide imaging of tissue oxygenation. The device is based on NIRS, as described, and it has recently received U.S. Food and Drug Administration (FDA) clearance. According to the manufacturer, it provides an approximate level of oxygen saturation and relative levels of oxyhemoglobin and deoxyhemoglobin in superficial tissue. Although clinical data are still lacking for this application, within the category of devices assessing tissue oxygenation using the NIRS methods, the Kent KD203 appears to set a good standard, applicable to the task of assessing tissue flap viability.

HyperView (HyperMed; Memphis, TN)

The HyperMed HyperView is also a portable device that measures the amount of tissue oxygenation by spectroscopy of oxyhemoglobin and deoxyhemoglobin. The main

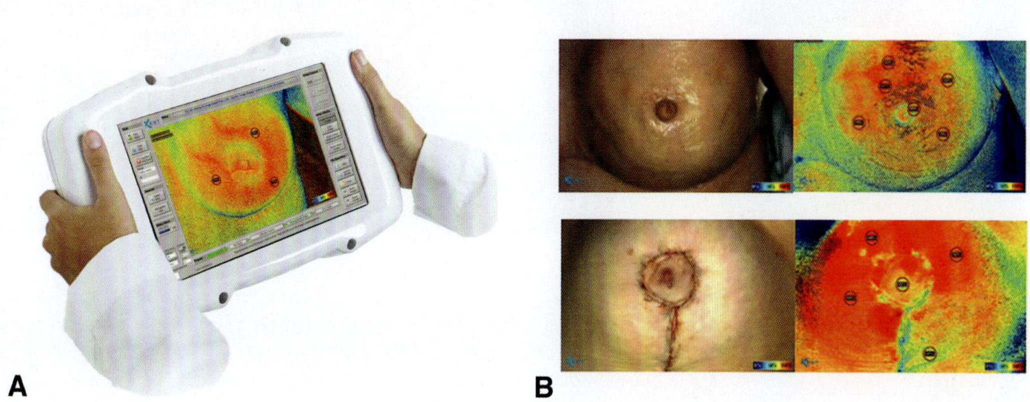

Figure 5.1 The KD203 from Kent Imaging. A, Photograph of the device itself. B, Representative image of breast flap oxygenation as assessed by the KD203.

difference of the HyperView system, compared to the Kent KD203 and other NIRS systems for other applications, is that the device seems to use only longer wavelengths of light in the visible spectrum. The manufacturer's current website remains somewhat opaque about this, but they do consistently speak of "visible spectrum light" and never of "near-infrared." Journal papers about OxyVue-1 (the progenitor device of HyperView) stated that it used light in the 500 to 660 nm range, thus effectively green, yellow, and orange light.[6] It is unclear whether this makes a meaningful difference for the assessment of tissue oxygenation in breast flaps, but HyperView is, in any case, FDA cleared (as are the other devices discussed in this chapter).

PERFUSION ASSESSMENT DEVICES

A different approach to assessing tissue viability is to visualize the amount of blood perfusion through the capillaries of the skin. Fluorescence angiography has become a well-established procedure for that in several fields of surgery.[7] The basic approach is that a radiopaque contrast dye is injected into the patient's circulation and then its flow through the capillary beds of the tissue can be imaged in real time.[7-9] Although sodium fluorescein has been used in the past and other contrast agents are still used in other applications, all currently available angiography devices for the assessment of tissue flaps in breast reconstruction surgery use the fluorescent dye, Indocyanine green, because of its superior performance and safety profile.[8,9] Indocyanine green bonds strongly to plasma proteins and lipoproteins, so it remains within the vascular and lymphatic systems.[8] The devices then project near-infrared light onto the tissue. Some uncertainty remains about the degree to which Indocyanine green is actually absorbing and emitting infrared lightwaves ("fluorescence") versus merely reflecting and scattering infrared lightwaves at altered wavelengths; but in either case, the spectra of infrared light detected in the presence of the dye is clearly different from that in its absence, thus enabling reliable assessment of perfusion.[8] Thus, all the devices provide real-time continuous imaging of tissue perfusion, down to a depth of about 1 cm. Reported side effects from Indocyanine green are rare and mild[7,8] (although formulations free of iodine should be preferred for patients allergic to iodine). Indocyanine green is eliminated only by the liver, so renal insufficiency is not a contraindication.[8]

SPY (Stryker; Mississauga, ON, Canada/Kalamazoo, MI)

The SPY-Elite system (**Figure 5.2**) from Stryker (Stryker acquired Novadaq in 2017) has been the established leader in the field, with numerous journal studies supporting

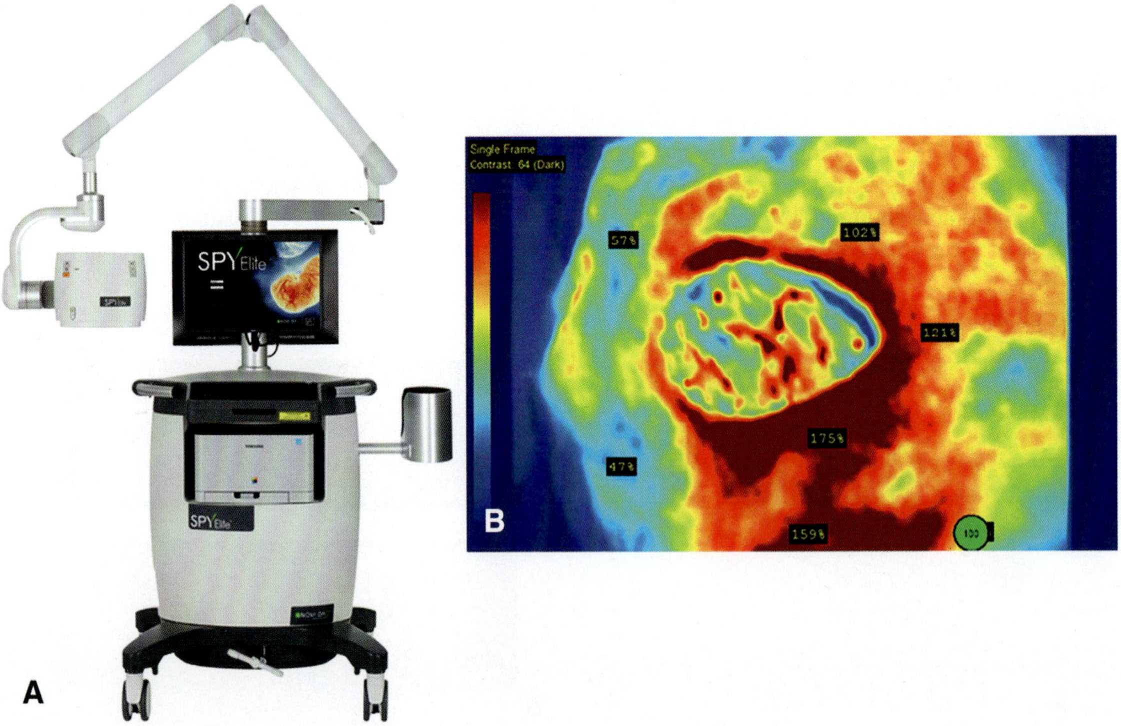

Figure 5.2 **The SPY-Elite from Stryker.** A, Photograph of the device itself. B, Representative image of breast flap perfusion as assessed by SPY-Elite.

its clinical usage. Images and data can be stored and analyzed with its SPY-Q software, both during and after the operation. The SPY system can display and analyze the intensity of the Indocyanine green signal in either of two modes: "complete" (brightness intensity of the signal is simply quantified on a fixed scale, although it does not account for the influence of signal confounding factors, such as tissue fat content, distance to camera, or ambient OR lighting) or "relative" (a point of maximum intensity chosen by the operator is defined as 100% and all other points are scaled relative to that reference point). One small study suggests that both modalities can accurately differentiate tissue that will have necrosis postoperatively, but the relative mode appears to make this differentiation more reliably, and the authors of that study recommended the relative mode preferentially.[10] Various SPY-Q quantitative thresholds for predicting necrosis have been proposed in the literature. The most apparent distinguishing characteristic of the SPY-Elite system is that it is a large piece of OR equipment (circa 2-m tall, 165 kg), not a portable handheld device. The more recently introduced SPY-PHI version is a more mobile handheld camera, but it must be powered by the Pinpoint endoscopic tower. The SPY-PHI does not offer a relative quantification mode, but it can be used with ambient lighting (**Figure 5.3**).

PhotonVue (Invuity; San Francisco, CA)

The PhotonVue device from Invuity, by contrast, is a quite compact and portable device, consisting of a camera unit connected by cable to the control box, which is then connected to a laptop computer that runs the PhotonVue clinical software. The camera unit, being small and handheld, can be quickly and easily moved around by the surgeon both inside and outside of the operating theater. Images and data can be stored and analyzed with its SPY-Q software, both during and after the operation. The system images in two modes: either in live mode or in relative quantification. In live imaging mode, the device measures the signal intensity and displays it in real time. In relative quantification mode, the device autocalculates the point of highest signal intensity, defines it as 100%, and then displays the rest of the imaged tissue in graytone or color scale relative to that point identified as 100%. This "relative" approach to visualization of perfusion has the advantage of maximizing the visual differentiation between areas of higher and lower perfusion, adjusted to each individual patient. This attenuates the influence of signal confounding factors, such as tissue fat content, distance to camera, or ambient OR lighting. In Europe, a very closely related device, the Fluobeam, is manufactured and distributed by Fluoptics (Grenoble, France).

PDE Neo-II (Hamamatsu; Hamamatsu, Japan)

The Photodynamic Eye (PDE) Neo-II device (**Figure 5.4**) from Hamamatsu similarly consists of a handheld camera unit that is roughly flashlight shaped, attached by a cable to a compact controller unit that is then connected to any compatible video monitor and/or recording units.

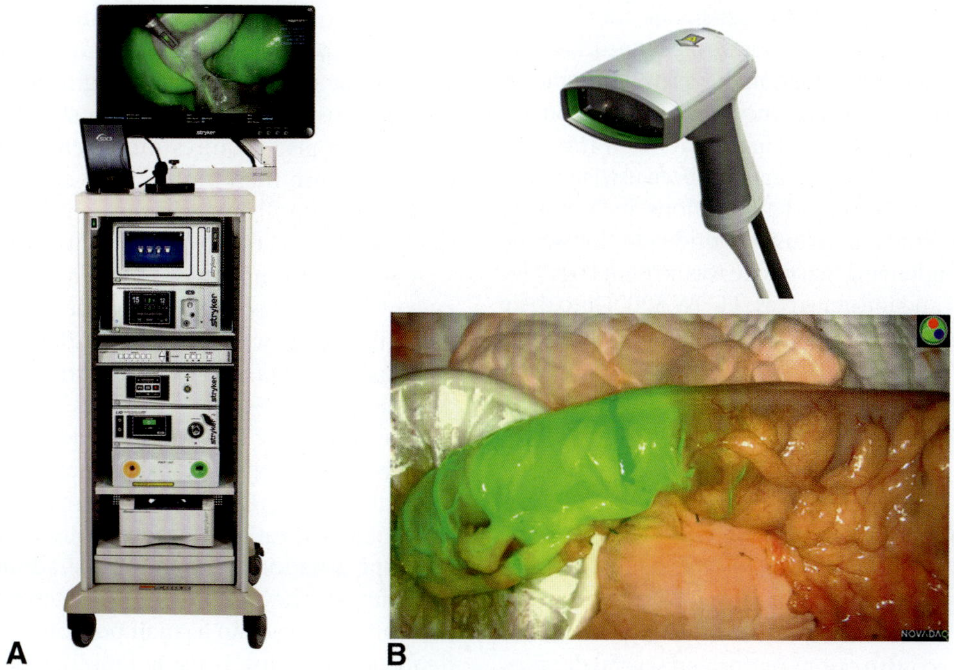

Figure 5.3 **The SPY-PHI from Stryker.** A, Photograph of the device itself. B, Representative image demonstrating tissue perfusion.

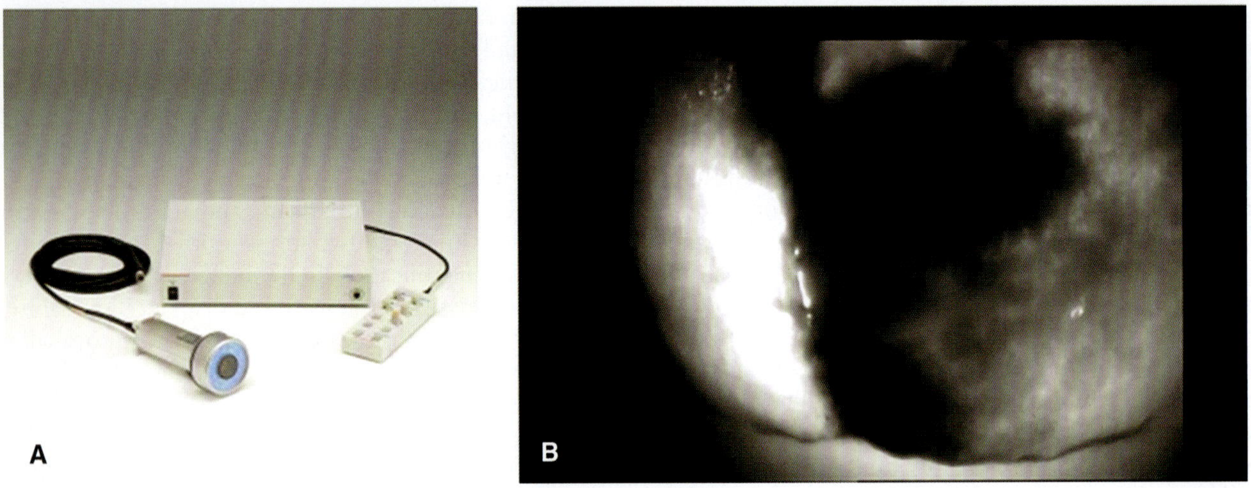

Figure 5.4 The PDE from Hamamatus. A, Photograph of the device itself. B, Representative image of breast flap perfusion as assessed by PDE. PDE, photodynamic eye.

The PDE system has been in existence longer than any other fluorescence angiography system, although earlier models (PDE) appear to still be available only outside the United States. The camera unit can be switched between fluorescence imaging and regular film imaging, to enable comparison of perfusion imaging to the actual anatomy. With that said, for the Hamamatsu PDE Neo-II system (and its predecessors) the output video imaging for the perfusion assessment mode is only in graytones (or monochrome green brightness intensity), not in full color scale. The system does not have a relative quantification mode.

Other Systems

Two other fluorescent angiographic systems are not currently available at the time of this writing but are mentioned, because reports about them can be found in the scientific literature and because it is conceivable that they could reappear on the market sometime in the future. First, the IC-View (Pulsion Medical Systems; Munich, Germany) had been used in many European studies in a variety of applications, including in skin flap assessment.[9] An exclusive worldwide license for the technology underlying that device was acquired by Zeiss (Jena, Germany) and integrated (as "FLOW 800") into their operating microscope systems for other surgical applications. Second, the FLARE system (Curadell; Marlborough, MA) has also been used in studies on breast cancer surgery.[9] It appears to remain in the R&D stage at this time.

SUMMARY

As mentioned in Chapter 1, prepectoral prosthetic breast reconstruction is not entirely novel—the original subcutaneous breast reconstructions performed several decades ago also placed the implant prepectorally. The advances in implant technology, availability of acellular dermal matrices for soft-tissue support, and better processing systems for fat grafting have brought back prepectoral reconstruction successfully; and depending on the long-term results, it is here to stay. In addition, one thing that is different between then and now is that in the past, the viability of skin flaps could really only be assessed by direct clinical observation, which was not always adequate. This often led to tissue necrosis, inadequate dermal healing, and other postoperative complications, which in turn contributed to the gradual replacement of subcutaneous techniques with subpectoral ones.

In the meanwhile, new technologies that allow for more reliable assessment of tissue viability have become available. This has been a key contributing factor to making prepectoral prosthetic breast reconstruction feasible again today with our new bioengineered approach. The skin flaps used in reconstruction should be viable, and this in turn also requires more sensitive assessment of their perfusion than in the past—something that again is better accomplished with the support of the currently available devices than with clinical observation alone.

A newly published study reported on the national usage rates of fluorescence angiography for breast reconstruction, using the Agency for Healthcare Review and Quality's National Inpatient Sample administrative database (a random sample of 20% of all inpatients in the United States).[11] For the years 2012 to 2014, they identified 110 320 adult women undergoing unilateral or bilateral mastectomy with immediate breast reconstruction (tissue expander, implant, or autologous) for breast cancer without metastases (thus implying a national annual rate of about 184 000 such procedures). They reported that fluorescence angiography has only been used in a small portion of women, but the frequency of its use is rising rapidly, from 1.9% of these patients in 2012 to 3.7% in 2014. The study did not assess

Specification	PhotonVue	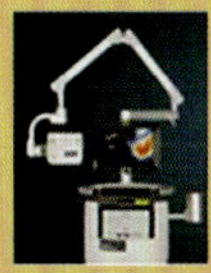 SPY-Elite	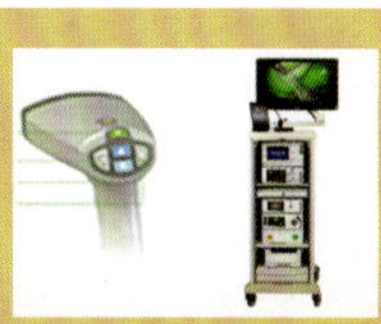 SPY-PHI (+ Pinpoint)	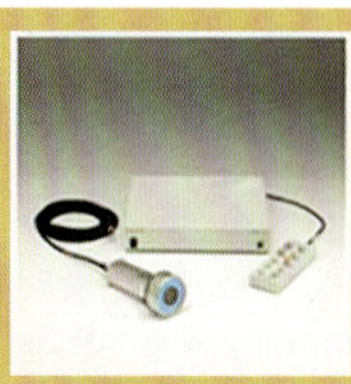 Hamamatsu

Footprint	**Small, portable**
	• 38 cm × 30 cm × 10 cm
	• 9 kg
		Large, not portable
		• 98 cm × 202 cm
		• 202 kg
			Large, not portable
			• Pinpoint Laparoscopic Tower:
			  • 75 cm × 175 cm
			  • 100kg
			• SPY-PHI Camera: hand piece
				Small, portable

Optical Safety	Class 1 Laser	Class 2 Laser	Class 2 Laser	Class 2 Laser
Maneuverability of Camera	**Yes** Autofocus	**No** Fixed camera placement	**Yes** Manual focus	**Yes** Autofocus
Image and Video Recording Capability	**Yes** Images and video	**Yes** Images and video	**No**	**?**
Relative Quantification	**Yes** Real Time	**Yes** At end of study	**No**	**No**
Color Mapping	**Yes** Real Time	**Yes** At end of study	**No**	**No**
Utilization	**• Preoperative** **• Intraoperative** **• Postoperative**	**• Intraoperative**	**• Intraoperative**	**• Preoperative** **• Intraoperative** **• Postoperative**

Figure 5.5 Comparison of all tissue assessment devices.

how often tissue flaps were assessed by other methods such as NIRS oxymetry or probes, but it seems safe to assume that all other technology-assisted methods combined probably did not exceed the rate of fluorescence angiography, thus suggesting that direct clinical assessment alone still remains standard practice. Unfortunately, we also know from recent meta-analyses[1,2] that the rate of postoperative tissue necrosis is about 5% or 30%, thus implying that there is still further room for improvement of the intraoperative assessment of tissue viability.[12] Several studies have shown that technologic assessment of tissue viability reduces the rate of postoperative necrosis compared to clinical assessment alone.[7,9,12]

This chapter has provided an overview of the different types of technologies (**Figure 5.5**) available to plastic surgeons today, and every surgeon will have his or her personal preferences for one or the other, according to how each device's various advantages and disadvantages match up with each individual surgeon's needs and preferences (**Figure 5.5**).

Personally, for immediate reconstruction procedures, this author prefers devices that assess perfusion. At present, the devices assessing oxygenation only provide static snapshots of the tissue at individual timepoints, and, therefore, require assessment of multiple images over time to understand perfusion. By comparison, the devices assessing perfusion provide a continuous dynamic video of the blood flow through the tissues.

Regardless of each surgeon's individual preferences, the current technologies for imaging of the flap enable us to better assess tissue viability, thereby better preventing possible postoperative necrosis and other complications. Assessing and ensuring tissue viability is therefore an essential component of our new bioengineered approach to prepectoral prosthetic breast reconstruction.

KEY REFERENCES

1. Chatterjee A, Nahabedian MY, Gabriel A, et al. Early assessment of post-surgical outcomes with pre-pectoral breast reconstruction: a literature review and meta-analysis. *J Surg Oncol.* 2018;117(6):1119-1130. doi:10.1002/jso.24938.
2. Heidemann LN, Gunnarsson GL, Salzberg CA, SØrensen JA, Thomsen JB. Complications following Nipple-Sparing Mastectomy and Immediate Acellular Dermal Matrix Implant-based Breast Reconstruction—A Systematic Review and Meta-analysis. *Plast Reconstr Surg Glob Open.* 2018;6:e1625.

3. Hampton DA, Schreiber MA. Near infrared spectroscopy: clinical and research uses. *Transfusion*. 2013;53:52S-58S.
4. Torella F, Haynes SL, McCollum CN. Cerebral and peripheral oxygen saturation during red cell transfusion. *J Surg Res*. 2003;110: 217-221.
5. Scheeren TWL, Schober P, Schwarte LA. Monitoring tissue oxygenation by near infrared spectroscopy (NIRS): background and current applications. *J Clin Monit Comput*. 2012;26:279-287.
6. Chin JA, Wang EC, Kibbe MR. Evaluation of hyperspectral technology for assessing the presence and severity of peripheral artery disease. *J Vasc Surg*. 2011;54:1679-1688.
7. Burnier P, Niddam J, Bosc R, Hersant B, Meningaud J-P. Indocyanine green applications in plastic surgery: a review of the literature. *J Plast Reconstr Aesthet Surg*. 2017;70:814-827.
8. Desmettre T, Devoisselle JM, Mordon S. Fluorescence properties and metabolic features of indocyanine green (ICG) as related to angiography. *Surv Ophthalmol*. 2000;45:15-27.
9. Griffiths M, Chae MP, Rozen WM. Indocyanine green-based fluorescent angiography in breast reconstruction. *Gland Surg*. 2016;5:133-149.
10. Newman MI, Jack MC, Samson MC. SPY-Q analysis toolkit values potentially predict mastectomy flap necrosis. *Ann Plast Surg*. 2013;70:595-598.
11. Chattha A, Bucknor A, Chen AD, Lee BT, Lin SJ. Indocyanine green angiography use in breast reconstruction: a national analysis of outcomes and cost in 110,320 patients. *Plast Reconstr Surg*. 2018;141:825-832.
12. Robertson SA, Jeevaratnam JA, Agrawal A, Cutress RI. Mastectomy skin flap necrosis: challenges and solutions. *Breast Cancer*. 2017;9:141-152.

CHAPTER 6

THE ROLE OF ACELLULAR DERMAL MATRIX AND PREPECTORAL BREAST RECONSTRUCTION

C. Coleman Brown, Maurice Y. Nahabedian, Allen Gabriel, and Steven R. Sigalove

KEY POINTS

- Role of ADM for prepectoral breast reconstruction has become an important consideration for prepectoral reconstruction.
- The incorporated ADM prevents inferior and lateral migration of the implant if adequate ADM is utilized.
- When the ADM is removed from the packaging, recommendations include minimal handling, with the ADM being treated as a sterile device.
- All ADMs require some degree of soaking when removed from the package to remove the preservative solutions and packaging antibiotics.
- Use of ADM for expander coverage is an essential component of prepectoral reconstruction, irrespective of the thickness of the flap or the amount of subcutaneous tissue present.

INTRODUCTION

Prepectoral breast reconstruction is unique in that by being in the subcutaneous space, there is no other structural anatomic component between the implant and the skin. Submuscular or partial-muscle coverage reconstruction utilizes the pectoralis muscle to cover, or at least, partially cover the implant, thereby maintaining a supportive structure between the implant and the skin. Despite this support, there are other long-term muscle-related issues to consider when performing implant-based breast reconstruction, namely, muscle animation, capsular contracture, radiation fibrosis, pain, and functional concerns. The use of an acellular dermal matrix (ADM) along with improvements in implant design and the widespread use of fat grafting have allowed the surgeon to bridge this gap between adequate support and improved aesthetics.

To view figures associated with this chapter, please access the eBook bundled with this book. Access instructions are found on the inside front cover.

ACELLULAR DERMAL MATRIX

Use of an ADM in breast reconstruction began in the early 2000s and has become the mainstay of modern implant-based reconstruction.[1,2] The addition of an ADM in this arena allowed for the advancement of implant-based breast reconstruction away from full-muscle coverage and into the realm of better aesthetics and more overall pocket control. Historically, subcutaneous placement of implants in breast reconstruction has demonstrated increased rates of capsular contracture and those studies were utilizing older generation implants and no ADM. We have learned a great deal over the years on how to handle devices, tissue, and meshes in a sterile manner for implantation utilizing appropriate antiseptic solutions. Although there are proponents of entirely subcutaneous implant reconstruction today,[3] utilizing ADM in breast reconstruction in the prepectoral space has been shown to be not only a viable technique but is also becoming the go-to method for initial implant-based breast reconstruction. Even though early and long-term follow up is needed, early results show that the addition of ADM has reduced the rates of capsular contracture to less than 1% as compared to 6.8% in prepectoral reconstruction without ADM.

The first use of ADM in breast reconstruction began as a means to bridge the gap between the leading edge of the pectoralis muscle and the inframammary fold. The traditional pre-ADM "dual-plane" technique was centered on releasing the pectoralis muscle and creating a subpectoral pocket, thereby allowing the expander to sit under the muscle. The muscle would not often cover the device entirely and, to prevent window shading of the muscle, it was tacked to the subcutaneous tissue and dermal surface. The device then sat partially in the subcutaneous plane. Although this afforded a better position of the expander with respect to the previously performed total muscle coverage technique, it did not relieve the patient of window shading or potential issues related to direct subcutaneous contact. With the advent of acellular dermal tissue and its application in the breast reconstruction arena, the ability to control the lower pole of the breast and the accurate positioning of the tissue expander became possible.

ADM is arguably one of the most important components of prosthetic reconstruction. In general, sterile ADMs are preferred to reduce the rate of infection.[4,5] Human ADM is preferred because of the inherent elasticity of the human skin, although porcine and bovine ADMs have also been used with success.[6,7] Fenestrated or perforated ADM is preferred to minimize the risk of seroma formation and to promote zones of adherence that can promote better incorporation of the ADM. With prepectoral reconstruction, thicker sheets of ADM in the range of 2 to 3 mm are preferred, to provide the additional tissue support needed.

When the ADM is removed from the packaging, recommendations include minimal handling, with the ADM being treated as a sterile device. All ADMs require some degree of soaking when removed from the package to remove the preservative solutions and packaging antibiotics. Failure to soak in a sterile solution may be responsible for the development of "red breast syndrome" that is typically located along the cutaneous distribution overlying the ADM.[5]

The characteristics of ADM are important and are briefly reviewed. Most ADMs are available in a rectangular or contoured form. The dimensions of the rectangular form typically used for prepectoral are 16 × 20 cm. The ADM should be trimmed appropriately such that it fits the device and covers the entire anterior surface. The posterior surface can also be covered depending on surgeon preference and the availability of the ADM. The orientation of the ADM is important because human ADMs are polarized with a dermal and basement membrane surface. The dermal surface should be in contact with the mastectomy skin flap to enhance soft-tissue incorporation. Typical sutures for the ADM include a mono- or multifilament absorbable that can be placed in a continuous or interrupted manner. Refer to Chapter 15 for a detailed approach of techniques utilized for prepectoral reconstruction.

Rationale for Prepectoral Reconstruction

During the time of what we now call the "dual-plane" technique, the success and improvement of implant-based breast reconstruction flourished. Although autologous tissue is still a mainstay of the reconstruction armamentarium, expander and, subsequently, direct-to-implant (DTI) reconstruction became the majority of reconstructions performed nationwide. With the advent of ADM use, DTI reconstruction became a viable alternative; and as genetic testing also increased and improved, it expanded. Using ADM in this realm offered patients the ability to quickly reach full-cup sizes that, during the total muscle era, were never possible. Because using an ADM allowed quicker expansion and also DTI reconstruction, the possibility of full-coverage ADM in the subcutaneous plane was entertained. When using ADM in DTI reconstruction, the surgeon often used the larger pieces available to not only attach the ADM to the inframammary fold but to also allow for larger volume implants to be inserted. As this practice expanded, many surgeons began to realize that with larger implant volumes coupled with the typical 30% or greater stretch of the ADM, the pectoralis muscle was essentially window shading cephalad and covering at best only 20% of the implant, depending on the size of the implant. This allowed us to question the viability of using the muscle at all. If the muscle is truly only covering a small percentage of the device, then what good does it provide?

Since 2010, utilization of the total ADM prepectoral implant-based reconstruction became a reality.[8-14] During this time, many options of dermal matrices became available and thus created issues with outcomes, complications, cost, reimbursement, and consistency of product. Because of this, the expansion of prepectoral full-coverage ADM reconstruction halted. Although still performed intermittently during that time, it was the introduction of better ADM material with ready-to-use options, perforations, and other advancements that allowed the rebirth of the prepectoral reconstruction. The ability to perform prepectoral reconstruction hinges on full-coverage ADM and its ability to resist capsular contracture integrate fully and reduce muscle-related consequences. ADM products today allow for better drainage, thus reducing the overall seroma rate; better integration, allowing for a more vascularized plane separating the implant from the surface; and less scar and contracture formation, allowing better long-term results. One concern that is always brought up is the cost of the products being utilized in these cases. Refer to Chapter 22 for the economic discussion. One argument can be made that no ADM utilization has a higher capsular contracture rate than the combined prepectoral evidence reported thus far (Hani).[8-10] These techniques all vary with the variety of coverage of the implants, but one commonality in these chapters includes the total anterior coverage. Is the posterior coverage necessary? That remains to be decided in the coming years. When cost is an issue, one can think of using the same ADM that is being utilized in current dual-plane reconstructions, where only the lower pole of the breast is covered in the prepectoral reconstruction. This has not been studied and we are not certain about the stability of the device placed and how this will play a role in future capsular contracture rates. One must imagine that the capsular contracture rate may be similar to our current dual plane with ADM evidence, but as of now is unknown.

TECHNIQUE

When performing prepectoral breast reconstruction, proper technique of ADM placement is important in obtaining better outcomes and minimizing complications. Once the type of reconstruction is decided upon (expander or DTI), preparation of the ADM is performed. There are many sizes and shapes of ADM available. Many surgeons will choose a 16 × 20 cm sheet of perforated ADM on the basis of ease of use and convenience. Occasionally, a shaped or contoured piece can provide the necessary coverage; ultimately, it will be the patient anatomy that will dictate the size and shape chosen. It is important to note that regardless of the piece of ADM chosen, it needs to match the surface area of the expander or implant desired and be able to fully cover the anterior surface of the device. In addition, it is recommended that the ADM not overlap itself to improve the tissue integration. Coverage of all or a portion of the posterior surface is occasionally considered and is dependent on surgeon preference.

TWO-STAGE PROSTHETIC RECONSTRUCTION

It is important to recognize that there are on-label and off-label techniques for ADM use in the setting of prosthetic reconstruction. The on-label techniques utilize ADM for soft-tissue support and are placed into the mastectomy space and sutured before implant insertion. The off-label techniques are where the ADM is placed around the tissue expander and wrapped, creating an ADM-tissue expander construct that is inserted into the prepectoral space. The other labeling aspect is the fill of the tissue expander with saline or air. Saline is considered on-label, whereas filling the tissue expander with air is considered off-label.

The author's preferred technique is to select the tissue expander based on biodimensional planning and then partially fill it with a known quantity of air. A 16 × 20 cm sheet of ADM is then draped evenly over the tissue expander. A perforated ADM is preferred; however, if the perforated variety is not available, then fenestrations are created using an 11-blade to make full-thickness slits throughout the entire surface of the ADM. This will allow for adequate drainage. The ADM is then draped over the expander, ensuring that the entire anterior surface is covered with a 3 to 4 cm cuff along the posterior aspect. This author prefers a 16 × 20 cm sheet in the "thick" variety of AlloDerm (Allergan, Irvine, CA). Alternatively, two "contour" sheets can be used after they have been sutured together along the short axis of the AlloDerm. Once the ADM has been oriented appropriately, it is then attached to the expander at the respective tabs using 3-0 Vicryl suture. Slits should be made in the ADM to allow the tabs to protrude through the ADM and to facilitate suturing to the chest wall. Excess ADM is trimmed to smooth the surface. Spanning sutures can be placed posteriorly to maximize contact between the expander surface and the ADM. Once the ADM/expander unit has been created, it is then set aside into a bath of antibiotic irrigation until ready to insert.

The mastectomy pocket is then evaluated, taking care to perform meticulous hemostasis and checking of the skin flaps. Drains are placed and typically include two 15-French hubless channel drains on every primary mastectomy/implant reconstruction. Both drains are placed between the ADM and the mastectomy skin flap, one coursing medially along the inferior border and the other laterally and superiorly. The drains may overlap and are not trimmed unless overly redundant. Drains are typically removed 7 and 10 days postoperatively. After securing the drains, the expander is deflated and then filled with the sterile saline-transfer set until the desired amount is reached. One should fill up to the point of maximal apposition of the ADM and mastectomy flap without applying tension to the tissue. If there is any concern with the viability of the skin flap, expansion should be delayed until the tissue is healthy.

The incisions are closed with 3-0 and 4-0 Monocryl and dressed with Dermabond, covered with gauze dressings and then Tegaderm is applied to the entire breast surface. The use of negative-pressure wound management systems can be considered.

ONE-STAGE PROSTHETIC RECONSTRUCTION

One-stage prosthetic reconstruction can be performed in the subpectoral or prepectoral position. There are significant differences in the technique comparing the two approaches. With the subpectoral implant placement, the ADM is used to compartmentalize the implant in the dual-plane position. The upper half of the implant is under the pectoralis major and the lower half is under the ADM. With prepectoral reconstruction, the entire anterior surface of the implant is under the ADM.

Salient features of the one-stage prepectoral technique are reviewed. Following the skin- or nipple-sparing mastectomy, it is absolutely essential that the perfusion of the mastectomy skin flaps be present and that the thickness of the skin flap be optimized to ensure adequate soft-tissue coverage. As with the two-stage technique, device selection is based on biodimensional planning. The selected ADM needs to cover the anterior surface of the implant and should be 2 to 3 mm in thickness. It is useful to use implant sizers to ensure that the desired implant volume will not place undue pressure on the mastectomy skin flaps. The ADM–implant construct can be created with the on- or off-label technique. When the on-label technique is selected, the initial sutures that anchor the ADM to the chest wall will depend on the location of the incision. When inframammary, the sutures are placed superiorly first; however, with a skin-sparing mastectomy, the ADM can be sutured inferiorly or superiorly first because visibility is facilitated. Once the suturing has covered 270°, the implant is inserted. With the off-label technique, the ADM is wrapped around the implant and sutured edge to edge. The ADM–implant construct is inserted and the base perimeter of the ADM is sutured to the chest wall. A closed suction drain is used in all cases.

SUMMARY

The role of ADM for prepectoral breast reconstruction has become an important consideration for prepectoral reconstruction. The ability of the ADM to adhere to the pectoral muscle and to the subcutaneous fat is well demonstrated and is the basis for the success of this procedure. The stability afforded by the ADM prevents inferior and lateral migration of the implant. The observation that capsular contracture is reduced has been noted in several studies.[8-10] The ability to fat graft between the ADM and the mastectomy skin flaps has facilitated the achievement of excellent outcomes and served to increase the thickness of the mastectomy skin flaps and reduce the incidence of rippling and wrinkling.

KEY REFERENCES

1. Salzberg CA. Nonexpansive immediate breast reconstruction using human acellular tissue matrix graft (AlloDerm). *Ann Plast Surg*. 2006;57:1-5.
2. Breuing K, Colwell AS. Inferolateral AlloDerm hammock for implant coverage in breast reconstruction. *Ann Plast Surg*. 2007;59:250-255.
3. Salibian AH, Harness JK, Mowlds DS. Staged suprapectoral expander/implant reconstruction without acellular dermal matrix following nipple-sparing mastectomy. *Plast Reconstr Surg*. 2017;139(1):30-39.
4. Lewis P, Jewell J, Mattison G, Gupta S, Kim H. Reducing postoperative infections and red breast syndrome in patients with acellular dermal matrix based breast reconstruction: the relative roles of product sterility and lower body mass index. *Ann Plast Surg*. 2015;74:1-3.
5. Weichman KE, Wilson SC, Saadeh PB, et al. Sterile "ready-to-use" AlloDerm decreases postoperative infectious complications in patients undergoing immediate implant-based breast reconstruction with acellular dermal matrix. *Plast Reconstr Surg*. 2013;132:725-736.
6. Bernini M, Calabrese C, Cecconi L, et al. Subcutaneous direct-to-implant breast reconstruction: surgical, functional, and aesthetic results after long-term follow-up. *Plast Reconstr Surg Glob Open*. 2015;3:e574.
7. Reitsamer R, Peintinger F. Prepectoral implant placement and complete coverage with porcine acellular dermal matrix: a new technique for direct-to-implant breast reconstruction after nipple-sparing mastectomy. *J Plast Reconstr Aesthet Surg*. 2015;68:162-167.
8. Woo A, Harless C, Jacobson SR. Revisiting an old place: single surgeon experience on post-mastectomy subcutaneous implant-based breast reconstruction. *Breast J*. 2017;23(5):545-553.
9. Sigalove S, Maxwell GP, Sigalove NM, et al. Prepectoral implant-based breast reconstruction: rationale, indications, and preliminary results. *Plast Reconstr Surg*. 2017;139:287-294.
10. Sbitany H, Piper M, Lentz R. Prepectoral breast reconstruction: a safe alternative to submuscular prosthetic reconstruction following nipple-sparing mastectomy. *Plast Reconstr Surg*. 2017;140(3):432-443.
11. Gabriel A, Maxwell A. Prepectoral breast reconstruction in challenging patients. *Plast Reconstr Surg*. 2017;140(suppl 6):14S-21S.
12. Nahabedian MY. Acellular dermal matrices in primary breast reconstruction: principles, concepts, and indications. *Plast Reconstr Surg*. 2012;130(suppl 2):44S.
13. Nahabedian MY. Prosthetic breast reconstruction with acellular dermal matrices: achieving predictability and reproducibility. *Plast Reconstr Surg Glob Open*. 2016;4:e698.
14. Nahabedian MY, Cocilovo C. Two-stage prosthetic breast reconstruction: a comparison between prepectoral and partial subpectoral techniques. *Plast Reconstr Surg*. 2017;140(suppl 6):22S-30S.

CHAPTER 7

PREPECTORAL BREAST RECONSTRUCTION: WHAT IS THE DATA?

John Hijawi

KEY POINTS

- The deleterious impact of pectoral muscle detachment has been noted for many years, but was never considered a contraindication to reconstruction.
- What many surgeons and patients have noted is the prevalence of an animation deformity in both total muscle coverage and dual-plane, ADM sling techniques.
- The evolution of prepectoral breast reconstruction has followed a typical course since its reintroduction.
- Larger studies show that the safety profile of prepectoral breast reconstruction is quite like that of dual-plane, ADM-assisted expander reconstruction.

Surgical techniques often evolve first in the operating room, to be followed later by retrospective and finally prospective analysis of results, complications, and outcomes. Prepectoral, implant-based breast reconstruction has had a rapid resurgence after several decades of being almost entirely ignored in the United States and much of the world. Early work in the 1980s by Gruber and colleagues demonstrated an advantage to total muscle coverage of prosthetic devices following mastectomy.[1] The concept of total or partial submuscular coverage in alloplastic breast reconstruction took firm hold and was even extended to cosmetic breast augmentation where the benefits were arguably less obvious.

The clinical reintroduction of the prepectoral technique in recent years has been followed, predictably, by literature ranging from retrospective analyses to, more recently, prospective comparisons of prepectoral to subpectoral techniques. The aim of this chapter is to review the most recent data regarding prepectoral breast reconstruction with an emphasis on the contribution each available manuscript makes to our overall understanding of this technique. It is important that as new techniques are developed, or in this case as old techniques are reintroduced and refined, we as surgeons take a stepwise approach in evaluating their utility and safety.

PROOF OF CONCEPT: MOVING FROM PARTIAL MUSCLE COVERAGE TO NO MUSCLE COVERAGE

The motivation for most surgical innovation remains a benefit to the patient. It is always desirable to improve the efficiency and predictability of surgery, to minimize the occurrence of complications and reoperations, and, in our current era of reconstructive breast surgery, to maximize the patient experience and the patient's outcomes. The demand for better results is driven not only by plastic surgeons but also by patients as they take to the Internet and social media to praise doctors who deliver great results and to demand more from those who do not.

REQUISITES FOR A NEW SURGICAL TECHNIQUE

1. Improve safety
2. Improve efficiency
3. Improve the patient's treatment experience
4. Reduce cost
5. Maintain or reduce complication rates
6. Improve long-term outcomes

The concept of prepectoral breast reconstruction is the logical next step once one realizes the benefits seen from the introduction of acellular dermal matrix (ADM)-supported dual-plane reconstruction. In the dual-plane technique, only the cranial portion of the tissue expander or implant is covered by muscle, with the lower pole of the device supported by an ADM. Early authors noted that when compared to total muscle coverage techniques, dual-plane coverage procedures required less operative dissection, less intraoperative blood loss, and subsequently resulted in less immediate postoperative pain.[2-4] In the recovery period, there was noted to be more rapid expansion with less tightness and pain reported by patients. In the months and years following reconstruction, surgeons noted significantly less capsular contracture.[5,6]

These benefits had also been seen when surgeons used partial muscle coverage techniques without the addition of ADMs, but in many of those cases window shading and loss of control of the inframammary fold was a problem.[7] It quickly became clear that the addition of ADM allowed the reduction in the amount of muscle coverage by maintaining the caudal border of the pectoralis muscle in the correct position (avoiding window shading) and by allowing control of the inframammary and lateral mammary folds, thus avoiding bottoming out. The reduction in the amount of muscle covering tissue expanders and breast implants was credited for most of these improvements. Also important was the ability to strictly control the placement of the inframammary and lateral mammary folds rather than relying on the anatomy of a particular patient's thoracic musculature. Once the clinical benefit of reducing muscle coverage and adding ADM support was recognized by surgeons, data on the early complications of a new technique began to be published.

Early literature looking at postoperative complications demonstrated that these benefits could generally be obtained without a significant increase in acute complications. When comparing traditional total muscle coverage to a dual-plane technique with partial pectoral coverage supported by an ADM, Spear and colleagues found that the newer dual-plane techniques resulted in nearly identical infection rates and extrusion rates.[4,6,8] Seroma rates were initially noted to be higher when ADMs were employed; but as better drain management developed and prehydrated products came into the market, these rates dropped. As follow-up moved past several months and into the range of years, it was also noted that capsular contracture rates were significantly lower than those seen with a total muscle coverage technique.[9]

THE IMPACT AND TREATMENT OF PECTORALIS DETACHMENT AND ANIMATION DEFORMITY

The deleterious impact of pectoral muscle detachment has been noted for many years, but was never considered a contraindication to reconstruction. In 2007, de Haan and colleagues from the Netherlands compared the Biodex strength profile measurements of 10 women who had undergone unilateral, subpectoral tissue expander breast reconstruction to 18 unoperated control patients.[10] The unoperated patients acted as baseline examples of the impact of hand dominance on strength. When controlling for hand dominance, the authors noted a 20% reduction in torque strength of the operated upper extremity versus the nonoperated control extremity. Further, 60% of the patients who had undergone reconstruction noted daily discomfort when performing activities of daily living with the operated extremity and 70% reported feeling significant pressure and displacement of the prosthesis with upper extremity movement.

What many surgeons and patients have noted is the prevalence of an animation deformity in both total muscle coverage and dual-plane, ADM sling techniques.[11,12] Nigro studied the impact of animation deformity on patient satisfaction following implant-based reconstruction.[13] In a group of 84 patients, Nigro noted that 75.6% of patients were aware of animation deformity, with 51.9% reporting they would have preferred an alternative technique if possible to avoid the deformity. A variety of techniques have been developed to denervate the pectoralis muscle either surgically or chemically, generally with little success. There is some irony in the idea of surgically elevating the pectoralis, increasing operative time and pain, and then struggling to denervate or render immobile the very muscle that was so carefully dissected.

Winocour and colleagues published a systematic review of seven published studies evaluating the efficacy of Botulinum toxin type A in alleviating postoperative pain in expander-based reconstructive patients in 2014.[14] This review demonstrated inconsistent results and moderate efficacy when Botox is used to chemically denervate the pectoralis following breast reconstruction. The significant expense of chronic Botox treatment of a large muscle like the pectoralis is also noted as a major limitation of this technique, and therefore it would be limited to alleviating pain in the immediate postoperative period rather than a solution to long-term animation deformity.

Hammond et al. published a small series of 19 breasts in which implants were repositioned from a subpectoral pocket to a prepectoral one to alleviate pain and animation deformity.[15] There was complete resolution of animation deformity in this group of patients. Interestingly, the authors chose not to add an ADM to the anterior surface of the implants following pocket conversion and noted a 21% rate of capsular contracture requiring surgery to correct. Given the significant literature on a reduction in capsular contracture with the use of ADMs, it would be interesting to know if the results could have been improved in regard to capsular contracture in this group.[9,16,17]

Gabriel and colleagues reported on a larger series of subpectoral to prepectoral conversions in those patients.[12] In this group of 102 breasts in 57 patients presenting with animation deformity after dual-plane reconstruction, they noted complete resolution of animation deformity. Gabriel employed additional ADM to cover the entire surface of all implants at revision surgery, and interestingly no cases of capsular contracture were noted during follow-up.

Efforts to denervate the pectoralis muscle at the time of subpectoral expander placement have also been described.[18,19] The significant branching of the pectoral nerves makes this a time-consuming undertaking with variable results. Even if the denervation of the muscle is successful, one loses the physiologic advantage of muscle preservation as well as the efficiency advantage of less complex surgery seen with prepectoral placement of prostheses.

If one follows the logic that the move from total muscle coverage to dual-plane coverage with ADM support improved pain and enhanced the recovery process, the next logical step is to eliminate muscle coverage entirely. The strategies to address the problems associated with the subpectoral placement of implants discussed are logical.[20] However, it does seem equally logical that avoiding the problem of pain and animation deformity from the outset by placing the devices in a prepectoral plane to begin with would be economically more efficient and place less of a negative impact on the lives of patients. In fact, in the study previously discussed by Nigro, although over 50% of patients would have preferred an alternative original technique to avoid animation deformity as an index operation, the percentage of patients who would accept revision surgery after initial reconstruction was much less. In other words, patients would simply like to avoid the problem of animation deformity from the outset and are somewhat reluctant to return to the operating room to fix it.

EARLY READOPTERS OF THE PREPECTORAL TECHNIQUE

In 2014, Berna and colleagues from Italy and the United Kingdom reported on their experience with a direct-to-implant (DTI), prepectoral technique in 19 patients.[21] Their group employed Braxon, a porcine ADM, wrapping the entire device before insertion in the reconstructive pocket. The fundamental motivation for the prepectoral innovation noted in this report is avoidance of the morbidity associated with dissection and detachment of the pectoralis muscle. With 12-month follow-up, they noted that acute complications were similar to those seen in total muscle coverage techniques. Chronic seroma was noted in 8% of patients, whereas infection was noted in 4% of patients. This resulted in a 12% implant loss rate. No animation deformity was noted in any patient, the reconstructed breasts remained soft even with arm movement and an earlier return to full activity was noted even without any physiotherapy. At 12 months, there were no cases of capsular contracture noted.

In 2014, Casella and colleagues reported on their direct comparison of a dual-plane, partial submuscular DTI technique in 34 breasts with a prepectoral DTI technique in 39 breasts using TiLoop, a titanium-coated polypropylene mesh as support.[22] The two groups were matched for extent of disease and the authors noted restrictive selection criteria regarding skin flap quality. This report, published in the European Journal of Plastic Surgery, noted no statistically significant difference in the two groups when evaluating infection, wound dehiscence, hematoma, or implant removal. None of the patients in this study were treated with radiation therapy before or during the study period.

Jacobson and colleagues from the Mayo Clinic reported on their experience with both two-stage and DTI prepectoral breast reconstruction at the American Society of Plastic Surgeons Meeting in 2015.[23] This study evaluated 135 consecutive breast reconstructions in a prepectoral plane. The authors noted that 3.8% of patients had a postoperative infection requiring explantation, 3.8% had a postoperative hematoma, and 3.8% had a seroma requiring treatment. There were no cases of implant extrusion or skin necrosis requiring operative debridement. Although this peer-reviewed abstract did not look at long-term results, it demonstrates very comparable short-term complications when compared to the more traditional dual-plane technique.

Becker and colleagues have reported on the use of remote-port, postoperative adjustable saline implants in a prepectoral plane for breast reconstruction.[24] The concept here is to use a remote fill port to gain some of the benefits of a DTI reconstruction while still having control over the expansion rate of the device. These devices were covered with either a Vicryl mesh or Flex HD, an ADM. As in other reports, the primary motivation for placing the devices in a prepectoral position was the avoidance of animation deformity and to reduce postoperative pain. With almost a 5-year follow-up, the authors noted a very low incidence of acute complications with a 1.6% rate of infection, seroma, and hematoma. Implant extrusion was 3% and capsular contracture was reported at 3.2%. Interestingly, the authors report a 29% reoperation rate specifically for patients wishing to have their saline implants exchanged for silicone gel devices.

Bettinger directly compared the results of prepectoral and dual-plane implant-based reconstructions in a retrospective study published in 2017.[11] A total of 294 consecutively reconstructed breasts were divided into three groups. A total of 165 breasts were reconstructed with a prepectoral technique, 77 with a dual-plane "ADM sling" technique, and 52 with a total muscular coverage technique. There were no differences noted in either infections or seroma incidence. Infections were noted to occur in 6.8% of the entire study group. Similarly, the authors found no difference in infection or seroma rates at the time of expander to implant exchange. The authors did not comment on the incidence of capsular contracture given the short follow-up duration of the study.

Downs and Hedges reported a retrospective review of 79 prepectoral breast reconstructions in 45 patients using either Alloderm or FlexHD for implant support.[25] These were all DTI reconstructions. The authors did not consider smoking or previous radiotherapy to be contraindications to a prepectoral technique, but did use clinically apparent mastectomy skin flap ischemia as a potential reason to abort reconstruction in favor of a delayed approach. The complications reported by this group were somewhat higher than those in other studies, possibly as a result of the inclusion of a high number, 75%, of patients being exposed to radiotherapy before mastectomy and reconstruction. Almost a third of patients experienced mastectomy flap necrosis and 10% had a postoperative infection. The overall implant failure rate was 18%, demonstrating that no technique will avoid the importance of standard selection criteria in alloplastic-based breast reconstruction. The authors note that avoiding smokers and women with large or very ptotic breasts is strongly advised.

The largest series to date is that of Sigalove and colleagues.[26] They reported on 353 consecutive prepectoral reconstructions with total anterior ADM coverage. Acute complications were all noted to be low, including infection of 4%, seroma of 2%, flap necrosis of 2% and capsular contracture rates of 0% with relatively early follow-up. Animation deformity is nonexistent in this large group of patients that continues to be followed up for more long-term evaluation of results.

The studies reviewed strongly suggest that the prepectoral technique can be undertaken in a range of patients without increasing the acute complication rate of implant- and expander-based breast reconstruction. Other studies have looked further at the results of prepectoral breast reconstruction with a focus on longer term results and patient-reported outcomes.

WHAT ARE THE OUTCOMES OF PREPECTORAL BREAST RECONSTRUCTION BEYOND ACUTE COMPLICATIONS?

The literature has continued to look closely at the acute complications of prepectoral device placement. Several studies have begun to look at patient-reported outcomes and longer term results as they become available. Bernini applied the Breast-Q patient-reported outcomes instrument to the same group of patients previously reported on by Casella et al.[27,28] The same two groups of patients, treated with either a dual-plane or prepectoral TiLoop supported implant, completed the Breast-Q questionnaire. In addition, the patients were evaluated by surgeons not involved in their surgical care for contracture, rippling, implant visibility, and aesthetic result using a Likert scale. As noted earlier, acute complications were statistically similar in the two groups, with all common complications occurring in less than 6% of patients. The surgeon-rated outcomes all demonstrated superiority of the prepectoral group in aesthetics, capsular contracture, and implant rippling. The incidence of capsular contracture was significantly less than that in the dual-plane group, with 100% of prepectoral patients demonstrating a Grade I or II Baker capsule. This is particularly interesting given the fact that 26% of the prepectoral group received radiotherapy, and so would be expected to have a higher rate of capsular contracture.

Patient-reported outcomes in the Bernini study were also superior in the prepectoral group, with overall satisfaction with the reconstruction being 98% in the prepectoral group and only 84% in the dual-plane group.[27] The authors postulate less discomfort after surgery and a more natural, ptotic appearance as the key factors in that superior satisfaction.

Jones and colleagues published a large series of 73 DTI breast reconstructions in 50 patients using an ADM anterior coverage technique.[29] This study included an almost even distribution of skin-sparing and nipple-sparing mastectomies. The authors note that the extirpative surgeons involved in the care of this patient group were limited to two full-time breast surgeons, both very aware of the importance of viable skin flaps to this technique's success. And, 97% of the patients included in this study achieved incident-free wound healing with a DTI approach by 8 weeks postoperatively. Rippling was noted in 12% of patients and that relatively low incidence was felt to be due to the use of highly cohesive gel implants. When rippling or implant visibility did occur, fat grafting was employed at a later stage. Infection with subsequent implant removal occurred in 2.7% of patients. The long follow-up of up to 32 months allowed the monitoring of the subset of patients who received postmastectomy radiotherapy (PMRT). Of the 10% of patients in the study group who received PMRT, only 1.3% developed a Grade III contracture, whereas all of the others maintained a Grade I or II capsule. When taken in combination with other studies noted in this review, those results are promising.

ARE ACELLULAR DERMAL MATRICES NECESSARY FOR THE SUCCESS OF THE PREPECTORAL TECHNIQUE?

Several of the studies discussed strongly suggest that the addition of an ADM is beneficial to the success of procedures in which implants are converted from a subpectoral to a prepectoral plane.[12,15] When comparing the results of the Hammond and Sigalove conversion procedures, it seems clear that there is a significant reduction in the risk of capsular contracture with the addition of an ADM covering the surface of the implant.

Salibian has reported on prepectoral implant-based reconstruction without the use of any adjunctive ADM.[30] That study, published in 2017, evaluated 250 breasts reconstructed over a 10-year period. All mastectomies in the series were done with both the plastic surgeon and breast surgeon present and the placement of all tissue expanders was delayed by 3 to 4 months after mastectomy regardless of plans for adjuvant therapy. The tissue expanders were placed in a prepectoral plane without the use of any adjunctive ADM or supportive mesh. With excellent follow-up of 55 months, 7.6% of patients were noted to have Grade III or Grade IV capsular contractures. Expander loss was as high as 6.8% in this study. What is not made clear is whether the patients experiencing these complications had undergone radiotherapy. The paper does note that patients undergoing radiotherapy were included in the study, but does not delineate the results into the groups of radiated and nonradiated patients. Regardless, the relatively high rates of pathologic capsules reported do suggest a benefit to the addition of ADM coverage in the prepectoral plane.

Sbitany has evaluated a subset of patients receiving PMRT in the setting of nipple-sparing mastectomy as part of a larger study of patients undergoing prepectoral reconstruction in the setting of nipple-sparing mastectomy.[31] In this comparison of dual-plane and prepectoral techniques published in 2017, he noted that in those patients getting PMRT those with the device placed in a dual-plane or partial submuscular manner had a higher incidence of device migration at the conclusion of radiotherapy. Consistent with this was the higher incidence of Baker Grade III capsules in the subpectoral group when compared to the prepectoral group. To be clear, both of the groups in this study had some amount of ADM included in the reconstruction, but the prepectoral group had total anterior coverage of the device with ADM, whereas in the dual-plane group a large a portion of the devices were in direct contact with the pectoralis muscle.

All studies are summarized in **Table 7.1**.

SUMMARY

The evolution of prepectoral breast reconstruction has followed a typical course since its reintroduction. The data available begin with scattered case reports and case series. As larger studies were published and the acute complications

TABLE 7.1 SUMMARY OF RELEVANT PREPECTORAL STUDIES

Author	Publication Year	Title	Journal	
Gruber et al	1981	Breast reconstruction following mastectomy: a comparison of submuscular and subcutaneous techniques	*Plast Reconstr Surg*	One of the first comparisons of subcutaneous and total muscle coverage alloplastic breast reconstructions
Saltzberg	2006	Nonexpansive immediate breast reconstruction using human acellular tissue matrix graft (AlloDerm)	*Ann Plast Surg*	One of the original descriptions of the dual-plane tissue expander breast reconstruction technique utilizing AlloDerm tissue reinforcement
Zienowicz et al	2007	Implant-based breast reconstruction with allograft	*Plast Reconstr Surg*	
Bindingnavele et al	2007	Use of acellular cadaveric dermis and tissue expansion in postmastectomy breast reconstruction	*J Plast Reconstr Aesthet Surg*	
Salzberg	2012	Direct-to-implant breast reconstruction	*Clin Plast Surg*	
Spear et al	2008	Acellular dermis-assisted breast reconstruction	*Aesthetic Plast Surg*	
Spear et al	2012	Focus on technique: supporting the soft-tissue envelope in breast reconstruction	*Plast Reconstr Surg*	

(*continued*)

TABLE 7.1 SUMMARY OF RELEVANT PREPECTORAL STUDIES (*continued*)

Author	Publication Year	Title	Journal	
Cordeiro et al	2006	A single surgeon's 12-year experience with tissue expander/implant breast reconstruction: part II. An analysis of long-term complications, aesthetic outcomes, and patient satisfaction	*Plast Reconstr Surg*	
Vardanian et al	2011	Comparison of implant-based immediate breast reconstruction with and without acellular dermal matrix	*Plast Reconstr Surg*	
de Haan et al	2007	Function of the pectoralis major muscle after combined skin-sparing mastectomy and immediate reconstruction by subpectoral implantation of a prosthesis	*Ann Plast Surg*	
Bettinger et al	2017	Comparative study of prepectoral and subpectoral expander-based breast reconstruction and Clavien IIIb score outcomes	*Plast Reconstr Surg Glob Open*	
Gabriel et al	2018	Prepectoral revision breast reconstruction for treatment of implant-associated animation deformity: a review of 102 reconstructions	*Aesthet Surg J*	A report of patients with previous dual-plane breast reconstruction undergoing conversion to a prepectoral plane with the addition of supplemental AlloDerm for anterior reinforcement. Early results demonstrated very low capsular contracture rates
Nigro et al	2017	Animation deformity in postmastectomy implant-based reconstruction	*Plast Reconstr Surg Glob Open*	This study reported the results of questionnaires given to 84 dual-plane breast reconstruction patients. Around 75% of patients reported being aware of animation deformity in their daily lives. And 51% noted that they would have preferred an alternative technique if it would eliminate animation deformity
Winocour et al	2014	A systematic review of the use of Botulinum toxin type A with subpectoral breast implants	*J Plast Reconstr Aesthet Surg*	

TABLE 7.1 SUMMARY OF RELEVANT PREPECTORAL STUDIES (*continued*)

Author	Publication Year	Title	Journal	
Hammond et al	2015	Treatment of breast animation deformity in implant-based reconstruction with pocket change to the subcutaneous position	*Plast Reconstr Surg*	A report of dual-plane breast reconstructions converted to a prepectoral plane without the addition of supplemental ADM. All animation deformity resolved. Around 21% of patients developed a Grade III or IV capsular contracture
Komorowska-Timek et al	2009	The effect of AlloDerm envelopes on periprosthetic capsule formation with and without radiation	*Plast Reconstr Surg*	A basic science study evaluating the impact of AlloDerm on the development of pathologic capsule formation in radiated tissue expanders. The authors demonstrate less inflammatory change and fibrosis in those expanders covered with AlloDerm versus those without
Stump et al	2009	The use of acellular dermal matrix to prevent capsule formation around implants in a primate model	*Plast Reconstr Surg*	
Bernini et al	2017	Selective pectoralis major muscle denervation in breast reconstruction: a technical modification for more effective and cosmetic results	*Gland Surg*	A report of a technique to treat animation deformity without adjustment of the implant position
Aszmann et al	2000	The anatomy of the pectoral nerves and their significance in brachial plexus reconstruction	*J Hand Surg Am*	
Sbitany et al	2009	Acellular dermis-assisted prosthetic breast reconstruction versus complete submuscular coverage: a head-to-head comparison of outcomes	*Plast Reconstr Surg*	
Berna et al	2017	Evaluation of a novel breast reconstruction technique using the Braxon® acellular dermal matrix: a new muscle-sparing breast reconstruction	*ANZ J Surg*	

(*continued*)

TABLE 7.1 SUMMARY OF RELEVANT PREPECTORAL STUDIES (*continued*)

Author	Publication Year	Title	Journal	
Casella et al	2014	TiLoop® Bra mesh used for immediate breast reconstruction: comparison of retropectoral and subcutaneous implant placement in a prospective single-institution series	*Eur J Plast Surg*	This prospective study compared a group of patients reconstructed with a dual-plane technique to a group reconstructed with a prepectoral technique. All patients were reconstructed with a direct-to-implant approach using TiLoop, a polypropylene mesh for coverage. The authors noted no significant differences in the acute complications of implant loss, seroma, infection, or hematoma with a 13-month follow-up
Woo et al	2015	Revisiting an old place: single surgeon experience on postmastectomy subcutaneous implant-based breast reconstruction	*Plast Reconstr Surg*	
Becker et al	2015	Immediate implant-based prepectoral breast reconstruction using a vertical incision	*Plast Reconstr Surg Glob Open*	This study reports on 62 prepectoral breast reconstructions performed in 31 patients using either an ADM or Vicryl mesh anterior reinforcement and a remote-port saline implant. With 4.6-year follow-up, the authors reported infection, seroma, and hematoma, all at 1.6%, capsular contracture at 3.2%, and implant loss at 3%. Total complications requiring reoperation were at 23%
Downs et al	2016	An alternative technique for immediate direct-to-implant breast reconstruction—A case series	*Plast Reconstr Surg Glob Open*	

TABLE 7.1 SUMMARY OF RELEVANT PREPECTORAL STUDIES (*continued*)

Author	Publication Year	Title	Journal	
Sigalove et al	2017	Prepectoral implant-based breast reconstruction: rationale, indications, and preliminary results	*Plast Reconstr Surg*	This study reports on the largest group of prepectoral reconstructions to date. The authors report 4% infection, 2% seroma, and flap necrosis, and no cases of capsular contracture in a group of 353 prepectoral breast reconstructions with AlloDerm reinforcement
Bernini et al	2015	Subcutaneous direct-to-implant breast reconstruction: surgical, functional, and aesthetic results after long-term follow-up	*Plast Reconstr Surg Glob Open*	This prospective study compared a group of patients reconstructed with a dual-plane technique to a group reconstructed with a prepectoral technique. The results of a Breast-Q analysis were reported in this study. The authors noted that the prepectoral group had a higher percentage of Grade I or II capsules, superior aesthetic outcomes and better patient satisfaction. All patients were reconstructed with a direct-to-implant approach using TiLoop, a polypropylene mesh for coverage.
Casella et al	2015	Subcutaneous tissue expander placement with synthetic titanium-coated mesh in breast reconstruction: long-term results	*Plast Reconstr Surg Glob Open*	
Jones et al	2017	Prepectoral Immediate Direct-to-Implant Breast Reconstruction with Anterior AlloDerm Coverage	*Plast Reconstr Surg*	

(*continued*)

TABLE 7.1 SUMMARY OF RELEVANT PREPECTORAL STUDIES (*continued*)

Author	Publication Year	Title	Journal	
Salibian et al	2017	Staged suprapectoral expander/implant reconstruction without acellular dermal matrix following nipple-sparing mastectomy	*Plast Reconstr Surg*	This is a report on 250 breasts, all reconstructed in delayed manner using subcutaneous tissue expanders with no ADM or mesh reinforcement. At nearly 5-year follow-up, the authors note an expander loss rate of 6.8% and an 8% incidence of Grade III or IV capsular contractures
Sbitany et al	2017	Prepectoral breast reconstruction: a safe alternative to submuscular prosthetic reconstruction following nipple-sparing mastectomy	*Plast Reconstr Surg*	This is a head-to-head comparison of patients undergoing nipple-sparing mastectomy and reconstruction with either a dual-plane technique or a prepectoral technique. The authors found no significant difference in acute complications. They also reported on the radiated cohort, separately finding significantly more problems with TE migration in the dual-plane group.
Chatterjee et al	2018	Early assessment of postsurgical outcomes with prepectoral breast reconstruction: a literature review and meta-analysis	*J Surg Oncol*	
Berna et al	2014		*ANZ J Surg*	This study presents 25 prepectoral breast reconstructions in 19 patients using a porcine ADM, Braxon. All cases were direct-to-implant and none of the patients were exposed to radiotherapy. With 14 months' average follow-up, the authors reported no cases of capsular contracture, implant loss of 12%, seroma rate of 16%, infection rate of 4%, and no cases of extrusion.

TABLE 7.1 SUMMARY OF RELEVANT PREPECTORAL STUDIES (*continued*)

Author	Publication Year	Title	Journal	
Woo et al	2015	Revisiting an old place: single surgeon experience on post-mastectomy subcutaneous implant based breast reconstruction	Abstract, American Society of Plastic Surgeons Annual Meeting, 2015	This abstract presented 135 prepectoral breast reconstructions in 79 patients. The report includes patients reconstructed with both a direct-to-implant approach and a two-stage approach. The authors reported a 3.8% incidence of implant loss, 3.8% seroma, 3.8% infection, and 3.8% hematoma. No cases of extrusion were seen in this patient group and there was no comment on capsular contracture.
Reitsamer et al	2015	Prepectoral implant placement and complete coverage with porcine acellular dermal matrix: a new technique for direct-to-implant breast reconstruction after nipple-sparing mastectomy	*J Plast Reconstr Aesthet Surg*	This study reports on 22 prepectoral breast reconstructions in 13 patients. All reconstructions were direct-to-implant and used Strattice porcine ADM for reinforcement. The authors noted no cases of infection, seroma, or implant loss and a hematoma rate of 4.5%. None of the patients in the study required discharge narcotics and there was no animation deformity noted at follow-up. The authors mention a large and growing number of patients presenting to their practice requesting a prepectoral reconstruction in the interest of preserving their muscle integrity.

Abbreviations: ADM, acellular dermal matrix; TE, tissue expander.

were reported, it became clear that the safety profile of prepectoral breast reconstruction is quite similar to that of dual-plane, ADM-assisted expander reconstruction. As of early 2018, we are beginning to see reports of the longer term issues and the results of this technique.[32] Although a small number of patient-reported outcome studies have begun to appear, the next few years are certain to bring more information on how this promising technique is impacting patients' lives, and what the issues will be decades after initial reconstruction.

KEY REFERENCES

1. Gruber RP, Kahn RA, Lash H, Maser MR, Apfelberg DB, Laub DR. Breast reconstruction following mastectomy: a comparison of submuscular and subcutaneous techniques. *Plast Reconstr Surg.* 1981;67:312-317.
2. Salzberg CA. Nonexpansive immediate breast reconstruction using human acellular tissue matrix graft (AlloDerm). *Ann Plast Surg.* 2006;57:1-5.
3. Zienowicz RJ, Karacaoglu E. Implant-based breast reconstruction with allograft. *Plast Reconstr Surg.* 2007;120:373-381.
4. Bindingnavele V, Gaon M, Ota KS, Kulber DA, Lee, D-J. Use of acellular cadaveric dermis and tissue expansion in postmastectomy breast reconstruction. *J Plast Reconstr Aesthet Surg.* 2007;60:1214-1218.
5. Salzberg CA. Direct-to-implant breast reconstruction. *Clin Plast Surg.* 2012;39:119-126.
6. Spear SL, Parikh PM, Reisin E, Menon NG. Acellular dermis-assisted breast reconstruction. *Aesthetic Plast Surg.* 2008;32:418-425.
7. Spear SL, Sher SR, Al-Attar A. Focus on technique: supporting the soft-tissue envelope in breast reconstruction. *Plast Reconstr Surg.* 2012;130:89S-94S.
8. Cordeiro PG, McCarthy CM. A single surgeon's 12-year experience with tissue expander/implant breast reconstruction: part II. An analysis of long-term complications, aesthetic outcomes, and patient satisfaction. *Plast Reconstr Surg.* 2006;118:832-839.
9. Vardanian AJ, Clayton JL, Roostaeian J, et al. Comparison of implant-based immediate breast reconstruction with and without acellular dermal matrix. *Plast Reconstr Surg.* 2011;128:403e-410e.
10. de Haan A, Toor A, Hage JJ, Veeger HE, Woerdeman LA. Function of the pectoralis major muscle after combined skin-sparing mastectomy and immediate reconstruction by subpectoral implantation of a prosthesis. *Ann Plast Surg.* 2007;59:605-610.
11. Bettinger LN, Waters LM, Reese SW, Kutner SE, Jacobs DI. Comparative study of prepectoral and subpectoral expander-based breast reconstruction and Clavien IIIb score outcomes. *Plast Reconstr Surg Glob Open.* 2017;5:e1433.
12. Gabriel A, Sigalove S, Sigalove NM et al. Prepectoral revision breast reconstruction for treatment of implant-associated animation deformity: a review of 102 reconstructions. *Aesthet Surg J.* 2018;38(5):519-526.
13. Nigro LC, Blanchet NP. Animation deformity in postmastectomy implant-based reconstruction. *Plast Reconstr Surg Glob Open.* 2017;5:e1407.
14. Winocour S, Murad MH, Bidgoli-Moghaddam M, et al. A systematic review of the use of Botulinum toxin type A with subpectoral breast implants. *J Plast Reconstr Aesthet Surg.* 2014;67:34-41.
15. Hammond DC, Schmitt WP, O'Connor EA. Treatment of breast animation deformity in implant-based reconstruction with pocket change to the subcutaneous position. *Plast Reconstr Surg.* 2015;135:1540-1544.
16. Komorowska-Timek E, Oberg KC, Timek TA, Gridley DS, Miles DA. The effect of AlloDerm envelopes on periprosthetic capsule formation with and without radiation. *Plast Reconstr Surg.* 2009;123:807-816.
17. Stump A, Holton LH III, Connor J, Harper JR, Slezak S, Silverman RP. The use of acellular dermal matrix to prevent capsule formation around implants in a primate model. *Plast Reconstr Surg.* 2009;124:82-91.
18. Bernini M, Casella D, Mariotti C. Selective pectoralis major muscle denervation in breast reconstruction: a technical modification for more effective and cosmetic results. *Gland Surg.* 2017;6:745-750.
19. Aszmann OC, Rab M, Kamolz L, Frey M. The anatomy of the pectoral nerves and their significance in brachial plexus reconstruction. *J Hand Surg Am.* 2000;25:942-947.
20. Sbitany H, Sandeen SN, Amalfi AN, Davenport MS, Langstein HN. Acellular dermis-assisted prosthetic breast reconstruction versus complete submuscular coverage: a head-to-head comparison of outcomes. *Plast Reconstr Surg.* 2009;124:1735-1740.
21. Berna G, Cawthorn SJ, Papaccio G, Balestrieri N. Evaluation of a novel breast reconstruction technique using the Braxon acellular dermal matrix: a new muscle-sparing breast reconstruction. *ANZ J Surg.* 2017;87:493-498.
22. Casella D, Bernini M, Bencini L, et al. TiLoop Bra mesh used for immediate breast reconstruction: comparison of retropectoral and subcutaneous implant placement in a prospective single-institution series. *Eur J Plast Surg.* 2014;37:599-604.
23. Woo A, Harless C, Jacobson SR. Revisiting an old place: single surgeon experience on post-mastectomy subcutaneous implant based breast reconstruction. *Plast Reconstr Surg.* 2015;136:83.
24. Becker H, Lind JG II, Hopkins EG. Immediate implant-based prepectoral breast reconstruction using a vertical incision. *Plast Reconstr Surg Glob Open.* 2015;3:e412.
25. Downs RK, Hedges K. An alternative technique for immediate direct-to-implant breast reconstruction—a case series. *Plast Reconstr Surg Glob Open.* 2016;4:e821.
26. Sigalove S, Maxwell GP, Sigalove NM, et al. Prepectoral implant-based breast reconstruction: rationale, indications, and preliminary results. *Plast Reconstr Surg.* 2017;139:287-294.
27. Bernini M, Calabrese C, Cecconi L, et al. Subcutaneous direct-to-implant breast reconstruction: surgical, functional, and aesthetic results after long-term follow-up. *Plast Reconstr Surg Glob Open.* 2015;3:e574.
28. Casella D, Calabrese C, Bianchi S, Meattini I, Bernini M. Subcutaneous tissue expander placement with synthetic titanium-coated mesh in breast reconstruction: long-term results. *Plast Reconstr Surg Glob Open.* 2015;3:e577.
29. Jones G, Yoo A, King V, et al. Prepectoral immediate direct-to-implant breast reconstruction with anterior Alloderm coverage. *Plast Reconstr Surg.* 2017;140:31S-38S.
30. Salibian AH, Harness JK, Mowlds DS. Staged suprapectoral expander/implant reconstruction without acellular dermal matrix following nipple-sparing mastectomy. *Plast Reconstr Surg.* 2017;139:30-39.
31. Sbitany H, Piper M, Lentz R. Prepectoral breast reconstruction: a safe alternative to submuscular prosthetic reconstruction following nipple-sparing mastectomy. *Plast Reconstr Surg.* 2017;140:432-443.
32. Chatterjee A, Nahabedian MY, Gabriel A, et al. Early assessment of post-surgical outcomes with pre-pectoral breast reconstruction: a literature review and meta-analysis. *J Surg Oncol.* 2018;117(6):1119-1130.

CHAPTER 8

PREPECTORAL RECONSTRUCTION WITHOUT ACELLULAR DERMAL MATRIX

Arthur H. Salibian

KEY POINTS

- Reduced capsular contracture is the predominant reason for using ADM in two-step NSM reconstruction.
- The use of "thick" mastectomy flap was one of the reasons why ADM was not utilized in non-ADM–based breast reconstruction.
- To prevent implant descent in thin patients with implants greater than 400 mL, chest wall skin is anchored to rib periosteum with nonabsorbable sutures along the inframammary fold in the second stage.

INTRODUCTION

The transition and evolution of prosthetic implantation from retropectoral to prepectoral space following nipple-sparing mastectomy (NSM) is a paradigm shift in implant-based breast reconstruction.[1-6] One of the factors that helped bring about this change is the use of acellular dermal matrix (ADM).

ADM, developed more than a decade ago, was used in dual-plane breast reconstruction after NSM to facilitate lower pole expansion and improve the shape of the breast at a time when total muscle coverage was not giving the desired aesthetic and functional results.[7-10] The benefits of ADM in dual-plane submuscular reconstruction have been used in prepectoral one- or two-stage implant reconstruction. These advantages include implant support, compartmentalization, and reduced capsular contracture.

My experience in prepectoral NSM reconstruction, reported previously, differed from that of others in that ADM was not used.[11,12] Another departure from the norm was the close surgical collaboration with an oncologic surgeon in all therapeutic/prophylactic inframammary NSM between 2005 and 2016. The goal of our collaboration in the operating room was to maintain oncologic safety while preserving subcutaneous fat following mastectomy in the setting of two-stage prepectoral implant reconstruction.

In this chapter, the reasons for not using ADM are discussed. Terms such as "thick" flaps and tissue "expander," commonly employed in NSM/reconstruction, are examined to avoid misrepresentation.

NSM: THIN VERSUS THICK FLAPS

In our previous reports, the use of "thick" mastectomy flap was one of the reasons why ADM was not utilized in breast reconstruction. The term "thick" flap can be misleading when applied to NSM. With "thick" flaps, NSM follows precise anatomic landmarks that remove glandular tissue with its encasing anterior mammary fascia and attached Cooper's ligaments while preserving the entire subcutaneous fat. The subareolar glandular tissue is also removed, leaving pigmented skin and nipple only.

Flaps with full-thickness subcutaneous fat are considered "thick" regardless of the patient's body mass index (BMI). Thus, thick flap refers to preserved subcutaneous vascular architecture and quality of skin perfusion, and not necessarily flap thickness in millimeters. As an example, a patient with BMI <20 with what appears to be a thin 5-mm flap in which the subcutaneous vasculature has been preserved (**Figure 8.1**), will have good skin perfusion and no flap loss. On the contrary, a patient with a BMI >35 in whom the normal 20-mm-thick subcutaneous fat is thinned down to 5 mm will more than likely have skin complications.

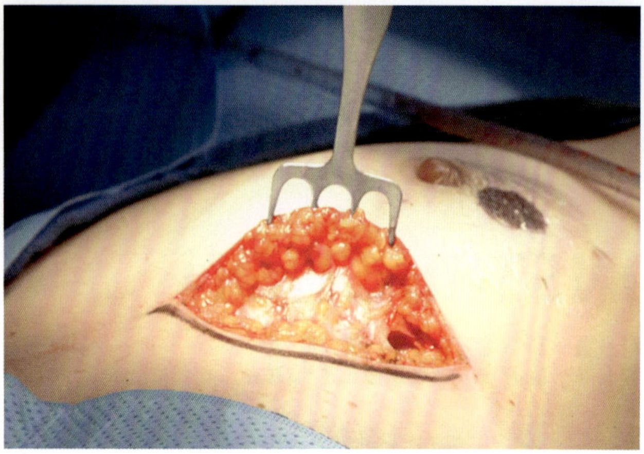

Figure 8.1 "Thick" flap in thin patient. Full-thickness subcutaneous fat superficial to the anterior mammary fascia (white) preserves the vascular architecture needed to optimally perfuse the skin. From Salibian AH, Harness JK, Mowlds DS. Staged suprapectoral expander/implant reconstruction without acellular dermal matrix following nipple-sparing mastectomy. *Plast Reconstr Surg*. 2017;139(1):30-39.

A thin flap and a *thinned out* flap with the same thickness will have different outcomes. Skin complications are more common when the entire subcutaneous fat is thinned and its vascular anatomy disrupted. In our experience, thin patients with thin flaps did not have more skin complications than did patients with greater BMI and thicker flaps.

Plastic surgeons are faced with complications of thinned out flaps on the basis of the oncologic surgeon's technique. To this end, ADM is used to "protect" the implant in the event of skin loss and implant exposure. Localized implant exposure after surgery is best treated with direct excision of the eschar and primary closure. Nonvascularized ADM in the immediate postoperative period does not have a role in protecting an exposed implant.

Preserving subcutaneous fat in thick flaps as described does not compromise the oncologic safety of the procedure, as some contend. The "thick" flaps used in our series are not the same as the thick subcutaneous mastectomy flaps practiced in the 1980s. Our tumor recurrence results for NSM after an average follow-up of more than 5 years has been 2.6%, which is comparable to other reports.[13,14]

TISSUE EXPANDER IN TWO-STAGE PREPECTORAL NSM RECONSTRUCTION

Tissue expanders were developed in the 1970s at a time when total mastectomy was the accepted surgical procedure for treating breast cancer.[15] Reconstruction required use of

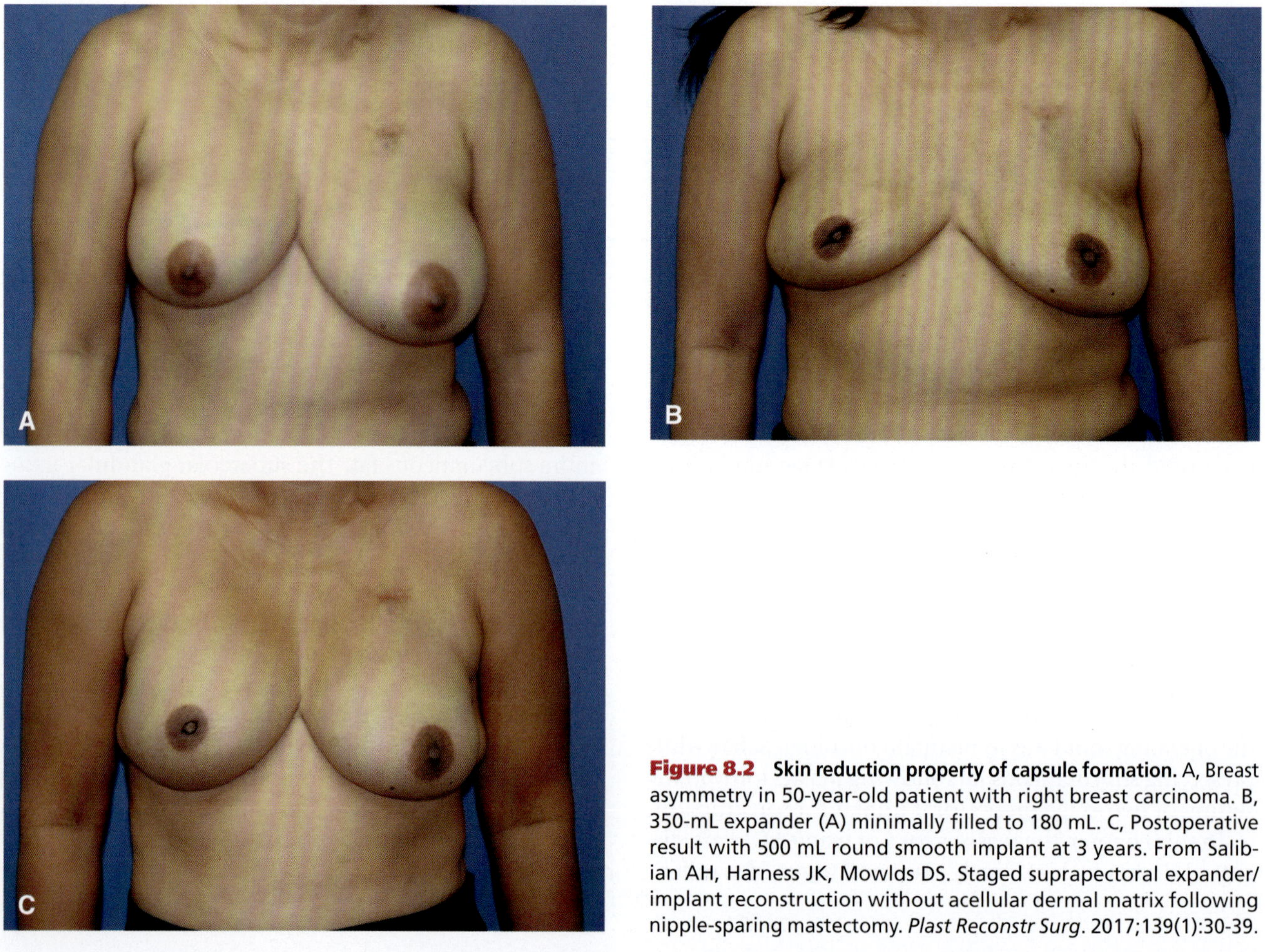

Figure 8.2 Skin reduction property of capsule formation. A, Breast asymmetry in 50-year-old patient with right breast carcinoma. B, 350-mL expander (A) minimally filled to 180 mL. C, Postoperative result with 500 mL round smooth implant at 3 years. From Salibian AH, Harness JK, Mowlds DS. Staged suprapectoral expander/implant reconstruction without acellular dermal matrix following nipple-sparing mastectomy. *Plast Reconstr Surg*. 2017;139(1):30-39.

an expander to stretch the skin and accommodate a breast implant. Because of increased incidence of skin complications, the expander was moved to the subpectoral space to protect against implant exposure. A subpectoral/subserratus expander was meant to expand both muscle and skin.

With the advent of NSM and the introduction of dual-plane reconstruction with ADM, the expander's role was limited to expanding the muscle rather than the skin. In two-stage prepectoral reconstruction, the expander continues to play an important role, although skin expansion beyond the preoperative surface area of the breast is rarely needed. Skin expansion is necessary only if small breasts, A cup or B cup, are increased two sizes to C cup or D cup, respectively. Single-cup enlargement often does not require skin expansion and there has to be adequate tissue perfusion for this step.

Tissue expanders are used to allow for soft-tissue contraction of the skin envelope to correct ptosis through capsule formation around an underinflated implant (**Figure 8.2**). In our patients, the average number of postoperative implant fill was 0.62, and the average postoperative fill volume was 248 mL. The average size of the final smooth round silicone gel implant was 515 mL, approximately twice the size of the final expander fill volume.

The advantage of a thick capsule that causes the skin to contract and raises the location of the silicone gel implant cannot be employed if ADM is used because of the inflammatory reduction properties of ADM.[16]

PREPECTORAL RECONSTRUCTION OF LARGE PTOTIC BREASTS WITHOUT ADM

The complication rates of two-stage breast reconstruction in large ptotic breasts increase with increasing BMI and breast size due to reduced skin perfusion, poor draping over an inflated expander, seromas, and infection.[17,18] Large ptotic breasts require surgical skin reduction using mastopexy techniques to prevent skin loss.[19] We have used the buttonhole mastopexy because of its flexibility, safety, and less visible scars.[20]

In primary buttonhole mastopexy, the mastectomy is performed through a U-shaped incision tangential to the areola to raise two thick mastectomy flaps. The broad-based inferior flap carrying the nipple-areola is deepithelialized and placed beneath the buttonholed superior flap (**Figure 8.3**). To minimize nipple-areola complications, a

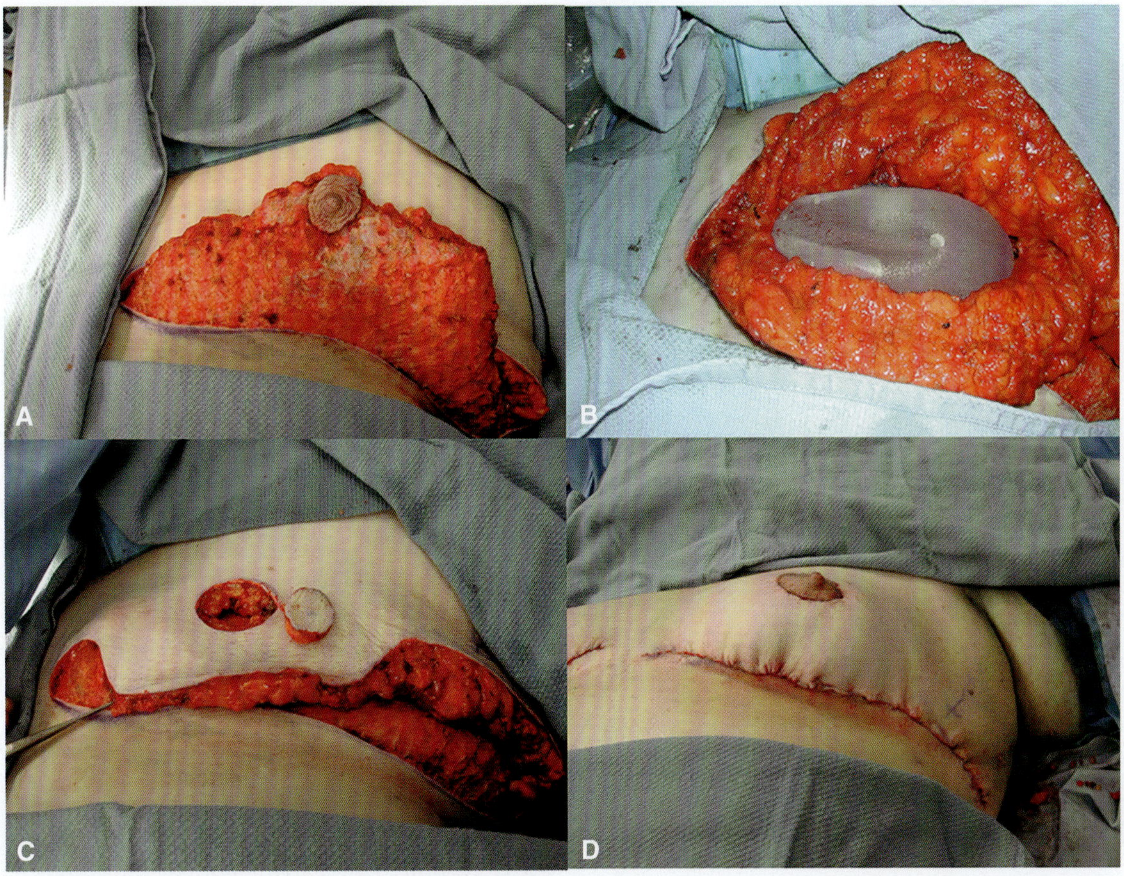

Figure 8.3 **Primary buttonhole mastopexy and nipple-sparing mastectomy.** A, Deepithelialized inferior flap carries nipple-areola to its new location within the superior flap. B, Tabbed expander fixed to pectoralis fascia without acellular dermal matrix. C, Buttonholed upper flap ready to receive nipple-areola. D, Upper flap retracted inferiorly and sutured along the inframammary fold. Exteriorized nipple-areola sutured in place. From Salibian AH, Harness JK, Mowlds DS. Primary buttonhole mastopexy and nipple-sparing mastectomy: a preliminary report. *Ann Plast Surg*. 2016;77(4):388-395.

thin layer of tumor-free subareolar breast tissue is retained in the first stage for removal in the second stage. Lower pole tumors close to the skin requiring flap thinning is a contraindication to primary buttonhole mastopexy-NSM.

Buttonhole mastopexy can be used in extremely large breasts without ADM if an expander is optimally situated and fixed in place to create the compartment for the final implant. If an expander is not used, the medial and lateral edges of the inferior pedicle are tacked down to the pectoralis and serratus muscles for compartmentalization and direct-implant insertion. Extremely large breasts may not require an implant for augmentation because of the large inferior flap (**Figure 8.4**).

For moderately large ptotic breasts, the buttonhole technique is modified to increase the vertical height of the proposed areola-to-fold distance (**Figure 8.5**). By rotating the excess horizontal upper flap skin into the central vertical plane, the height of the lower pole is increased, placing the nipple at the apex of the breast mound. Redundant lower pole skin is deepithelialized, buried, and flap margins approximated for inverted T-closure (**Figure 8.6**). This modification differs from the Wise keyhole-pattern technique in that excess flap centrally is not excised to avoid creating two separate medial and lateral flaps with diminished circulation at the corners of the inverted T-closure.

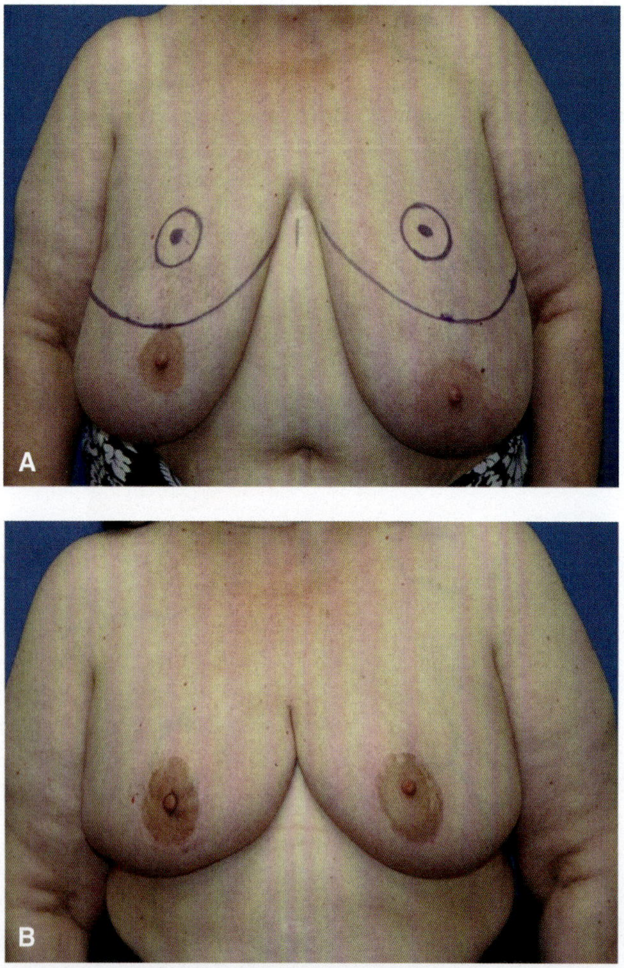

Figure 8.4 **Buttonhole mastopexy.** A, A 53-year-old patient with carcinoma of right breast showing markings to raise the nipple 16 cm. B, Result at 3 years. Left breast did not require an expander or an implant; right implant 450 mL.

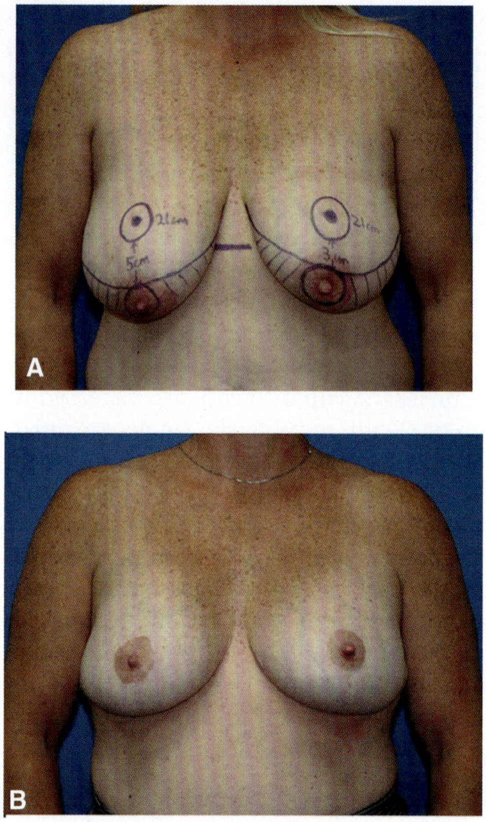

Figure 8.5 **Modified buttonhole mastopexy.** A, Preoperative markings in a 44-year-old patient with carcinoma of left breast. Short 3-cm left lower pole height requires lengthening with a modified buttonhole technique to match the opposite side. B, Postoperative result at 3 years. From Salibian AH, Harness JK, Mowlds DS. Primary buttonhole mastopexy and nipple-sparing mastectomy: a preliminary report. *Ann Plast Surg*. 2016;77(4):388-395.

SECONDARY MASTOPEXY AFTER PREPECTORAL RECONSTRUCTION WITHOUT ADM

Breast or nipple asymmetry after completion of two-stage breast reconstruction may require correction and implant exchange.[21-23] We have described a modified keyhole-pattern mastopexy to correct residual nipple/breast asymmetry and contour deformities related to capsular contracture (**Figures 8.7 and 8.8**).[24]

Secondary mastopexy is performed by modifying the Wise keyhole-pattern to incorporate the nipple-areola into a 4- to 5 cm-wide bipedicle dermal-fat flap. Adjacent skin flaps are undermined several centimeters for mobilization and closure (**Figure 8.9**). The nipple may be raised 2 to 6

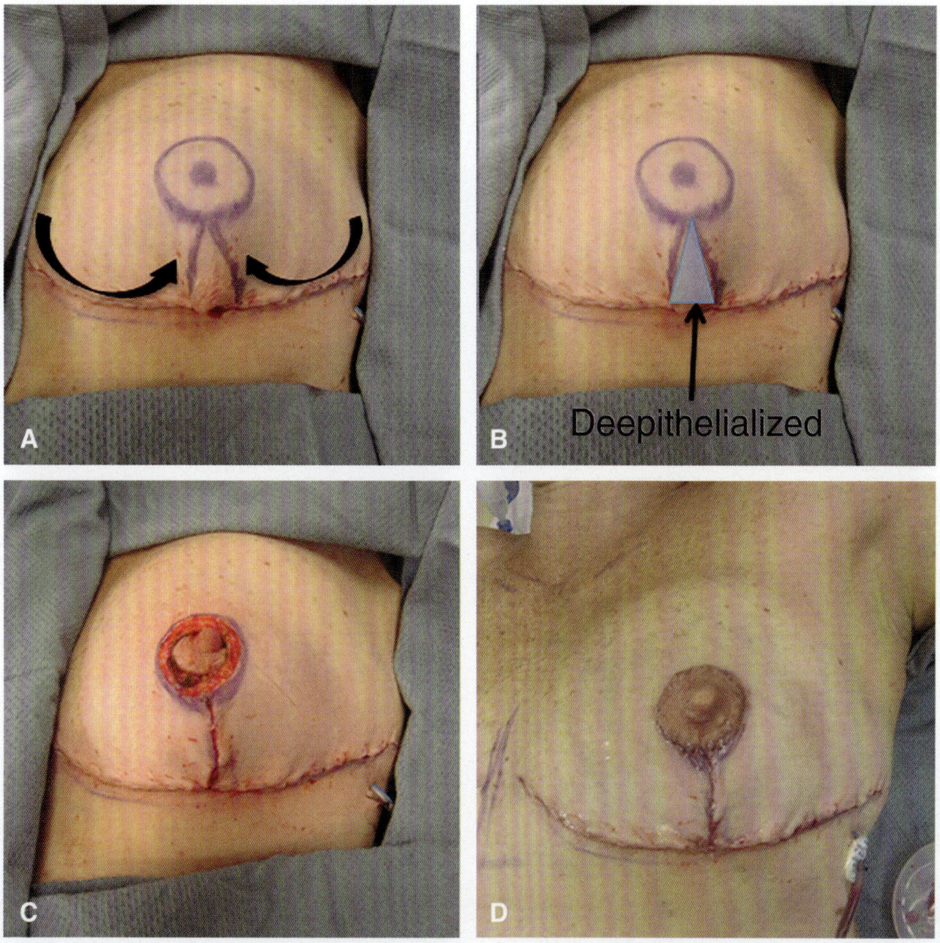

Figure 8.6. **Modified buttonhole mastopexy.** A, Upper flap margin rotated into vertical plane to increase the height of the lower pole, creating a dog-ear centrally. B, Dog-ear (blue triangle) deepithelialized and (C) buried for (D) final closure. From Salibian AH, Harness JK, Mowlds DS. Primary buttonhole mastopexy and nipple-sparing mastectomy: a preliminary report. *Ann Plast Surg*. 201677(4):388-395.

cm depending on the thickness of the flaps. Thicker flaps are undermined more for greater lifts.

The bipedicle flap will support the nipple-areola for mastopexy because of improved subdermal and subcutaneous circulation over several months after insertion of the expander. An additional source of collateral circulation to the nipple-areola is through the capsule. A mature capsule on histologic examination shows independent blood supply with vessels running along the superficial surface of the capsule.[25] The presence of a capsule beneath the nipple-areola allows collateral circulation to develop between the two structures, enhancing skin circulation. Although collateral capsular circulation has not been verified experimentally, it is well accepted that collateral circulation invariably develops between adjacent vascularized tissues.

The use of ADM minimizes capsule formation because of its anti-inflammatory properties. If ADM is used, it is theorized that in the absence of an important source of collateral circulation, skin complications may occur if a secondary mastopexy is attempted. Secondary mastopexy for minor lifts no greater than 2 cm may be tried initially in patients with ADM to determine whether the dermal-fat flap will support the nipple-areola.

SURGICAL COLLABORATION

The multidisciplinary team approach in management of breast cancer is the basis for improving outcomes.[26] Oncologic and plastic surgeons collaborate in the perioperative management of patients, but their collaboration in performing NSM is rarely practiced. The advantages of two surgeons working at the same time across the operating room table to perform the NSM, optimize tumor clearance without compromising skin circulation, and expedite the procedure has been reported by us.[27]

Operating in sequence with oncologic surgeons, and unaware of the details of flap thinning and status of skin perfusion, plastic surgeons depend on skin perfusion assessment technology (Spy Elite imaging system—Novadaq Inc., Mississauga, Canada), to decide whether to proceed with the reconstruction.[28,29] We have not used tissue perfusion devices because, as an onco-plastic surgical team,

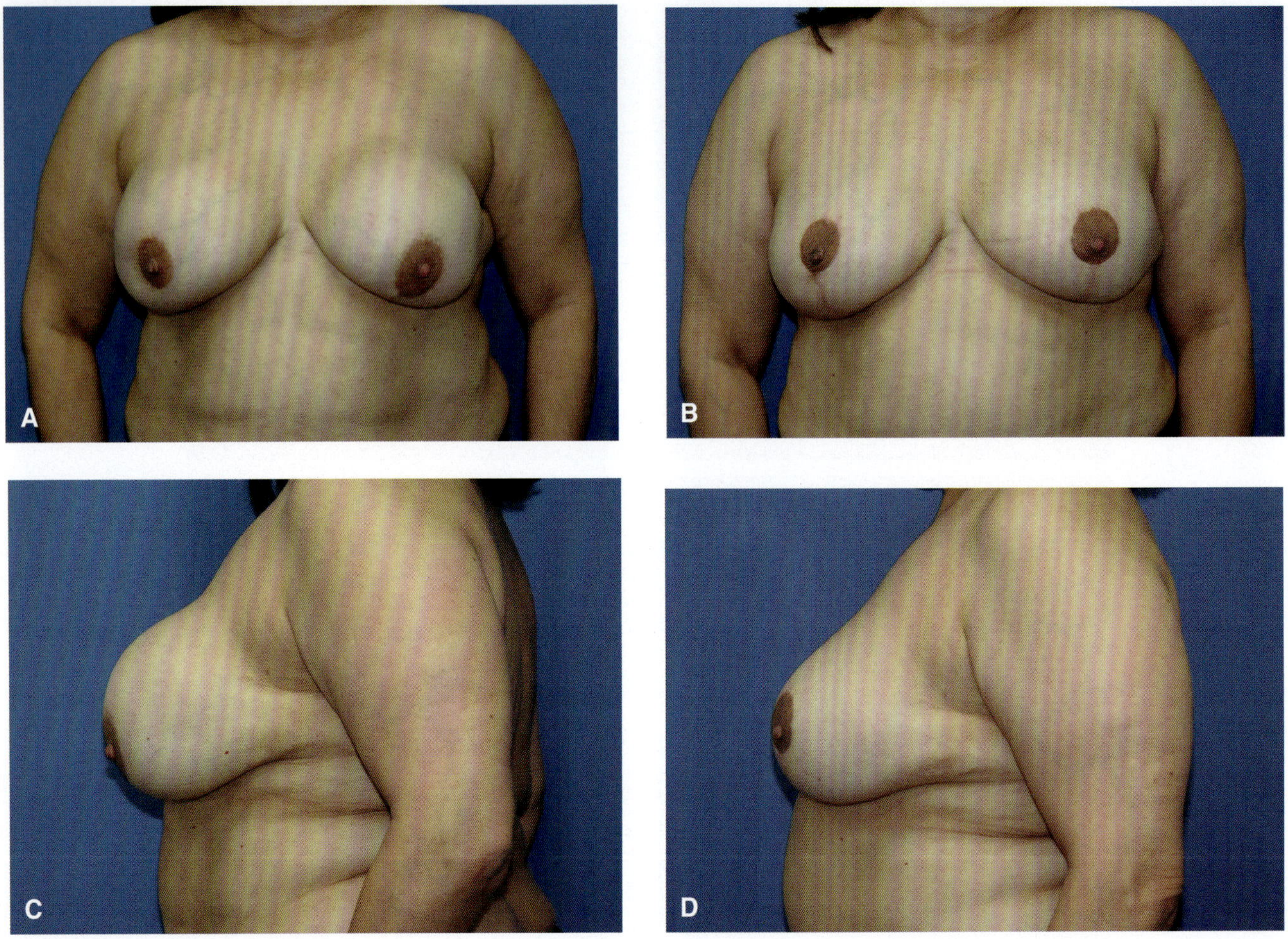

Figure 8.7 Secondary mastopexy for capsular contracture and implant downsizing. A, Grade IV capsular contracture in 50-year-old patient 3 years following completion of staged expander/implant reconstruction. B, Postoperative result at 1 year after secondary modified Wise pattern mastopexy (nipple raised 6 cm) and implant downsizing from 650 to 475 mL. C, Lateral preoperative view. D, Postoperative view.

we rely on thick flaps for optimal perfusion. In two-stage reconstruction we have not changed plans or postponed reconstruction because of skin perfusion concerns.

DISCUSSION

ADM is universally used in implant-based breast reconstruction following NSM. The reasons for the use of ADM in one- or two-stage prepectoral reconstructions are flap protection, support, defining and maintaining the pocket and inframammary fold, and reducing the incidence of capsular contracture.

Flap protection with ADM has been emphasized because of skin complications related to thinning of NSM flaps. Skin complications increase proportionately to increased flap thinning. Our experience with thick flaps has shown that skin complications are rare.

Generalized thinning of NSM flaps will not support the nipple-areola. Localized thinning of flaps may also cause skin loss if certain guidelines are not followed. Localized flap thinning can be done safely if the following are taken into consideration: (1) depth of thinning, (2) thinned out area, and (3) its proximity to the areola. Flap thinning down to the dermis is limited to no more than 14 cm^2. Partial subcutaneous fat thinning may be performed up to 25 cm^2. Periareolar subcutaneous fat should not be thinned so as not to compromise areolar dermal circulation. If a superficial tumor is located close to the areola, the flap may be thinned to reach the dermis for tumor clearance provided a 5-mm tumor-free subareolar breast tissue is preserved for complete excision several months later in the second stage. In large areolae with diameters greater than 5 cm, removing the entire subareolar breast tissue may cause skin loss. Localized areola necrosis is treated with excision and primary closure (**Figure 8.10**).

All patients are considered candidates for NSM using thick flaps except those with direct nipple-areola involvement, locally advanced tumor involving skin, and inflammatory breast cancer. Preoperative radiation is not

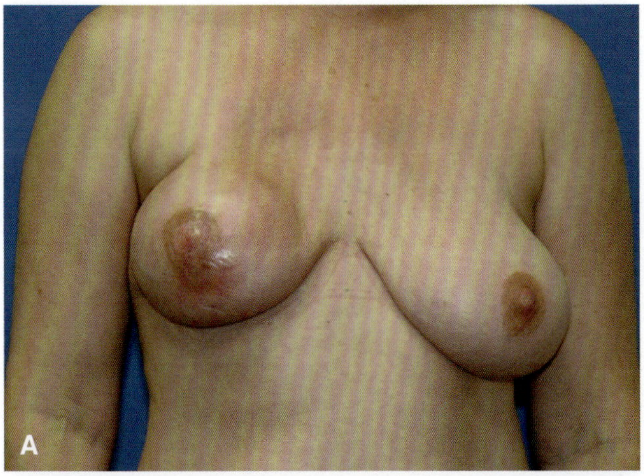

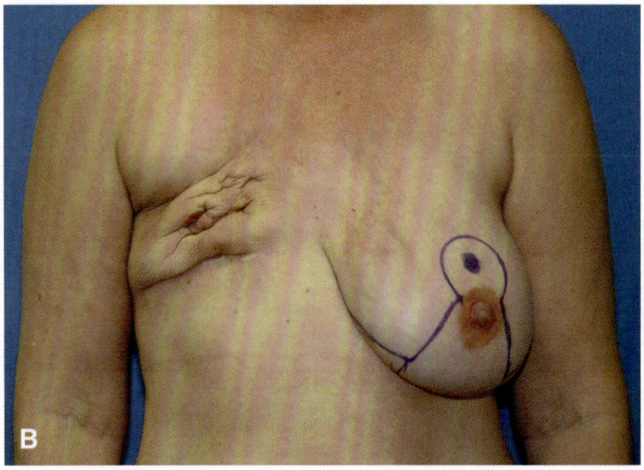

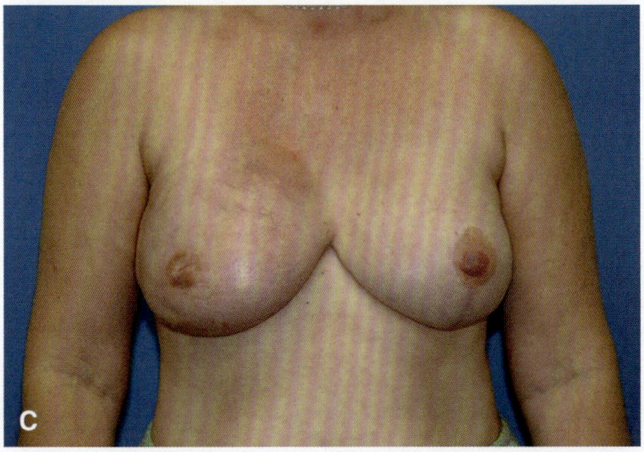

Figure 8.8 Secondary mastopexy for symmetry after contralateral radiation. A, Expander infection after radiotherapy requiring removal of the expander in a 43-year-old patient with recurrent right breast carcinoma who underwent bilateral two-stage reconstruction after nipple-sparing mastectomy. The left side has been reconstructed with a 650-mL silicone gel implant. B, Secondary mastopexy markings to raise the nipple 4 cm and reduce implant size to 450 mL. Right side will be reconstructed with a latissimus dorsi myocutaneous flap and 500-mL implant. C, Postoperative result at 1-1/2 years. Left inframammary fold raised 3 cm by anchoring chest wall skin to rib periosteum. From Salibian AH, Harness JK, Mowlds DS. Staged suprapectoral expander/implant reconstruction without acellular dermal matrix following nipple-sparing mastectomy. *Plast Reconstr Surg*. 2017139(1):30-39.

a contraindication to two-step reconstruction. Localized dermal involvement away from the nipple-areola is treated with elliptical skin excision in continuity with the rest of the breast. Tumors in proximity to pectoralis fascia are resected en bloc with a full-thickness segment of the underlying muscle.

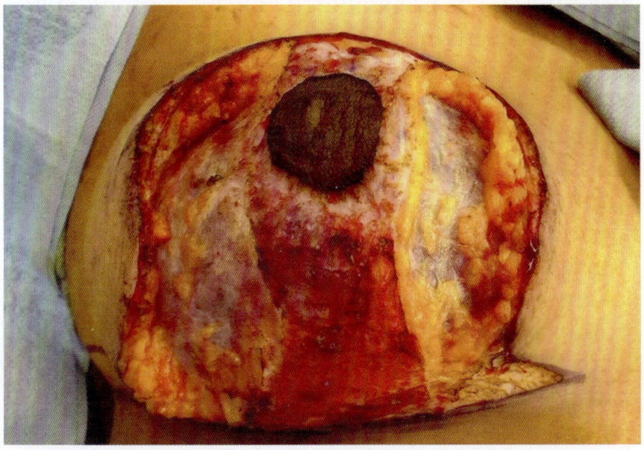

Figure 8.9 Bipedicle dermal-fat flap and capsule (light purple) supports the circulation to the nipple-areola. The medial and lateral flaps have been undermined 4 cm for mobilization and closure.

The use of ADM in one- or two-stage prepectoral reconstruction has been advocated to define the location of the pocket and the inframammary fold. Because present-day tabbed expanders (Mentor Worldwide, Irvine, CA) can be fixed (**Figure 8.11**) to maintain the location of the pocket, the role of ADM in positioning the pocket and inframammary fold is less important.

A mature capsule after first-stage healing prevents implant dystopia much the same as ADM. We have observed implant dystopia in prepectoral reconstruction without ADM in two thin patients (0.8%) who had relatively large implants (425 mL, 500 mL). To prevent implant descent in thin patients with implants greater than 400 mL, the chest wall skin is anchored to the rib periosteum with nonabsorbable sutures along the inframammary fold in the second stage.

In direct-implant prepectoral reconstruction, ADM is used for implant positioning and stabilization, particularly in large breasts where pocket size is greater than the implant. With thick flaps, lateral implant migration can be controlled without ADM by placing several subcutaneous-to-serratus/pectoralis tacking sutures at the level of the anterior axillary fold. The pocket in small- and medium-sized breasts will accommodate a matching or slightly larger implant without ADM stabilization.

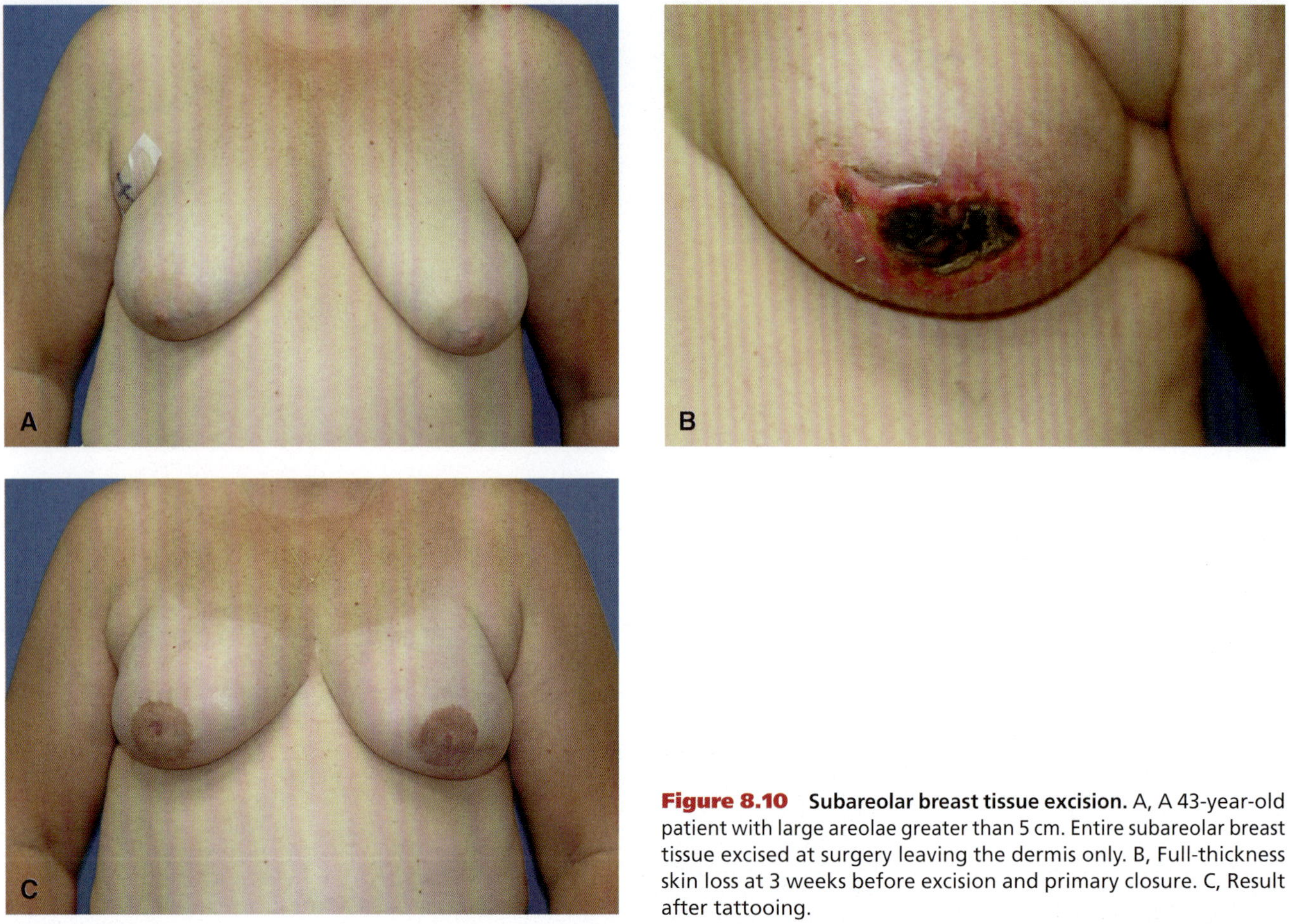

Figure 8.10 **Subareolar breast tissue excision.** A, A 43-year-old patient with large areolae greater than 5 cm. Entire subareolar breast tissue excised at surgery leaving the dermis only. B, Full-thickness skin loss at 3 weeks before excision and primary closure. C, Result after tattooing.

Total implant coverage, "hand-in-glove" manner, and fixation with ADM prevent upward implant mobility, creating a depression along the upper border of the implant that may require lipofilling. This phenomenon is not seen in two-stage reconstruction without ADM where the capsule is released up to the infraclavicular area in the second stage. We have not used lipofilling for upper pole contour deformity.

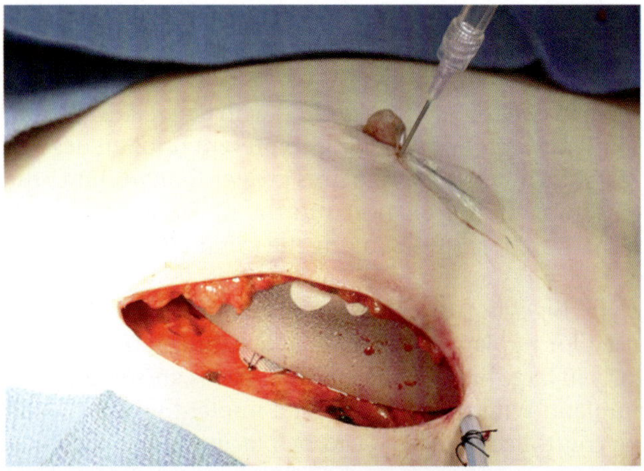

Figure 8.11 Suprapectoral expander fixation above inframammary fold with minimal inflation. From Salibian AH, Harness JK, Mowlds DS. Staged suprapectoral expander/implant reconstruction without acellular dermal matrix following nipple-sparing mastectomy. *Plast Reconstr Surg*. 2017139(1):30-39.

ADM is advocated for implant support in one-stage prepectoral reconstruction to reduce the pressure on the skin. Although this may be true for implants greater than 500 mL, smaller implants placed directly in the pocket will rarely cause pressure ischemia in well-perfused thick flaps.

Direct prepectoral implant reconstruction, with or without ADM, is preferable to obviate a second operation. Under certain circumstances, such as preoperative or postoperative radiation, patients may benefit from staged reconstruction. The effects of radiation on skin circulation differ, with each patient requiring caution in choosing the implant size and timing of implantation. Minimal expander inflation in patients with previous radiation, rather than direct large implant insertion, reduces skin complications. For patients undergoing postoperative radiotherapy, capsulotomies performed 6 months after completion of radiotherapy affords more flexibility in controlling the pocket and choosing the correct implant size for symmetry (**Figure 8.12**). In our series, 31% of patients ($N = 48$) underwent preoperative (9%) and postoperative (22%) radiation therapy. Of these patients, 73% ($N = 35$) had very good/good results.

If cleavage and upper pole fullness is desired, it is safer to perform the reconstruction in two stages, undermining

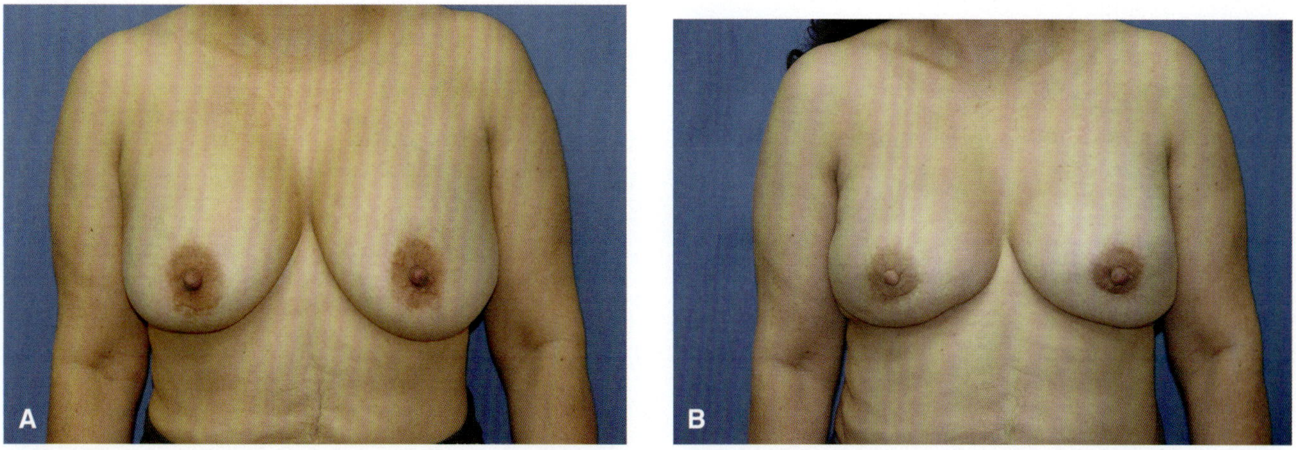

Figure 8.12 Postoperative radiation therapy in staged prepectoral breast reconstruction. A, Bilateral carcinomas in 49-year-old patient with previous bilateral augmentation (350 mL). B, Result 3 years after completion of radiation therapy and staged reconstruction with 550-mL smooth round silicone gel implant.

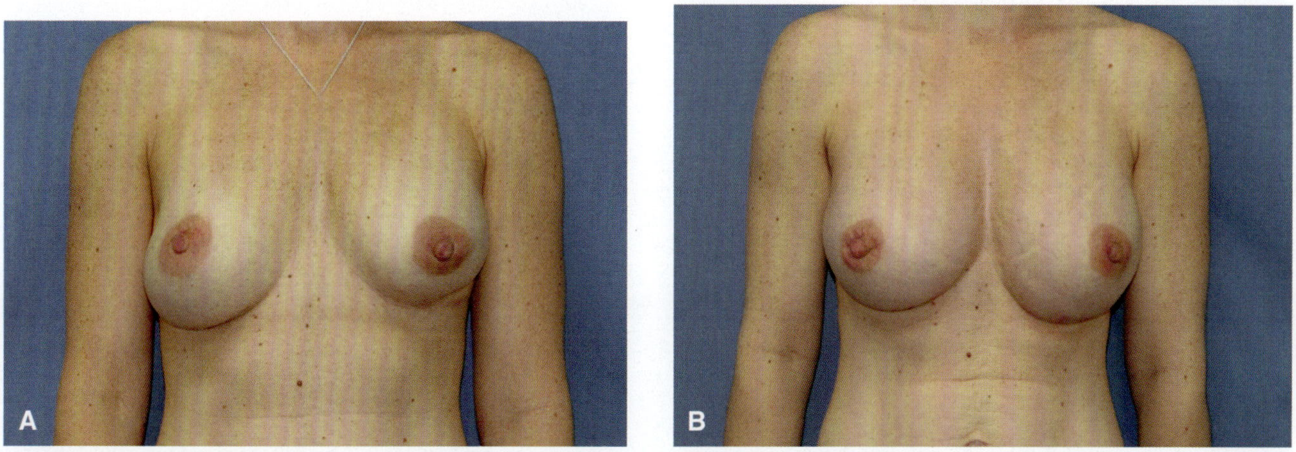

Figure 8.13 Staged prepectoral reconstruction. A, First-stage bilateral expander reconstruction (fill volume 270 mL) in 40-year-old patient with right breast carcinoma. B, Postoperative view showing improved cleavage with 550-mL implant.

the pocket medially and superiorly beyond the confines of the mastectomy pocket at a later date after skin circulation has improved (**Figure 8.13**). Patients with very large ptotic breasts are also better served with two-stage primary buttonhole mastopexy to avoid skin complications.

The role of ADM in minimizing capsule formation, reported extensively in retropectoral reconstruction, has shown similar results in prepectoral reconstruction over short-term follow-up.[6] Our experience in two-stage reconstruction without ADM has shown continued changes in capsular contracture after 3 years. The incidence of grade III and IV capsular contractures was 7.6%, with 4.4% requiring capsulotomy within 3 years.

Breast firmness and contour deformity due to capsular contracture after reconstruction is evaluated by patient's history, physical examination, photographic analysis, and breast tonometry.[30] Prospective studies for at least 3 years after prepectoral ADM reconstruction, including lateral photographs of the breast, are needed to more accurately assess the true incidence of grades III to IV capsular contracture.

In spite of ADM's advantage in minimizing capsular contracture, we prefer not to use ADM in two-stage reconstruction because of the overriding benefits of capsular skin reduction properties to correct ptosis, tailoring the pocket in the second stage for medial and upper pole fullness, management of very large ptotic breasts, and secondary mastopexy after reconstruction to improve symmetry. ADM, in our experience, has not been a prerequisite for prepectoral reconstruction.

SUMMARY

Reduced capsular contracture is the predominant reason for using ADM in two-step NSM reconstruction. Controlled prospective studies for more than 3 years are needed to determine the incidence of grades III and IV capsular contracture in prepectoral ADM reconstruction. On the basis of these studies, the advantages of each method, reconstruction with or without ADM, have to be evaluated to decide on one's own preference.

KEY REFERENCES

1. Rohrich RJ. The "prepectoral breast reconstruction" supplement. *Plast Reconstr Surg*. 2017;140:1S-2S.
2. Vidya R, Iqbal FM. A guide to prepectoral breast reconstruction: a new dimension to implant-based breast reconstruction. *Clin Breast Cancer*. 2017;17:266-271.
3. Sbitany H, Piper M, Lentz R. Prepectoral breast reconstruction: a safe alternative to submuscular prosthetic reconstruction following nipple-sparing mastectomy. *Plast Reconstr Surg*. 2017;140:432-443.
4. Reitsamer R, Peintinger F. Prepectoral implant placement and complete coverage with porcine acellular dermal matrix: a new technique for direct-to-implant breast reconstruction after nipple-sparing mastectomy. *Br J Plast Surg*. 2014;68:162-167.
5. Becker H, Lind JG, Hopkins EG. Immediate implant-based prepectoral breast reconstruction using a vertical incision. *Plast Reconstr Surg Glob Open*. 2015;3:e412.
6. Sigalove S, Maxwell GP, Sigalove NM et al. Prepectoral implant-based breast reconstruction: rationale, indications, and preliminary results. *Plast Reconstr Surg*. 2017;139:287-294.
7. Rawlani V, Buck DW II, Johnson SA, Heyer KS, Kim JY. Tissue expander breast reconstruction using prehydrated human acellular dermis. *Ann Plast Surg*. 2011;66:593-597.
8. Namnoum JD. Expander/implant reconstruction with AlloDerm: Recent experience. Plast Reconstr Surg. 2009;124:387–394.
9. Spear SL, Parikh PM, Reisin E, Menon NG. Acellular dermis-assisted breast reconstruction. *Aesthetic Plast Surg*. 2008;32:418-425.
10. Sbitany H, Sandeen SN, Amalfi AN, Davenport MS, Langstein HN. Acellular dermis-assisted prosthetic breast reconstruction versus complete submuscular coverage: a head-to-head comparison of outcomes. *Plast Reconstr Surg*. 2009;124:1735-1740.
11. Salibian AH, Harness JK, Mowlds DS. Inframammary approach to nipple-areola-sparing mastectomy. *Plast Reconstr Surg*. 2013;132:700e-708e.
12. Salibian AH, Harness JK, Mowlds DS. Staged suprapectoral expander/implant reconstruction without acellular dermal matrix following nipple-sparing mastectomy. *Plast Reconstr Surg*. 2017;139:30-39.
13. Adam H, Bygdeson M, de Boniface J. The oncological safety of nipple-sparing mastectomy - A Swedish matched cohort study. *Eur J Surg Oncol*. 2014;40:1209-1215.
14. Shimo A, Tsugawa K, Tsuchiya S, et al. Oncologic outcomes and technical considerations of nipple-sparing mastectomies in breast cancer: experience of 425 cases from a single institution. *Breast Cancer*. 2016;23:851-860.
15. Radovan C. Breast reconstruction after mastectomy using the temporary expander. *Plast Reconstr Surg*. 1982;69:195-208.
16. Basu CB, Leong M, Hicks MJ. Acellular cadaveric dermis decreases the inflammatory response in capsule formation in reconstructive breast surgery. *Plast Reconstr Surg*. 2010;126:1842-1847.
17. Gabriel A, Maxwell GP. Prepectoral breast reconstruction in challenging patients. *Plast Reconstr Surg*. 2017;140:14S-21S.
18. Chen CL, Shore AD, Johns R, Clark JM, Manahan M, Makary MA. The impact of obesity on breast surgery complications. *Plast Reconstr Surg*. 2011;128:395e-402e.
19. Caputo GG, Marchetti A, Dalla Pozza E, et al. Skin-reduction breast reconstructions with prepectoral implant. *Plast Reconstr Surg*. 2016;137:1702-1705.
20. Salibian AH, Harness JK, Mowlds DS. Primary buttonhole mastopexy and nipple-sparing mastectomy: a preliminary report. *Ann Plast Surg*. 2016;77:388-395.
21. Takayanagi S. Transposition of the malpositioned nipple-areola complex in breast reconstruction with implants. *Aesthetic Plast Surg*. 2010;34:52-58.
22. Small K, Kelly KM, Swistel A, Dent BL, Taylor EM, Talmor M. Surgical treatment of nipple malposition in nipple-sparing mastectomy device-based reconstruction. *Plast Reconstr Surg*. 2014;133:1053-1062.
23. Spear SL, Albino FP, Al-Attar A. Classification and management of the postoperative high-riding nipple. *Plast Reconstr Surg*. 2013;131:1413-1421.
24. Salibian AH, Harness JK, Mowlds DS. Secondary mastopexy after nipple-sparing mastectomy and staged subcutaneous expander/implant reconstruction. *Ann Plast Surg*. 2018;80:475-480.
25. Tomita K, Yano K, Nishibayashi A, Hosokawa K. Effects of subcutaneous versus submuscular tissue expander placement on breast capsule formation. *Plast Reconstr Surg Glob Open*. 2015;3:e432.
26. Storm-Dickerson T, Sigalove N. Prepectoral breast reconstruction: the breast surgeon's perspective. *Plast Reconstr Surg*. 2017;140:43S-48S.
27. Salibian AH, Harness JK. Operative approaches to nipple-sparing mastectomy. Switzerland: Springer International Publishing; 2017.
28. Jones G, Yoo A, King V, et al. Prepectoral immediate direct-to-implant breast reconstruction with anterior AlloDerm coverage. *Plast Reconstr Surg*. 2017;140:31S-38S.
29. Komorowska-Timek E, Gurtner GC. Intraoperative perfusion mapping with laser-assisted indocyanine green imaging can predict and prevent complications in immediate breast reconstruction. *Plast Reconstr Surg*. 2010;125:1065-1073.
30. Mosahebi A, Ramakrishnan V, Gittos M, Collier J. Aesthetic outcome of different techniques of reconstruction following nipple-areola-preserving envelope mastectomy with immediate reconstruction. *Plast Reconstr Surg*. 2007;119:796-803.

CHAPTER 9

THE ROLE OF FAT GRAFTING IN PREPECTORAL BREAST RECONSTRUCTION

Hani Sbitany

KEY POINTS

- Autologous fat grafting is a safe, autologous method for volume augmentation in prosthetic breast reconstruction.
- Autologous fat grafting is especially important in prepectoral breast reconstruction, given the need for greater volume over the upper pole of the implant, without the pectoralis major muscle covering this area.
- The use of fat grafting as an adjunct procedure in prepectoral breast reconstruction will help reduce the risk of visible rippling.
- Autologous fat grafting can be performed at the time of prepectoral tissue expander to implant exchange, or as a staged procedure.
- In prepectoral patients, the upper pole of the breast has only one layer to inject with fat (between skin and ADM), but this can be safely cannulated and can accept fat.
- Fat must be injected in long and thin strands, all contacting surrounding vascularized tissue, to maximize fat take rate, and to prevent fat necrosis.
- Fat is best processed through filtration and light washing, to maximize graft take rates; overprocessing of fat results in higher rates of fat necrosis.
- Autologous fat that is grafted into the breast will survive and restore soft-tissue volume to the upper pole, in the area where the pectoralis major muscle would have been used in traditional subpectoral techniques.

INTRODUCTION

Prepectoral implant-based breast reconstruction carries significant benefits for patients, including reduced pain, elimination of animation deformity, and full maintenance of strength because of complete muscle preservation.[1] However, with the elimination of pectoralis major muscle harvest for upper pole implant coverage, there is a greater need for volume augmentation of the upper pole skin flaps, to eliminate contour deformities such as rippling and implant palpability. This need for increased volume is further necessary in cases of thin mastectomy skin flaps.

Autologous fat grafting provides an excellent solution for upper pole volume augmentation. The ability to harvest and inject autologous fat allows for long-lasting, healthy tissue to mask the upper pole of the prosthesis, with low infection rates and proven oncologic safety.[2] Furthermore, this is a safe and minimally invasive technique at the donor site, with the fat being harvested through liposuction techniques. Because of these characteristics, autologous fat grafting has become an essential component of prepectoral breast reconstruction for many surgeons.[3] When combined with proper implant selection (ie, cohesive, full capacity) and underexpansion of the skin envelope, this technique can help prevent contour deformities in the majority of reconstructive cases.[4]

Autologous fat also carries the benefit of being a rich source of stem cells. Although the majority of surgeons does not concentrate or potentiate proliferation of these stem cells, this does allow fat grafting to result in improved tissue quality in the reconstructed skin envelope. In radiated skin envelopes, fat grafting has been shown to reverse some of the damaging characteristics of radiation fibrosis, such as fibrosis and vessel depletion.[5] Clinically, this translates as softer skin envelopes with potential for improved healing.

For all these reasons, fat grafting has allowed many patients to successfully complete prepectoral breast reconstruction with the highest quality aesthetic outcome, and with minimal morbidity. The patients who benefit most from the volume augmentation are the thinnest, low-BMI patient population. Given their minimal soft-tissue coverage, these patients are at high risk for visible implant edges, rippling, and a hollow upper pole appearance. For this category of patients, fat injection allows for maximal prevention of these aesthetic problems (**Figure 9.1A-C**). Without fat grafting, this group of patients would likely be a contraindication for prepectoral breast reconstruction, because they would require the soft-tissue coverage of the pectoralis major muscle over the upper pole of their implant.

The key to achieving long-lasting fat survival, with minimal complication rates (ie, fat necrosis and oil cysts), is the proper technique for fat harvest, processing, and reinjection. The fat must be harvested from proper donor sites, using techniques that do not physically damage fat cells. Similarly, processing must be done thoroughly enough to eliminate excessive blood and oil, but not so excessive that fat is damaged. Finally, the method of fat injection must ensure that all injected fat is directly contacting surrounding recipient bed vascularized tissue. Recommended techniques for all these steps are presented in the following sections.

PREOPERATIVE PLANNING

In assessing a patient for autologous fat grafting, the surgeon must first select the correct donor sites for fat harvest. The lower abdomen and thighs are the most commonly chosen donor sites when performing autologous fat grafting to the breast. This is due both to their ease of access with a patient in the supine position and to the relatively high volume of fat in these locations, in most patients.

In addition to these factors, it has been shown that fat from both the infraumbilical abdomen and the medial

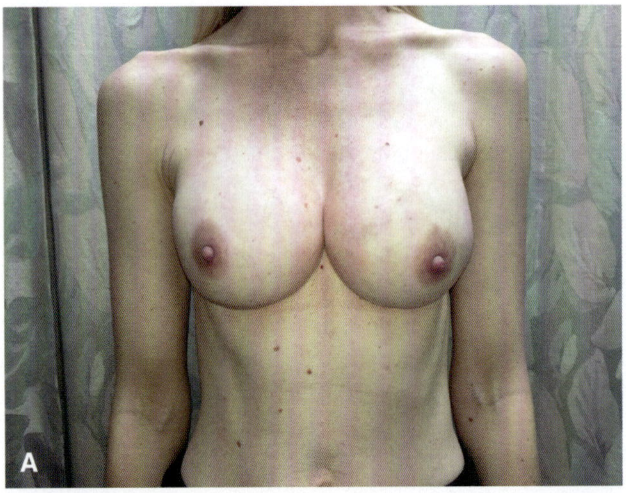

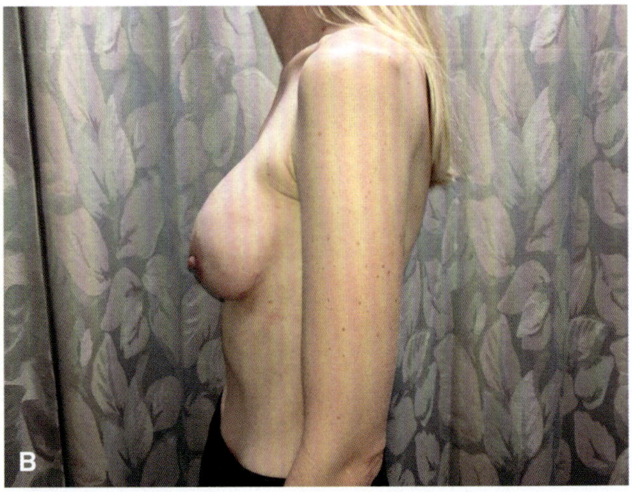

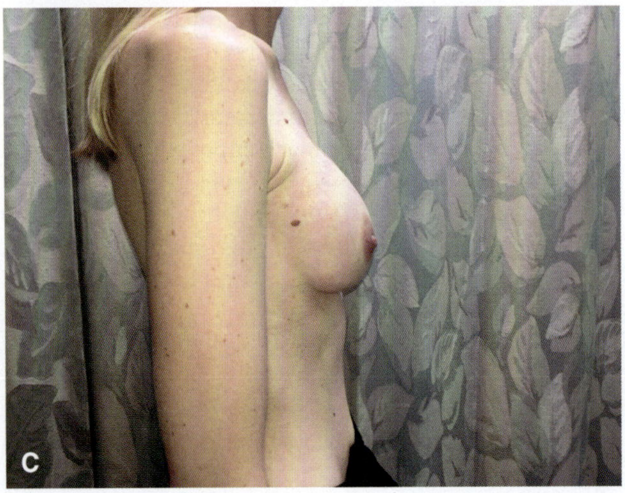

Figure 9.1 A-C, A 37-year-old female, 2 years postoperative result from bilateral nipple-sparing mastectomies and bilateral prepectoral breast reconstruction. Despite an extremely thin frame, and thin mastectomy skin flaps, the patient has no rippling on clinical examination. This is due to aggressive fat grafting at the time of expander-to-implant exchange operation, resulting in thicker upper pole breast skin flaps.

thighs tend to have the highest concentration of viable adipocytes.[6] Thus, in most instances, it is advisable that these areas be used for fat harvest when available.

Preoperatively, the surgeon must carefully mark the zones of planned liposuction, such that all areas are used equally and symmetrically, to avoid a donor site defect. The most frequent cause of patient dissatisfaction with autologous fat grafting comes when patients experience donor site defects, such as hollowing or deflation, from excessive liposuction. To avoid this, the surgeon should harvest conservatively and equally from multiple sites.

SURGICAL MANAGEMENT

Recipient Site Preparation

Intraoperatively, the donor sites must first be prepared for fat harvest. Each area should be infused with tumescent solution, consisting of epinephrine and lidocaine at safe concentrations. This allows for harvest of lipoaspirate with minimal blood content. The injection of this mixture has been shown to have no alteration on fat graft take rates or adipocyte viability, in subsequent fat grafting.

Fat Harvest

Harvest of fat can be performed with a multitude of techniques, depending on surgeon's preference. Safe and effective methods include conventional liposuction, power-assisted liposuction, and handheld syringe liposuction. All of these techniques have been shown to result in harvest of viable adipocytes, with maintained normal fat histologic structure.[7]

It is not recommended that ultrasonic liposuction techniques be used for fat harvest. This type of liposuction works through lysis of fat cells, before suctioning. Thus, it does not produce healthy and viable adipocytes for reinjection.

With all the recommended techniques, a blunt tip cannula should be used for harvest. In addition, larger harvest cannulas produce larger concentrations of viable adipocytes than do smaller cannulas.[8] This is a result of less physical trauma to fat cells during harvest, which is greater when they must pass through a smaller diameter tube. It is the author's preference to use a 5-mm or 6-mm blunt tip cannula for harvest of lipoaspirate. Once this is complete, the donor site can then be further aesthetically modified with a smaller cannula if necessary. With all cannula types, a suction harvest pressure of 250 mmHg or less should be used. Pressures higher than this have been shown to result in greater adipocyte damage.

Fat Processing

Following harvest, the lipoaspirate is then processed, to reduce the amount of oil, blood, collagen strands, and lysed cells. Traditionally, many techniques have been utilized, including decanting, filtration, and centrifugation. There is clear evidence showing that minimal processing results in more viable adipocytes. For example, filtration techniques (light wash, light spin) for lipoaspirate processing have been shown to result in higher concentrations of viable fat cells compared to centrifugation.[9] Regardless of the surgeon's exact preferred technique, it should be one that involves minimal processing, to avoid fat disruption.

When properly harvested, the fat will have a golden yellow color, without visible oil or blood contamination. When injected onto an operating room towel, there should not be excessive leakage of fluid leaching out from the fat cells. This indicates pure fat content, without contaminants.

Fat Injection

Following processing, the fat is then loaded into syringes for injection. Fat is often loaded into 1- or 3-cc syringes. This allows for improved control of injection volume per pass of the syringe. Those surgeons with greater experience performing fat injection may wish to load fat into 10-cc syringes, for efficiency.

The approach during injection is to infiltrate many thin strands of fat, dispersed equally throughout the soft-tissue envelope. This allows for maximal contact of all injected fat with surrounding vascularized tissue, and thus, maximal fat take rates. This also reduces the risk of complications such as fat necrosis. Injection of large boluses or clumps of fat will result in central fat necrosis within these injection areas.

Similar to fat harvest, it has been shown that using wider diameter cannulas for injection will result in improved fat graft survival and reduced fat graft resorption. This is due to less physical trauma to fat cells as they pass through wider diameter cannulas. Thus, cannulas in the 2- to 2.5-mm diameter range are recommended for fat injection. Each pass of the syringe with these cannulas should infiltrate 0.5 to 1 cc of fat, in an attempt to avoid fat necrosis.

To properly inject fat into the prepectoral skin envelope, the surgeon must cannulate the area between the skin and the underlying acellular dermal matrix (ADM). The majority of techniques for prepectoral breast reconstruction involve covering the entire anterior surface of the prosthesis with ADM, at the time of initial placement.[10] Thus, successful injection to increase soft-tissue thickness in this upper pole will require injection between the skin and ADM. This space will be well adhered, but can be cannulated with a blunt tip injection cannula.

Once the correct plane is established, one layer of fat can be injected into this area per grafting session. More than one layer will not be possible, given that some fat will not be in contact with the vascularized skin envelope, and will thus not survive. It is recommended that this injection be performed with an implant sizer, in place, to avoid risk of puncturing the permanent prosthesis.

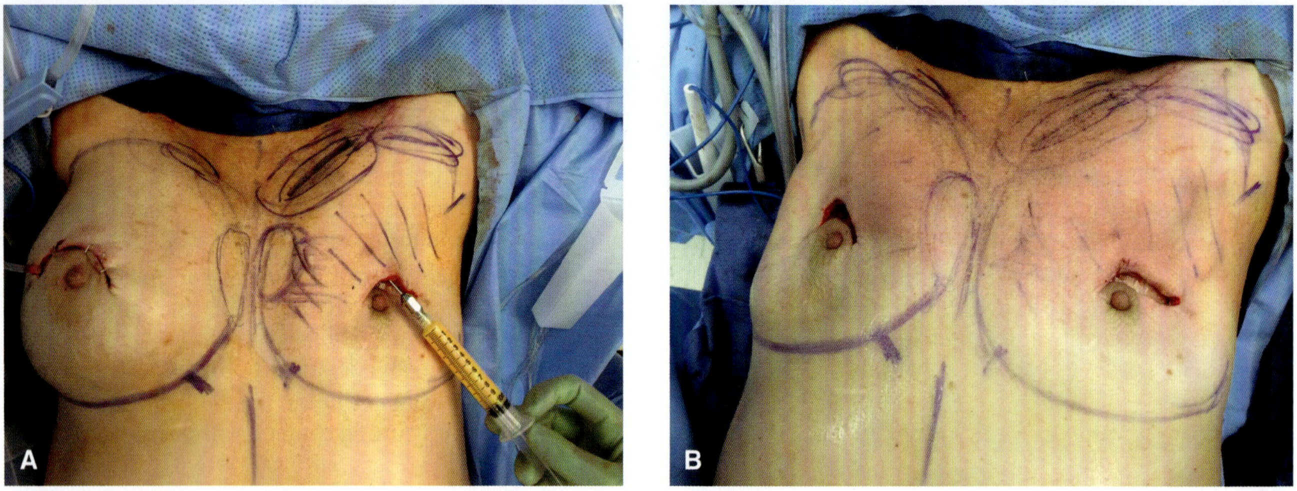

Figure 9.2 A and B, Autologous fat grafting at the time of expander-to-implant exchange. After marking the areas for upper pole grafting, with the patient upright and the sizer in place, the sizer is removed. Fat is injected at this point, into the flat skin surface (A). Following completion of fat injection, the skin is bruised but still healthy and viable (B). At this point, the pocket is irrigated, and the permanent implant is placed.

Another option, which is the author's preference, is to inject fat at the time of tissue expander to implant exchange, before permanent implant placement. This technique involves marking the patient for grafting while in the upright position in the table and with temporary sizers in place. Following this, the patient is placed back in supine position, the sizer removed, and the fat injected at this point (**Figure 9.2A-B**). Without an implant in place, the fat injection on the flat surface is easy and efficient and can be done with one hand in the pocket to ensure the ADM is not punctured with the cannula. Furthermore, because there is only one layer to inject under the prepectoral skin, the areas already injected are readily visible. Following completion of fat injection, the permanent implant is placed and the skin closed.

CLINICAL OUTCOMES

Autologous fat grafting in the setting of prepectoral breast reconstruction is a mandatory procedure in the majority of patients, to prevent minor degrees of rippling and contour deformity, particularly in the upper pole of the patient's reconstructed breast. Furthermore, this helps achieve a natural upper pole breast slope, in the absence of pectoralis major muscle sacrifice. This technique has proved to be extremely powerful in this setting, because it allows for autologous tissue correction and prevention of these deformities. Furthermore, the result is permanent, because the fat revascularizes and persists in this area.

Those patients in whom the benefits of fat grafting are most evident are in those with thin skin envelopes, and the implant surface or edges are visible. Oftentimes, these patients also happen to be of low BMI, accounting for the thin fat layer on the underside of their mastectomy skin envelope. Despite the thin stature of such patients, they often have enough subcutaneous tissue on their bodies for the purposes of fat grafting.

Figure 9.3A illustrates a 40-year-old patient following left breast two-stage prepectoral reconstruction, and a right breast augmentation for symmetry. The patient declined autologous fat grafting at the time of expander-to-implant

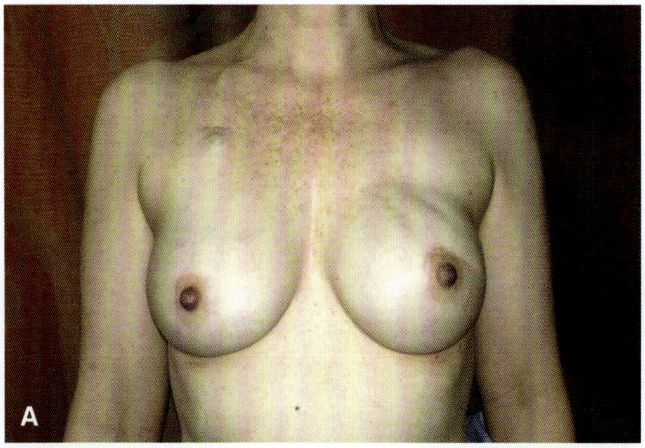

Figure 9.3 A-E, A 40-year-old female, who underwent left breast nipple-sparing mastectomy and left breast prepectoral breast reconstruction, along with right breast augmentation (A). Patient declined autologous fat grafting at the time of expander-to-implant exchange, and returned 9 months later with left breast upper pole rippling and hollowing. She then underwent 100 cc of autologous fat grafting to left breast, along with right breast crescent mastopexy (B). Postoperatively, 1 year after revisionary procedure, the patient maintains rippling correction and natural appearing slope of left breast upper pole, after fat grafting (C-E).

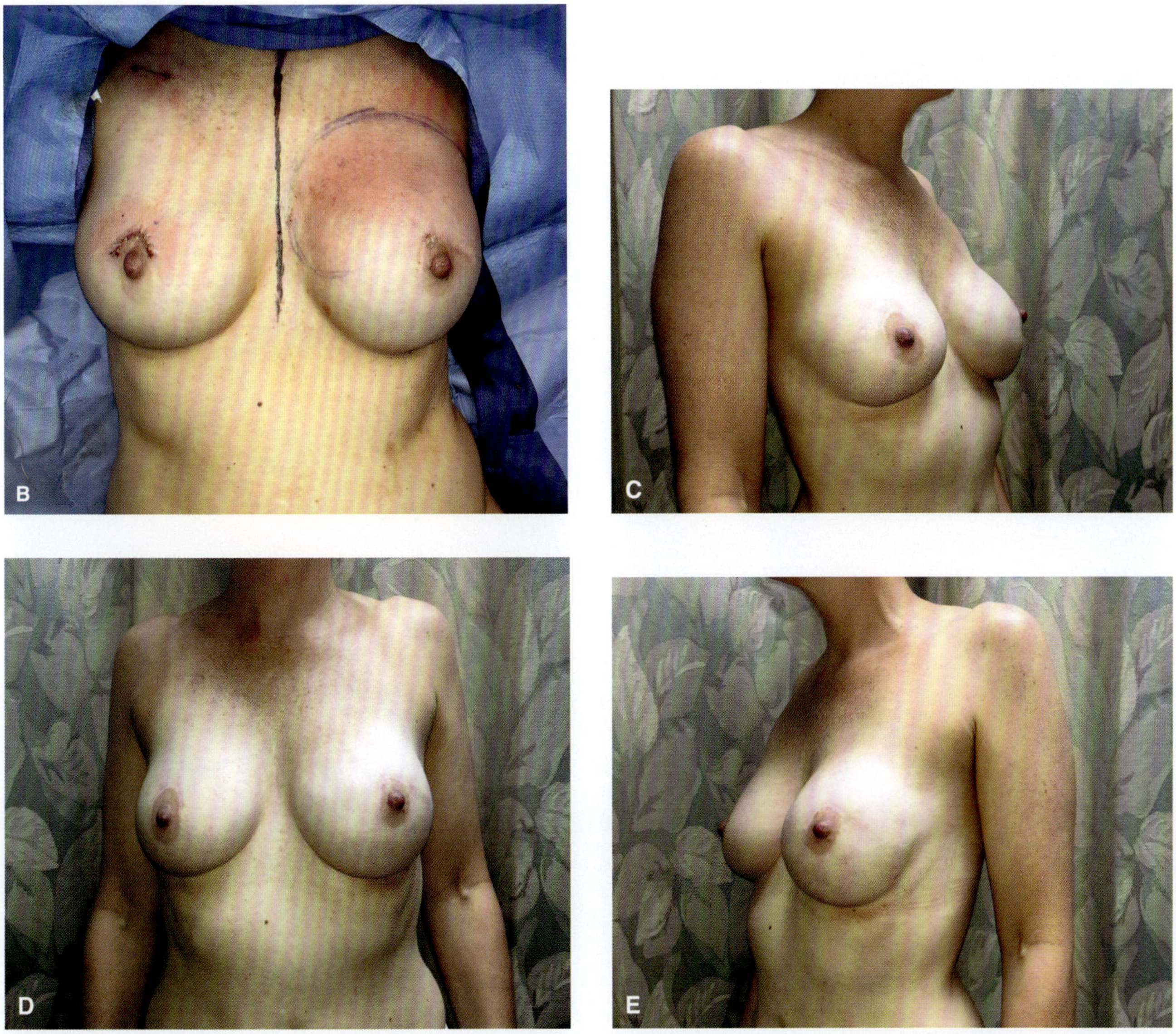

Figure 9.3 *(continued)*

exchange, and returned with visible rippling and breast asymmetry 9 months later. She then underwent one fat grafting session to the left breast, along with a right breast crescent mastopexy for symmetry (**Figure 9.3B**). At this operation, she underwent injection of 100 cc of autologous fat to the entire left breast upper pole skin envelope, and left upper chest area above the breast. No breast implant exchange was performed.

Postoperatively at 1 year, the patient's fat grafting session corrected the majority of her rippling and implant visibility (**Figure 9.3C-E**). Pinch test examination reveals a clinically thicker upper pole breast skin envelope, and rippling is not evident on examination. An estimated 75% of the injected fat has persisted and survived as a vascularized graft.

As evidenced, patients such as this one benefit tremendously from autologous fat grafting, and the ability to enhance skin thickness and coverage. This offers an entirely safe and autologous option for aesthetic enhancement.

SUMMARY

Autologous fat grafting is a critical adjunct procedure in prepectoral breast reconstruction, to help prevent upper pole rippling and contour deformities, and achieve a natural appearing slope to the upper pole, in the absence of a pectoralis major muscle over the implant. Fat grafting is often performed at time of expander-to-implant exchange operation. Fat harvest, processing, and reinjection must all be performed with minimal trauma, and while adhering to techniques that minimize fat cell damage. Once injected fat has revascularized, the aesthetic enhancement is permanent.

KEY REFERENCES

1. Sigalove S, Maxwell GP, Sigalove NM, et al. Prepectoral implant-based breast reconstruction: rationale, indications, and preliminary results. *Plast Reconstr Surg*. 2017;139(2):287-294.
2. Kronowitz SJ, Mandujano CC, Liu J, et al. Lipofilling of the breast does not increase the risk of recurrence of breast cancer: a matched controlled study. *Plast Reconstr Surg*. 2016;137(2):385-393.
3. Sbitany H, Piper M, Lentz R. Prepectoral breast reconstruction: a safe alternative to submuscular prosthetic reconstruction following nipple-sparing mastectomy. *Plast Reconstr Surg*. 2017 Sep;140(3):432-443.
4. Sbitany H. Important considerations for performing pre-pectoral breast reconstruction. *Plast Reconstr Surg*. 2017;140(6 suppl):7S-13S.
5. Garza RM, Paik KJ, Chung MT, et al. Studies in fat grafting: Part III. Fat grafting irradiated tissue–improved skin quality and decreased fat graft retention. *Plast Reconstr Surg*. 2014;134:249-257.
6. Padoin AV, Braga-Silva J, Martins P, et al. Sources of processed lipoaspirate cells: influence of donor site on cell concentration. *Plast Reconstr Surg*. 2008;122:614-618.
7. Pu LL, Coleman SR, Cui X, Ferguson RE Jr, Vasconez HC. Autologous fat grafts harvested and refined by the Coleman technique: a comparative study. *Plast Reconstr Surg*. 2008;122:932-937.
8. Erdim M, Tezel E, Numanoglu A, Sav, A. The effects of the size of liposuction cannula on adipocyte survival and the optimum temperature for fat graft storage: an experimental study. *J Plast Reconstr Aesthet Surg*. 2009;62:1210-1214.
9. Fisher C, Grahovac TL, Schafer ME, Shippert RD. Marra KG, Rubin JP. Comparison of harvest and processing techniques for fat grafting and adipose stem cell isolation. *Plast Reconstr Surg*. 2013;132(2):351-361.
10. Becker H, Lind JG II, Hopkins EG. Immediate implant-based prepectoral breast reconstruction using a vertical incision. *Plast Reconstr Surg Glob Open*. 2015;3(6):e412.

CHAPTER **10**

PATIENT SELECTION FOR PREPECTORAL RECONSTRUCTION

Allen Gabriel, Steven R. Sigalove, Noemi M. Sigalove, Toni Storm-Dickerson, G. Patrick Maxwell, and Maurice Y. Nahabedian

KEY POINTS

Prepectoral immediate oncologic contraindications include the following:

- Inability to obtain clear margins
- Extensive skin involvement
- Chest wall involvement
- Inflammatory breast cancer

Prepectoral immediate reconstructive contraindications include the following:

- Poorly vascularized/ischemic flaps
- HbA_{1c} >7.5%

Active smokers

INTRODUCTION

Modern techniques of prosthetic breast reconstruction continue to evolve. Reasons for this evolution include the availability of adjunct methods such as fat grafting and acellular dermal matrices (ADMs) as well as the desire of patients to have a quick recovery with optimal aesthetic outcomes. The current option that many patients desire and that more plastic surgeons are delivering is prepectoral reconstruction. Prepectoral implant-based breast reconstruction is a muscle-sparing procedure that simplifies the reconstructive process. By placing the implant above the pectoralis major muscle, the attendant problems associated with pectoralis muscle elevation are avoided.[1] The success of this approach rests on the bioengineered breast concept wherein highly cohesive, form-stable, and/or higher filled implants are utilized in combination with regenerative scaffold and regenerative cells to augment the soft-tissue envelope of the reconstructed breast.[2] The immediate prepectoral procedure, however, is not suitable for all patients, and the subsequent sections focus on both reconstructive and oncologic criteria of patient selection.

INDICATIONS FOR PREPECTORAL PLACEMENT

Reconstructive Indications

Although the prepectoral approach presents an alternative muscle-sparing reconstructive approach, not all patients are candidates for this approach. Critical to this approach is the availability of adequately vascularized skin flaps. Because of the proximity of the implant to the mastectomy skin flap, any skin-related complications can potentially compromise the reconstruction; hence, the absolute indication for adequately vascularized flaps. To ensure integrity of skin flap perfusion, close collaboration with general/breast surgeons is recommended to minimize overly aggressive mastectomies. In addition, objective assessment for tissue perfusion utilizing devices available for this purpose before prepectoral reconstruction is recommended. Even though clinical examination may not demonstrate any compromise with perfusion, Indocyanine green, imaging will show at-risk areas. These risks can be minimized using incisional negative pressure wound therapy to enhance perfusion and minimize the risk of delayed healing.[3]

Active smoking is an absolute contraindication for prepectoral reconstruction because of the adverse events associated with nicotine. In these patients, closure of the mastectomy without reconstruction is recommended. Delayed prepectoral reconstruction is a good alternative for these patients. Maneuvers before delayed prepectoral reconstruction include autologous fat grafting of the mastectomy skin flaps as well as the central incision area to ensure adequate thickness before approaching the reconstruction. For further details, refer to Chapter 17 focusing on delayed prepectoral reconstruction.

Diabetes mellitus (DM) has been reported to be a risk factor for surgical site occurrences and infections, which is a serious complication following prosthetic reconstruction. Although DM does not rule out prepectoral reconstruction, it does warrant that the hemoglobin A_{1c} (HbA_{1c}) level be less than 7.5%. The higher this value, the higher the risk of complications and therefore adequate blood glucose control is warranted.[4] If a patient is unable to maintain good control of her blood glucose at the time of mastectomy, then a delayed prepectoral reconstruction is typically recommended after the HbA_{1c} level is below the critical value.

Historically, patients are linked to higher complication rates during immediate reconstruction and the debate regarding whether these patients should undergo delayed reconstruction has persisted. There is a chapter dedicated to this topic; refer to Chapter 11 for further details. In short, for a patient with an elevated body mass index (BMI) to have an immediate prepectoral reconstruction, the patient should not have any other comorbidities (such as poorly controlled DM or tobacco use). If the patient is otherwise healthy, then an immediate reconstruction can be performed. In preparation for patients with high BMI, thinner ADMs are recommended given that the fat in these patients is not as vascular as in a patient with a lower BMI given the globule size. This also holds true for patients with high BMI who undergo delayed reconstructions.[5] If delayed, these patients undergo a delayed first-stage reconstruction, which includes fat grafting under the mastectomy focusing on raising the central mastectomy scar in preparation for the second stage of prepectoral reconstruction. Elevation of the central scar helps in minimizing complications in a prepectoral placement, given the tendency for thin flaps around old scarred incisions.

Another highly debated topic is prior radiation therapy such as in a failed breast conservation therapy patient or in a delayed patient who has had chest wall radiation. One option in these patients considering delayed prepectoral reconstruction is to begin with autologous fat grafting as a means of improving the quality and thickness of the radiated mastectomy skin flaps. Because these patients already lack an adequate soft-tissue envelope, it may be beneficial to have an autologous tissue flap with a skin paddle to further improve the shape of the breast long term. A latissimus flap is often used in these patients by placing the flap in the prepectoral space following chest wall radiation. Patients who have undergone prior lumpectomy and radiation therapy should be evaluated on a case-by-case basis. If the lumpectomy scar is in the upper inner or outer quadrants where there will be less expansion, and the soft-tissue envelope is not constricted, then prepectoral expander/implant-based reconstruction can be attempted. There should be low tolerance to adding an autologous tissue if there are any signs of early complications. Patients who have been previously radiated must understand that they are at high risk for complications. If the lumpectomy scar is in the lower pole of the breast, then an autologous tissue is often recommended to augment the soft-tissue envelope and the pocket for expansion and creating the aesthetically pleasing lower pole. For further details on this topic, refer to Chapter 18 in this book. Please refer to **Table 10.1** for complete summary of contraindications

Oncologic Guidelines and Indications

The oncologic guidelines for the prepectoral approach remain to be defined. As a multidisciplinary treatment plan is most optimal for the comprehensive care of the patient with breast cancer, a combined effort is needed to balance the safest oncologic care with the most desirable aesthetic outcome. The oncologic treatment plan is frequently configured on the basis of the availability of resources and the willingness of each discipline to embrace and be able to safely adapt to changes brought about by new techniques.

We have identified a number of oncologic contraindications for the prepectoral reconstructive approach (**Table 10.2**). Patients with late-stage breast cancer, posterior tumors near to or involving the pectoralis major muscle, and patients at high risk of recurrence are poor candidates for prepectoral placement. It is important to note that the oncologic safety of this procedure is yet to be determined. As with subpectoral reconstruction, extreme

TABLE 10.1 SUMMARY OF RECONSTRUCTIVE CONTRAINDICATIONS

Absolute reconstructive contraindications for *immediate* prepectoral reconstruction

- Poorly vascularized/ischemic flaps
- Hemoglobin A_{1c} >7.5%
- Active smokers

Questionable reconstructive contraindications for *immediate* prepectoral reconstruction

- Body mass index >35 kg/m^2
    - With associated comorbidities
- H/O Premastectomy radiation therapy
    - Unless latissimus is utilized

TABLE 10.2 SUMMARY OF ONCOLOGICAL CONTRAINDICATIONS

Absolute oncologic contraindications for *immediate* prepectoral reconstruction

- Inability to obtain clear margins
- Extensive skin involvement
- Chest wall involvement
- Inflammatory breast cancer

Questionable oncologic contraindications for *immediate* prepectoral reconstruction

- Palpable or matted axillary nodes
- Stage III, IV
- High risk of recurrence (based on multidisciplinary approach)

caution should be exercised for large tumors, and for clinically positive lymph nodes. An attempt can be made to downstage the tumor using neoadjuvant chemotherapy, whereby prepectoral reconstruction is deemed safe after a favorable clinical and radiographic response.

Because the prepectoral approach has been performed consistently for fewer than 5 years, oncologic guidelines will continue to undergo evolution as with any new technique. We feel that it is prudent to err on the side of caution until data from randomized, prospective clinical trials and results of oncologic outcomes become available.

Patient selection should be approached from a multidisciplinary standpoint and should involve the entire care team. Reconstructive and oncologic surgeons, medical oncologists, and radiation oncologists should understand and be comfortable with the implementation of the prepectoral technique. As long as oncologic safety criteria are upheld, prepectoral implant-based reconstruction can be used for both skin- and nipple-sparing mastectomies.

The common topic that is asked by breast surgeons and other specialties is how to monitor these patients for recurrence. Monitoring for cancer recurrence following prepectoral prosthetic reconstruction is approached in a manner similar to that of autologous reconstructions. Autologous flaps are routinely placed in a prepectoral location and these flaps are regularly monitored for cancer recurrence by clinical examinations and at times by radiologic screening. Similarly, in prepectoral reconstruction with implants, clinical and monthly self-breast examinations are important, because breast cancer recurrence in the majority of the cases occurs under the mastectomy flap. We have instituted a follow-up protocol of our prepectoral reconstructions using the U.S. Food and Drug Administration criteria for implant surveillance, which includes magnetic resonance imaging (MRI), with and without contrast, beginning at 3 years after reconstructive surgery and every other year thereafter. MRI not only monitors the implant but also helps monitor the overall chest.

It is important to note that not all immediate reconstructive contraindications pertain to delayed reconstructions because the delayed prepectoral reconstruction does not rely on viability of flaps; but the overall health of the patient should be considered for moving forward with a delayed reconstruction because ADM incorporation can be affected. The oncologic contraindications remain the same for immediate and delayed reconstruction.

SUMMARY

Patients undergoing skin- or nipple-sparing mastectomy can have prepectoral placement as long as they do not have the identified contraindications listed in this chapter. Prepectoral placement can be performed in single- or two-stage procedures. Given our early experience (less than 10 years) with this technique, we originally adopted a conservative cautious approach to indications; and since the original report, we already have modified and minimized the contraindications on the basis of patient outcome and continuous work with breast surgeons to minimize contraindications. When there is ever a question whether this procedure should be performed, a close discussion with the breast surgeon and other treating physicians can be made.

KEY REFERENCES

1. Sigalove S, Maxwell GP, Sigalove NM, et al. Prepectoral implant-based breast reconstruction: rationale, indications, and preliminary results. *Plast Reconstr Surg*. 2017;139(2):287-294.
2. Maxwell GP, Gabriel A. Bioengineered breast: concept, technique, and preliminary results. *Plast Reconstr Surg*. 2016;137(2):415-421.
3. Willy C, Agarwal A, Andersen CA, et al. Closed incision negative pressure therapy: international multidisciplinary consensus recommendations. *Int Wound J*. 2017;14(2):385-398.
4. Yang L, Sun Y, Li G, Liu J. Is hemoglobin A1c and perioperative hyperglycemia predictive of periprosthetic joint infection following total joint arthroplasty?: A systematic review and meta-analysis. *Medicine (Baltimore)*. 2017;96(51):e8805.
5. Nahabedian MY. Acellular dermal matrices in primary breast reconstruction: principles, concepts, and indications. *Plast Reconstr Surg*. 2012;130(5)(suppl 2):44S-53S.

CHAPTER 11

PREPECTORAL RECONSTRUCTION IN THE HIGH BODY MASS INDEX PATIENT

Allen Gabriel, Steven R. Sigalove, Maurice Y. Nahabedian, and G. Patrick Maxwell

KEY POINTS

- Obesity is associated with an elevated risk of postoperative complications; risk increases with increasing BMI.
- BMI alone is not a contraindication for immediate prepectoral reconstruction.
- Patient selection criteria for immediate reconstruction are identical in all patients, irrespective of BMI.
- Managing skin redundancy and minimizing pocket size are important reconstructive challenges in patients with obesity.
- Fat grafting may be needed, despite presence of thick subcutaneous tissue, especially at the upper pole to improve step-off.

INTRODUCTION

High body mass index (BMI) is a global epidemic and a significant public health concern. Over 50% of the world's adult population is overweight or obese (BMI >30 kg/m^2).[1] In the United States, more than 30% of adults are obese, with prevalence higher in women than in men.[2] Obesity is associated with significant morbidity and casts a heavy fiscal burden on health care systems.[3] With a rising trend of breast cancer rates and more women opting for mastectomy and reconstruction, reconstructive surgeons are likely to encounter an increasing number of obese patients. Prepectoral breast reconstruction in this patient population can be challenging and reconstructive surgeons need to be cognizant of the nuances and technical difficulties.

OBESITY AND INCREASED RISK OF POSTOPERATIVE COMPLICATIONS

It is well established that obesity is associated with an increased risk of postoperative complications following breast reconstruction.[4,5] BMI is an independent predictor of postoperative complications, with every unit increase in BMI increasing the odds of complication by 5.9% and reconstructive failure by 7.9%.[6] Complications of impaired wound healing, incision dehiscence, skin necrosis, infections, and seroma are all elevated with progressive increase in BMI.

Obesity interrupts normal physiological processes, which may explain the higher complication rate.[5] Obesity impairs collagen deposition, collagen maturation, and myofibroblast activity, all of which are important for normal wound healing. Impaired collagen deposition, in addition, weakens the mechanical strength of the skin. The mastectomy skin flap of obese patients has a relative reduction in collagen content and strength compared to the skin flap of normal-weight patients. The chronic, low-grade systemic inflammation present in obese individuals is implicated in decreased mastectomy skin flap survival. Flap survival is also linked to malperfusion that is usually due to the increased tissue volume and a limited vascular supply. Hypoxia resulting from inadequate perfusion of flap edges furthest from the vascular source can lead to skin necrosis and infection. Hypoxia also impedes collagen synthesis and contributes to impaired wound healing. Seromas commonly are the result of excessive dead space in the mastectomy pocket following parenchymal removal.

The current published literature on implant-based breast reconstruction in obese patients primarily involves the subpectoral approach and there is very little data with the prepectoral approach.[7] However, the elevated risk of postoperative complications will likely remain, irrespective of the reconstructive approach.

IMMEDIATE VERSUS DELAYED PREPECTORAL RECONSTRUCTION

Obesity, as an isolated factor, is not a contraindication for implant-based prepectoral breast reconstruction. The timing of reconstruction, immediate or delayed, is guided by flap perfusion and viability, patient comorbidities (uncontrolled diabetes and current tobacco use), and patient preference. A well-perfused, viable mastectomy skin flap; controlled diabetes ($HbA_{1c} < 7.5\%$); and avoidance of tobacco products are absolute requirements for immediate prepectoral reconstruction and applies to all cases, irrespective of BMI.[8] It should be emphasized that flap thickness should not be taken as an indication of flap vascularity. This is of particular importance in obese patients who often have thick mastectomy flaps. Assessment of flap vascularity should be performed objectively, preferably with a tissue perfusion device or clinically in its absence, in all cases before proceeding with immediate reconstruction. Because type 2 diabetes is highly prevalent among obese individuals,[9] HbA_{1c} status should be routinely assessed in all obese patients before reconstruction. In the event of $HbA_{1c} > 7.5\%$, reconstruction should be delayed until after blood glucose is controlled with treatment. In obese patients who use tobacco products, cessation of smoking for at least 2 months is required before reconstruction can be considered.

RECONSTRUCTIVE CONSIDERATIONS

The basic principles of preoperative reconstruction remain the same across the BMI strata. The challenge in obese patients involves managing skin redundancy as well as the excessive dead space in the postmastectomy pocket. Obese patients have an oversized pocket with a generous amount of subcutaneous tissue (**Figure 11.1**) that is displaced when breast tissue is removed. The challenge involves repositioning the subcutaneous tissue so as to collapse and minimize the pocket size for a snug fit of the future implant. Repositioning of subcutaneous tissue also reinforces the pocket providing additional support to the future implant, eliminates dead space, and minimizes the risk of seroma formation.

With the removal of breast tissue, the lateral anterior subcutaneous tissue naturally descends to the posterior axillary line. This tissue is repositioned and anchored to the anterior axillary line with closure sutures (0-Vicryl on CT-1) (**Figure 11.2A**). Removal of breast tissue also retracts the cephalad-subcutaneous tissue, which is repositioned more caudally (**Figure 11.2B**). Repositioning of the cephalad-subcutaneous tissue further collapses the pocket and renders a smoother transition of the mastectomy pocket to the implant, which is an additional benefit of prepectoral reconstruction. With a smoother transition zone, fat grafting may not be needed at the upper pole in some instances, depending on the final outcome of the breast form following the second-stage reconstruction. In dual-plane reconstruction, the cephalad area is ignored because all pocket work is limited to under the pectoralis major muscle.

Prepectoral reconstruction is typically performed as a two-staged, expander/implant procedure. Although obese patients have adequate subcutaneous tissue, direct-to-implant reconstruction is rarely performed because complication and revision rates have been demonstrated to be increased with increasing patient BMI following direct-to-implant reconstruction.[10] Poor breast projection and contour irregularities are common in this population and the second stage provides an opportunity to address these problems and improve the overall appearance of the breast. The expander is inflated with air intraoperatively to 50% to 70% of maximum capacity. Underfilling alleviates the pressure on the overlying flap and reduces the risk of ischemia, whereas the use of air alleviates the pressure on the inferior mastectomy flap and minimizes

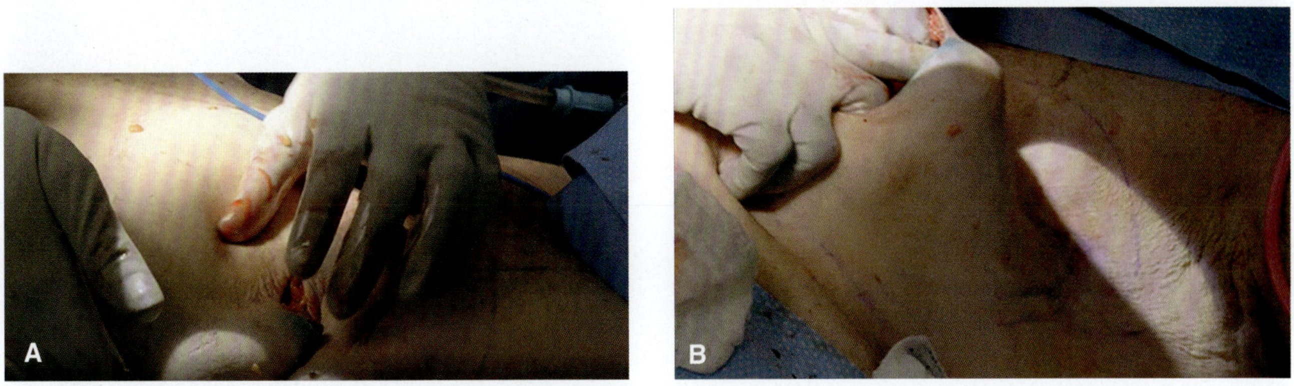

Figure 11.1 Oversized mastectomy pocket and excess subcutaneous tissue.

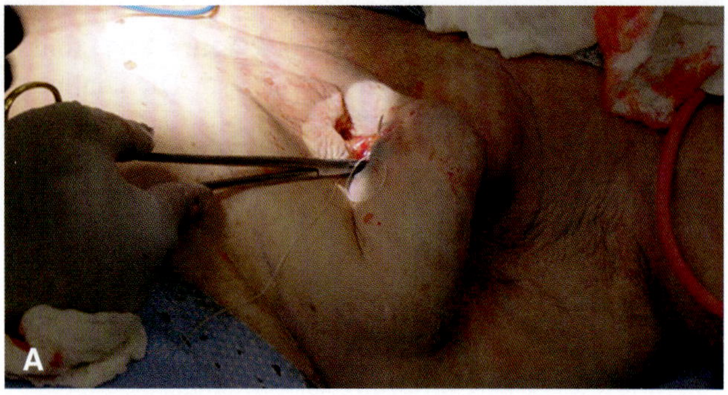

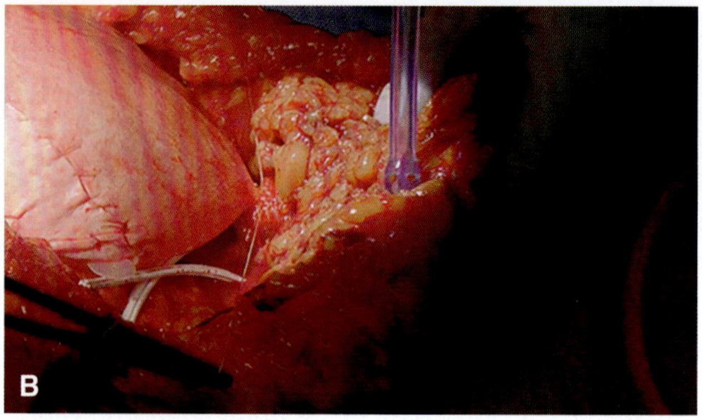

Figure 11.2 **Repositioning of subcutaneous tissue.** A, Repositioning of the lateral anterior subcutaneous tissue from the posterior axillary line to the anterior axillary line. B, Caudal repositioning of the cephalad-subcutaneous tissue.

suture pull-through. Use of acellular dermal matrix (ADM) for expander coverage is an essential component of prepectoral reconstruction, irrespective of the thickness of the flap or the amount of subcutaneous tissue present (*Refer to Chapter 6 for a discussion on The Role of ADM and Prepectoral Breast Reconstruction*).

Management of skin redundancy is a critical aspect of breast reconstruction in obese patients. Redundant skin flap is utilized as much as possible in reconstructing the new breast; however, only adequately vascularized tissue is utilized. Poorly vascularized flap tissue is excised. Excess skin flap can be reduced by closing the central mastectomy incision horizontally by extending laterally to the anterior and, at times, to the posterior axillary line (**Figure 11.3**). Although the excess skin can be addressed in this manner, the result is a long scar in an unnatural location that is inconsistent with aesthetic principles of breast surgery. In addition, the central flattening and the extenuation of the lateral chest-wall tissue make this an unpreferable approach. Alternatively, given the large size of the breasts, excessive skin envelope can be managed similarly to an aesthetic procedure. A skin-reducing procedure similar to a mastopexy can be performed, which is detailed here.

Preoperatively, the breast meridian and the highest point of the vertical incision on the breasts that matches the contralateral side are marked on the patient (**Figure 11.4**). These are the only two preoperative markings that are done in collaboration with the breast surgeon. The mastectomy approach is discussed with the breast surgeon, which involves a circumareolar approach with nipple–areolar complex (NAC) removal in all cases. The circumareolar approach allows the reconstructive surgeon maximum flexibility to manage the skin envelope. As in aesthetic breast surgery when mastopexy augmentation is performed, the implant is first placed and the skin envelope is addressed by tailor tacking that leads to removal of the excess skin. In the reconstructive approach, following completion of mastectomy through the circumareolar incision with NAC removal, the expander/ADM construct is placed and filled with air so the skin envelope can be addressed appropriately. The breast meridian is re-marked as well as the position of the cephalad vertical tip while matching it to the contralateral side (**Figure 11.5A**). Then the inframammary fold on the skin flap is marked (**Figure 11.5B**). The central flap is tailor tacked vertically to help assess the extent of skin reduction that will be needed (**Figure 11.6**). At this point, there is the option to proceed with definitive vertical closure, depending on the extent of lower pole excess skin that remains or to proceed with converting the vertical closure to an inverted T. In both cases, there is

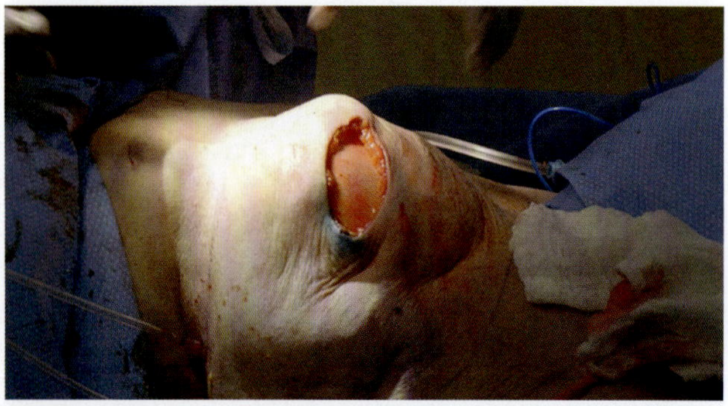

Figure 11.3 Skin reduction closure utilizing the horizontal central mastectomy incision.

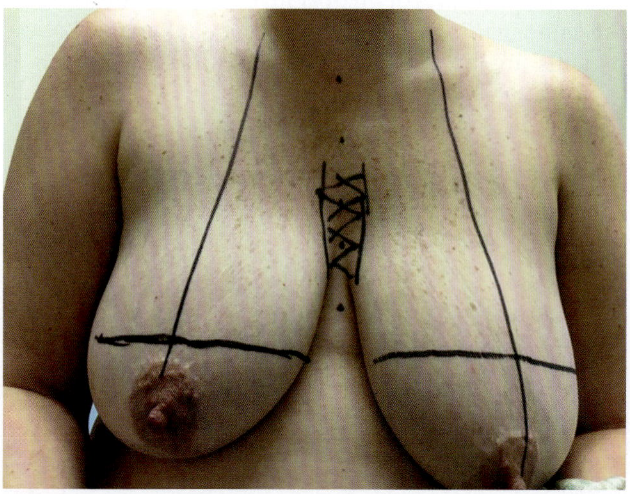

Figure 11.4 Preoperative markings.

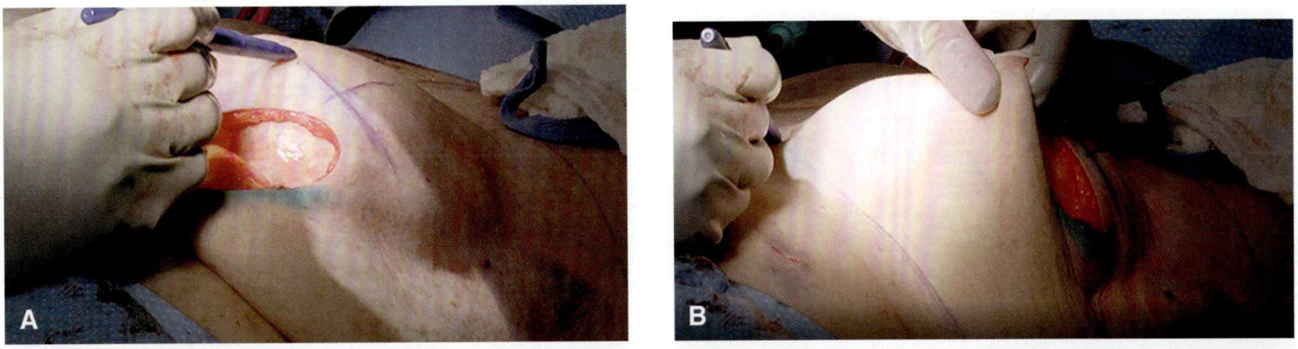

Figure 11.5 **Skin reduction markings for mastopexy-like procedure.** A, Position of breast meridian and cephalad vertical tip. B, Position of inframammary fold.

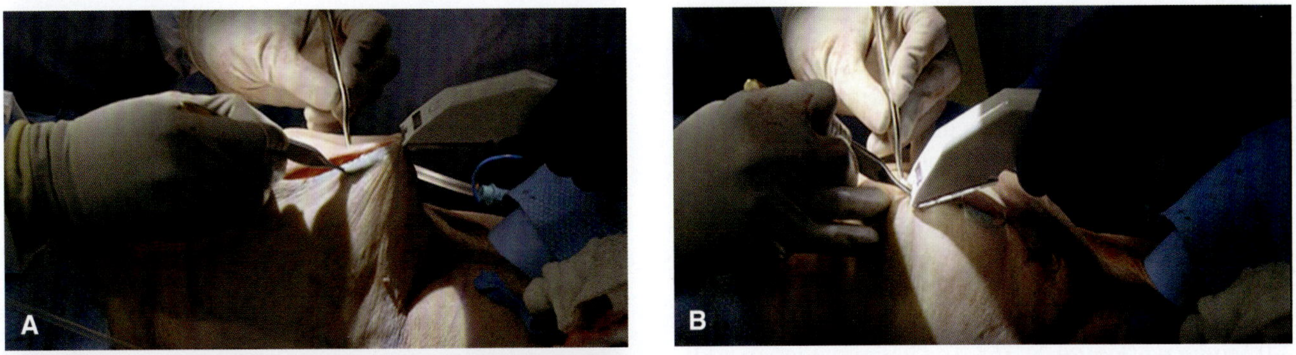

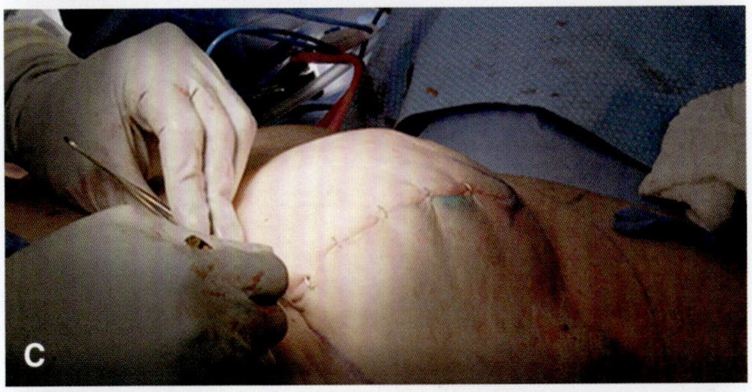

Figure 11.6 Tailor tacking the central flap.

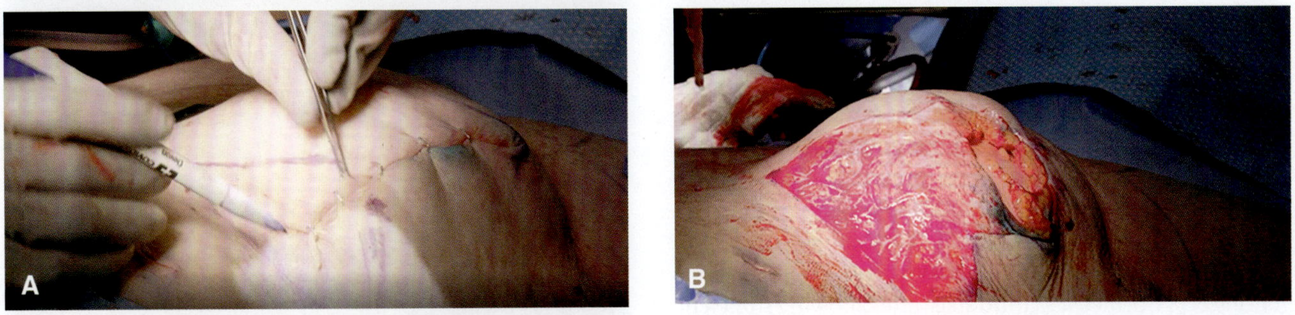

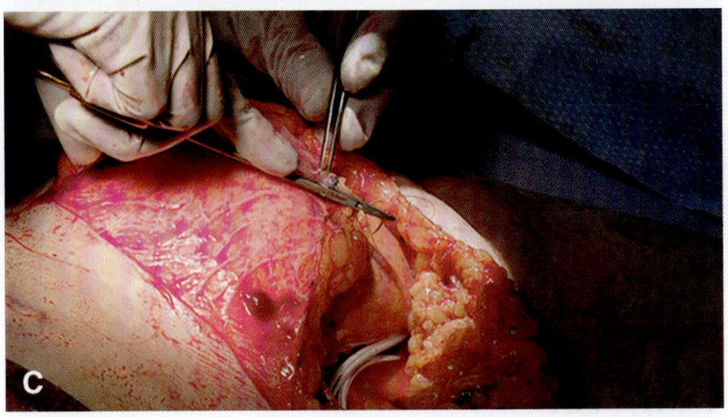

Figure 11.7 **Lower dermal flap creation.** A, Marking of flap. B, Deepithelialized flap. C, Deepithelialized flap tacked down over the acellular dermal matrix.

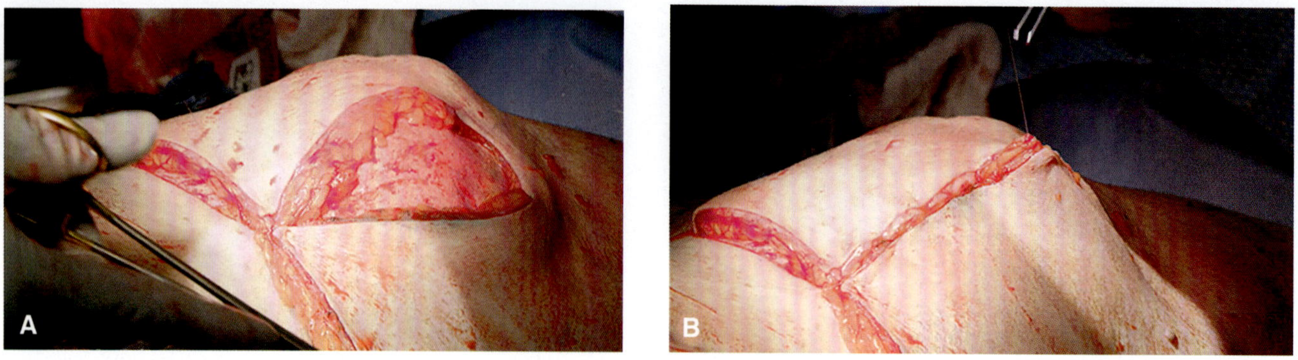

Figure 11.8 **Skin closure.** A, First stitch securing the medial and lateral skin flap to the inframammary fold. B, Vertical closure over the central breast.

excess skin under the tailor tacked portion and this leads to the creation of the dermal flap at the lower pole. If the length of the vertical closure is more than 9 to 10 cm and there is too much excess lower pole tissue that cannot be addressed with only the vertical approach, an inverted T is added. The area of the lower dermal flap is marked (**Figure 11.7A**) and the skin over the dermal flap surface is deepithelialized (**Figure 11.7B**). The deepithelialized flap is arranged over the ADM and is tacked down with 3-0 Monocryl (**Figure 11.7C**). The flap provides an additional layer of soft-tissue coverage, supports the incision, and prevents expander exposure in the event of incisional dehiscence. It also adds additional projection, which may be needed in some cases. Skin closure over the dermal flap begins with securing the medial and lateral flaps to the inframammary fold (**Figure 11.8A**) followed by vertical closure over the breast mound (**Figure 11.8B**), and then horizontal closure at the inframammary fold.

FAT GRAFTING

Fat grafting is an important adjunct to prepectoral reconstruction. Some patients will require fat grafting to enhance breast aesthetics in spite of having a thick subcutaneous layer. Obese patients typically require fat grafting at the upper pole to improve the step-off that is present at the transition zone between the upper pole and the implant unless the rotation of tissue from the cephalad portion of the pocket was successful to blunt the transition zone. If needed, fat grafting is performed as a third stage after allowing sufficient time for the reconstructed breast to recover from surgery.

BENEFIT OF PREPECTORAL RECONSTRUCTION IN OBESE PATIENTS

Obese individuals lack core body strength and rely on their upper body strength using their arms to help them rise from a seated position.[7] Chest wall muscles, including the pectoralis major muscles, are enlisted for this maneuver. In a patient who has undergone subpectoral breast reconstruction, in the immediate postoperative period, repeated use of the pectoralis major muscle could potentially have a shearing effect on the overlying skin flap and the underlying ADM. The shearing effect on the dermal matrix could potentially compromise the incorporation of the matrix and lead to seroma formation (**Figure 11.9**). The prepectoral approach eliminates this shearing effect and may be a particularly beneficial

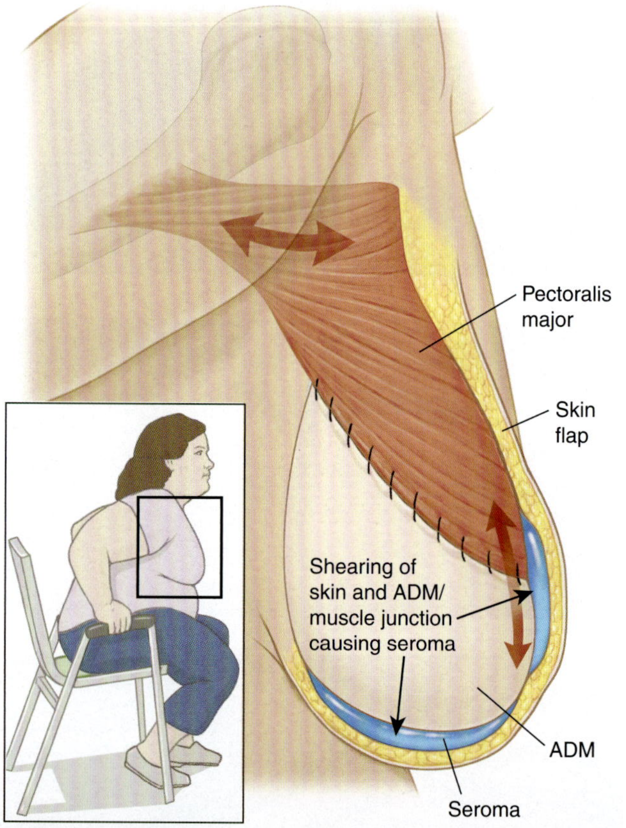

Figure 11.9 Schematic demonstration of a patient using her upper extremity for daily activity due to lack of abdominal core strength. These movements cause the activation of the pectoralis major and subsequent shearing of ADM, leading to non-incorporation, placing the patient for increased risk of seroma formation. ADM, acellular dermal matrix.

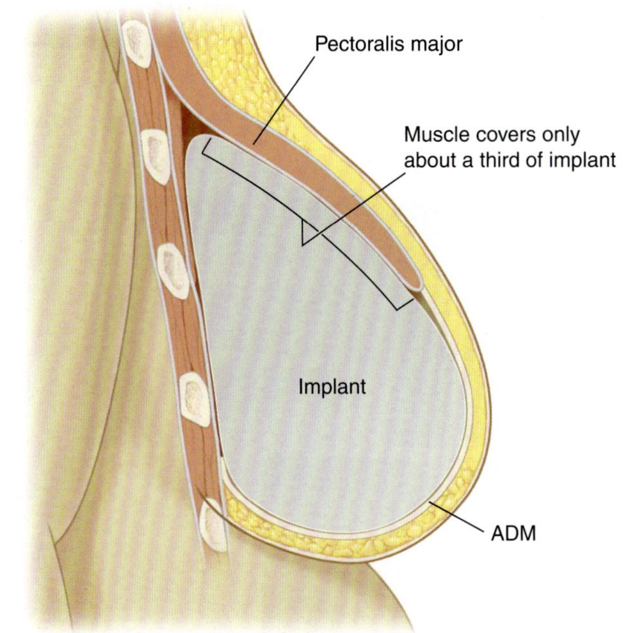

Figure 11.10 About one-third the surface of a higher projecting implant in a dual plane reconstruction is covered by the pectoral major muscle, leading to the question of why even use the muscle in these cases. ADM, acellular dermal matrix.

approach in obese patients. In addition, majority of these patients require a higher projecting implant given the depth of the chest that is present. With a higher projecting implant, generally only less than a third of the implant is covered by the muscle in dual plane + ADM reconstructions (**Figure 11.10**). This is only in the upper pole; and in this population, fat grafting can be performed to camouflage any implant visibility, if any. In addition, subpectoral reconstruction generally minimizes the projection of the implant and by staying over the muscle, gives the surgeon the opportunity to create the maximally projecting breast without any compression from the pectoralis major (**Figure 11.11**).

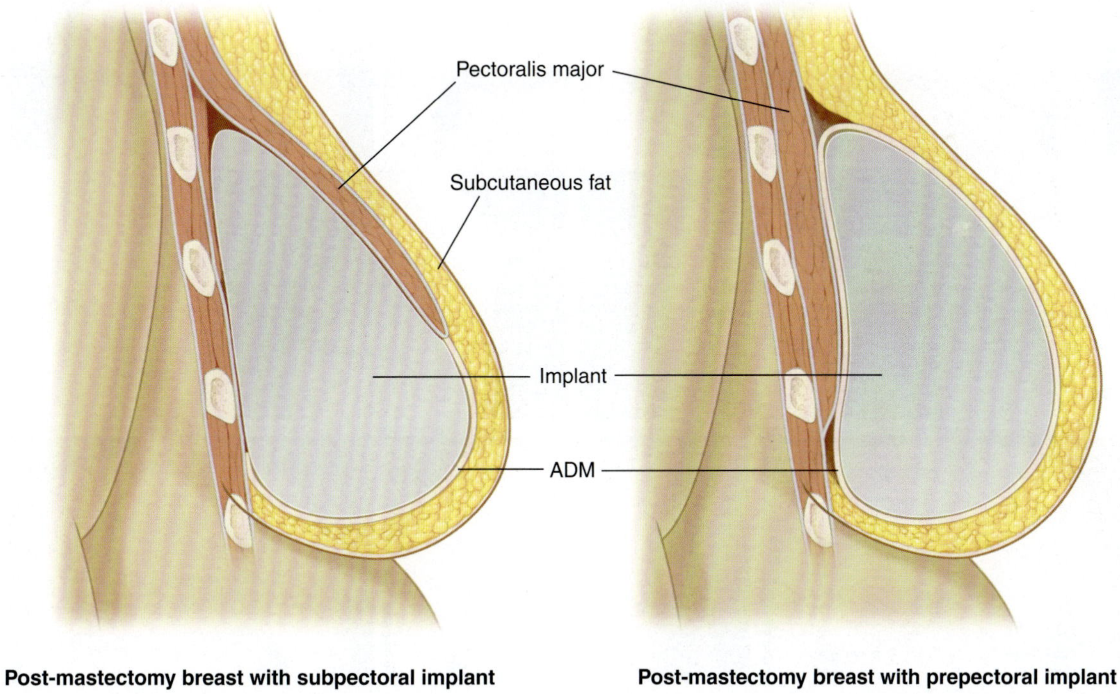

Figure 11.11 The final projection of the reconstructed breast form varies by which plane the implant is placed. The same implant located in a dual vs prepectoral plane can have different projections as a result of compression of pectoralis major on the surface of the implant leading to less projection overall. ADM, acellular dermal matrix.

CASE EXAMPLES

CASE 1

A 45-year-old female with left breast invasive ductal carcinoma, a BMI of 43 kg/m^2, and no other comorbidities. Her HbA_{1c} was 5.8% (**Figure 11.12**).

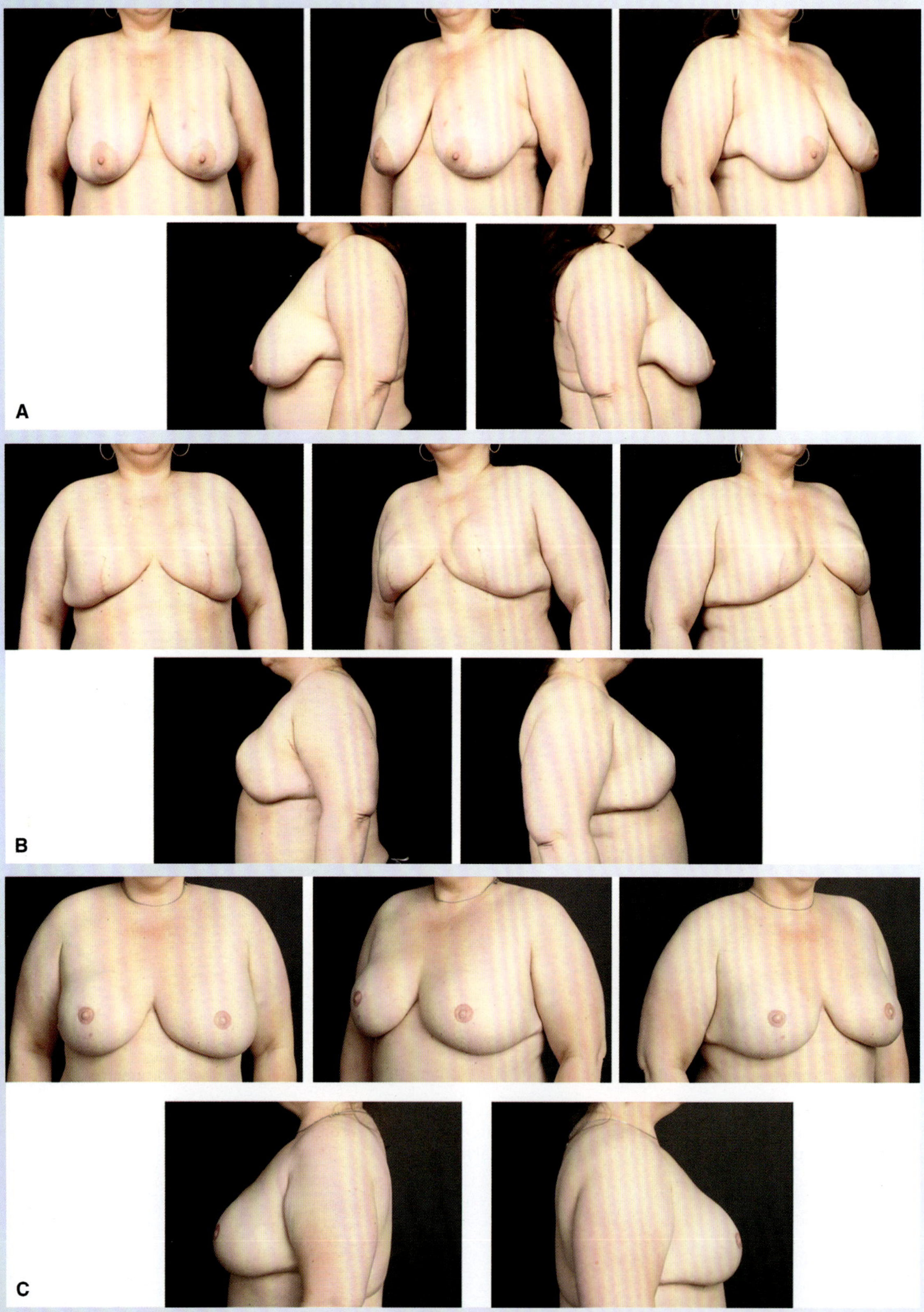

Figure 11.12 A, Preoperative views. B, At 6 weeks after bilateral skin-reducing mastectomy and prepectoral reconstruction with 133MV 500-cc expanders and AlloDerm. C, At 4 years after bilateral breast reconstruction with style 20 800-cc implants, one session of fat grafting, areolar tattooing, and nipple reconstruction.

CASE 2

A 59-year-old female with left breast invasive ductal carcinoma, a BMI of 35 kg/m^2, and no other comorbidities. Her HbA_{1c} was 5.5% (**Figure 11.13**).

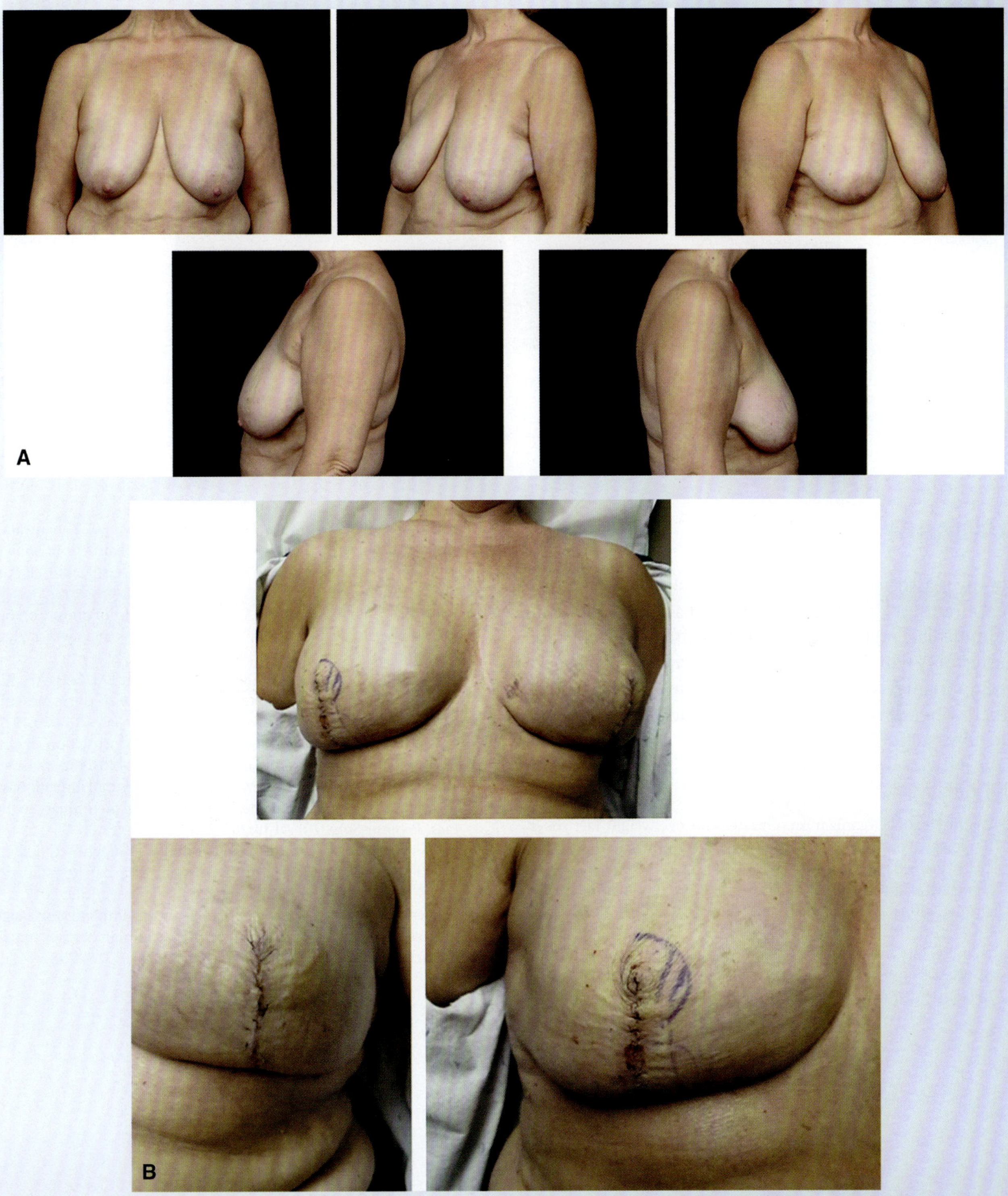

Figure 11.13 A, Preoperative views. B, Bilateral skin-reducing mastectomy and prepectoral reconstruction with 133 FV 550-cc expanders and AlloDerm. Patient is shown at postoperative day 7 following removal of negative pressure incision management device.

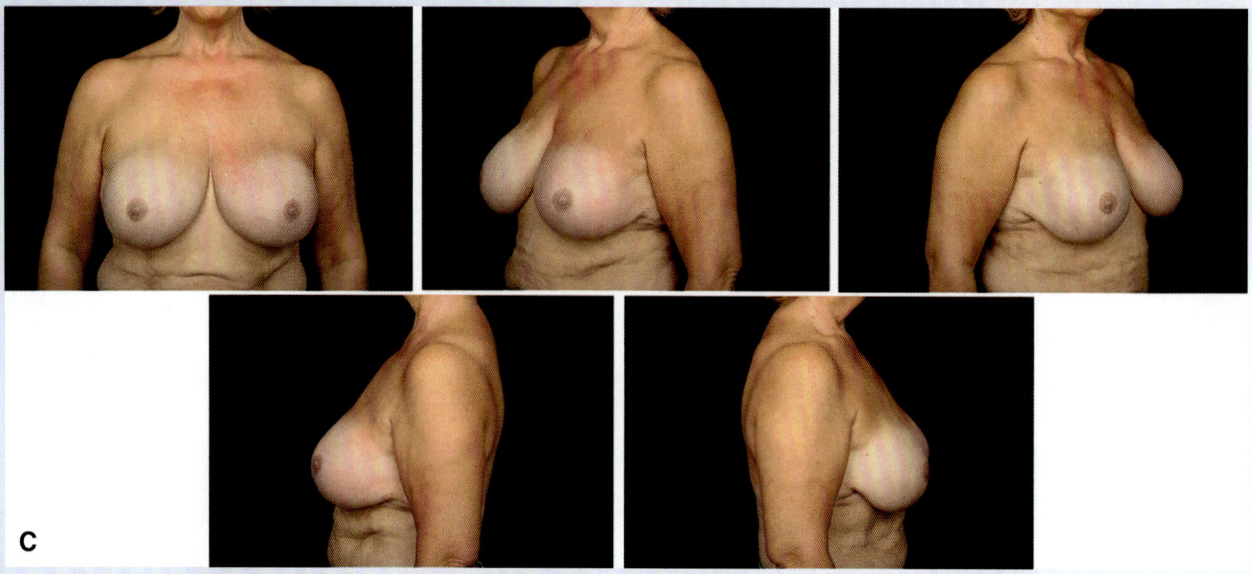

Figure 11.13 (*continued*) C, At 3 years following bilateral breast reconstruction with SRX 800-cc implants, one session of fat grafting, and 3-D nipple tattooing.

SUMMARY

Obesity is associated with an elevated risk of postoperative complications. High BMI in itself is not a contraindication for immediate prepectoral breast reconstruction. Managing mastectomy flap redundancy and minimizing pocket size are important reconstructive challenges in this population, which, when properly addressed, can lead to acceptable and consistent outcomes.

KEY REFERENCES

1. World Health Organization. Obesity and overweight fact sheet. Reviewed February 2018. http://www.who.int/mediacentre/factsheets/fs311/en/
2. Ogden CL, Carroll MD, Fryar CD, Flegal KM. Prevalence of obesity among adults and youth: United States, 2011-2014. *NCHS Data Brief*. 2015;219:1-8.
3. Tremmel M, Gerdtham UG, Nilsson PM, Saha S. Economic burden of obesity: a systematic literature review. *Int J Environ Res Public Health*. 2017;14(4):435.
4. Fischer JP, Nelson JA, Kovach SJ, Serletti JM, Wu LC, Kanchwala S. Impact of obesity on outcomes in breast reconstruction: analysis of 15,937 patients from the ACS-NSQIP datasets. *J Am Coll Surg*. 2013;217:656-664.
5. Panayi AC, Agha RA, Sieber BA, Orgill DP. Impact of obesity on outcomes in breast reconstruction: a systematic review and meta-analysis. *J Reconstr Microsurg*. 2018;34(5):363-375.
6. Nguyen KT, Hanwright PJ, Smetona JT, Hirsch EM, Seth AK, Kim JY. Body mass index as a continuous predictor of outcomes after expander-implant breast reconstruction. *Ann Plast Surg*. 2014;73:19-24.
7. Gabriel A, Maxwell GP. Prepectoral breast reconstruction in challenging patients. *Plast Reconstr Surg*. 2017;140:14S-21S.
8. Sigalove S, Maxwell GP, Sigalove NM, et al. Prepectoral implant-based breast reconstruction: rationale, indications, and preliminary results. *Plast Reconstr Surg*. 2017;139:287-294.
9. Center for Disease Control. Maps of trends in diagnosed diabetes and obesity—April 2017. https://www.cdc.gov/diabetes/statistics/slides/maps_diabetesobesity_trends.pdf. Accessed June 2017.
10. Gdalevitch P, Ho A, Genoway K, et al. Direct-to-implant single-stage immediate breast reconstruction with acellular dermal matrix: predictors of failure. *Plast Reconstr Surg*. 2014;133(6):738e-747e.

CHAPTER 12

TWO-STAGE PREPECTORAL RECONSTRUCTION USING TISSUE EXPANDERS

Maurice Y. Nahabedian and Allen Gabriel

KEY POINTS

- Indications for two-stage prepectoral reconstruction include patients who have skin deficiency and will require expansion before permanent implant as well as patients with postmastectomy skin quality that is insufficient for a direct-to-implant reconstruction.
- Two-stage prepectoral prosthetic reconstruction allows for gradual inflation of the post-mastectomy pocket.
- Two-stage prepectoral reconstruction can be safely performed in women with a BMI < 40.
- Prerequisites for prepectoral reconstruction include careful assessment of the mastectomy skin flap to ensure adequate thickness and perfusion.
- Two-stage prepectoral reconstruction is commonly performed with the assistance of acellular dermal matrices.

INTRODUCTION

Prosthetic breast reconstruction can be performed as a one-stage or as a two-stage procedure. According to statistics compiled by the American Society of Plastic Surgeons, the majority of prosthetic breast reconstruction is performed in two stages for a variety of reasons (**Table 12.1**). For many surgeons, the most important reason is that the second stage allows for maximal aesthetic control of the reconstruction based on optimizing permanent implant selection and modification of the periprosthetic space. There are a myriad of permanent implants available for the second stage that include sizes ranging from 100 to 800 cc, silicone gel versus saline implants, round versus shaped implants, and smooth versus textured surface implants. In addition, the ability to perform a capsulotomy or capsulorrhaphy at the second stage will allow for optimal control of the breast footprint and position of the implant.

The benefits of prepectoral breast reconstruction are now well appreciated on the basis of several recent publications.[1-6] Benefits include no animation with pectoral muscle contraction, less pain based on the absence of muscle spasm, and natural breast aesthetics. Factors conducive for success include well-perfused mastectomy skin flaps, minimal undermining of the mastectomy skin flaps, and the absence of visible dermis following the mastectomy. As with partial or total muscle coverage,

TABLE 12.1 REASONS FOR TWO-STAGE PROSTHETIC BREAST RECONSTRUCTION
• Mastectomy skin flaps are too thin • Mastectomy skin flap are poorly perfused • Ability to use a partially filled device • Two opportunities for optimal aesthetics • Ability to fine tune during second stage • Myriad of permanent implants to choose from at the second stage

prepectoral breast reconstruction can be performed in one or two stages. This chapter reviews the salient aspects of two-stage prepectoral breast reconstruction with and without bioprosthetic materials.

PREOPERATIVE PLANNING

Preoperative planning for prepectoral breast reconstruction in two stages is much like partial or total muscle coverage techniques and includes a thorough history and physical examination. First and foremost, it is important to assess patient expectation and to ensure that they are realistic. It is also important to assess comorbidities such as diabetes mellitus, hypertension, and cardiac disease.[7] In patients with poorly controlled diabetes mellitus with blood glucose levels > 200 or HbA_{1c} levels > 7.5, immediate prosthetic reconstruction is discouraged because of the increased incidence of delayed healing. Active tobacco use is considered by many to be a contraindication for prosthetic breast reconstruction because of the increased incidence of delayed healing, infection, and mastectomy skin flap necrosis. Obesity in and of itself is not considered a contraindication for immediate prosthetic reconstruction unless the patient has confounding comorbidities such as poorly controlled diabetes mellitus or cardiac disease. In women with a BMI > 40, most plastic surgeons will forego immediate breast reconstruction and perform it on a delayed basis or following sufficient weight loss. Women who have had previous radiation following mastectomy or breast conservation therapy should be advised that there is an increased incidence of infection, capsular contracture, distortion, pain, and premature removal in this setting.[8,9]

Women who are good candidates for the two-stage procedure typically include those who have skin deficiency and will require expansion before permanent implant as well as patients with postmastectomy skin quality that is insufficient for a direct-to-implant reconstruction. The role of the tissue expander is to stretch or maintain the periprosthetic space. The two-stage technique is preformed most often because it will provide a second opportunity to optimize breast contour, volume, and position. It is the goal of all surgical procedures to provide results that are predictable and reproducible and associated with high patient satisfaction.

The initial physical examination is critically important and will provide the necessary measurements by which to select the appropriate tissue expanders using the principles of biodimensional planning.[2,6] The most important measurement is the base width of the breast because this correlates with the base diameter of the tissue expander to be used. Other important breast parameters include the degree of breast ptosis, elasticity of the skin, location of scars, and the position of the nipple–areolar complex on the breast. The concept of the footprint, conus, and skin envelope are important to understand and can assist in determining the nature of the mastectomy, location of the incisions, and the type of prosthetic device used.[10]

Women who are good candidates for prepectoral reconstruction are similar to those who are candidates for partial or total muscle coverage. In the authors' practice, prepectoral reconstruction is discussed with all women choosing to have prosthetic breast reconstruction. The decision as to whether the final reconstruction is prepectoral or partial subpectoral is ultimately made in the operating room and principally based on the quality of the mastectomy skin flaps. If the flaps are of sufficient thickness and well-perfused, prepectoral reconstruction is performed. It is estimated that prepectoral reconstruction is performed in 50% to 90% of patients who are deemed candidates preoperatively. Prepectoral reconstruction is performed more commonly when breast surgeons and plastic surgeons have a close working relationship.

SURGICAL MANAGEMENT

The surgical technique of two-stage prepectoral reconstruction has several variations based on surgeon preference. Some surgeons will use a bioprosthetic mesh and others will not. Of those who use the bioprosthetic mesh, some will cover the anterior and posterior surface of the tissue expander and others will cover the anterior surface only. All three of these variations are reviewed.

PREPECTORAL RECONSTRUCTION WITH BIOPROSTHETIC MESH

There are a variety of bioprosthetic mesh materials that can be used for prepectoral prosthetic reconstruction. These include human acellular dermal matrix (ADM), porcine ADM, titanium-coated polypropylene mesh, and Vicryl mesh.[2,3,5,6,11] The primary indication to use a bioprosthetic mesh is to provide tissue support for the mastectomy skin flaps and to compartmentalize the space in which the tissue expander is placed.

When bioprosthetic materials are used, it is important to carefully assess the mastectomy skin flap to ensure that adequate thickness and perfusion are present. This may be performed visually by evaluating arterial and venous bleeding from the mastectomy incision, capillary refill of the mastectomy skin flaps, color of the mastectomy skins flaps, or perfusion assessment using fluorescence angiography. When tissue perfusion is compromised to the degree that viability is questionable, options include tissue debridement or delaying the reconstruction for 2 to 4 weeks.[12] When postmastectomy clearance to proceed with immediate two-stage prepectoral reconstruction is deemed safe, the methods by which bioprosthetic material can be used include anterior and posterior coverage of the tissue expander as well as the anterior coverage alone.

The authors' choice for bioprosthetic mesh is to use an ADM (AlloDerm, LifeCell Corporation, an Allergan affiliate, Branchburg, NJ). The reasons for this include biocompatibility, a collagen and elastin–based matrix, and scientific evidence demonstrating regenerative potential. The mesh materials are made in various sizes, shapes, and thicknesses. Commonly used shapes include rectangular (16 × 20 cm) or contoured (small, medium, large). Thickness varies from 1 to 3 mm; however, for prepectoral reconstruction, the 2- to 3-mm thickness is preferred as this provides better thickness. Perforations within the ADM are desirable to minimize the incidence of fluid accumulation and to promote incorporation of the ADM to the surrounding mastectomy skin flaps by creating zones of adherence.

The U.S. Federal Drug Administration has provided labeling information on the proper use of ADM when used clinically and is based on providing additional tissue support when necessary. Thus, there are on-label and off-label techniques by which ADM can be used. Both are safe and effective on the basis of the authors' experience and will be reviewed.

PREPECTORAL RECONSTRUCTION WITH BIOPROSTHETIC MESH (STAGE 1)

The salient aspects of the first and second stage of prepectoral prosthetic breast reconstruction are reviewed.

Technique—Getting Started

- Preoperative markings include the sternal midline, inframammary folds (IMFs), and the upper border of the breast (**Figure 12.1**). Nipple-sparing mastectomy is usually performed via an inframammary incision or a laterally or inferiorly based radial incision. Skin-sparing mastectomy is performed via an obliquely oriented elliptical incision that includes the nipple–areolar complex. In women with mammary hypertrophy, an inverted T mastectomy with preservation on an inferior dermal flap is designed.
- Following the mastectomy, the operative field is reprepped and draped and new surgical instruments are obtained. The mastectomy site is copiously irrigated to remove free fat and blood products. Hemostasis is ensured.
- Careful assessment of the mastectomy skin flaps for thickness and perfusion is critical. With nipple-sparing mastectomy via an IMF or a radial approach, the incision should be 8 to 10 cm in length. With skin-sparing mastectomy, incision length can be adjusted as needed. If the mastectomy flaps are poorly perfused or suboptimal, prepectoral reconstruction should not be performed with strong consideration for delayed reconstruction.
- Selection of the appropriate tissue expander is based on biodimensional planning. The width of the tissue expander should approximate the width of the mastectomy defect.
- Selection of the appropriate sheet or sheets of ADM is important. Options include one or two 16 × 20 sheets (**Figure 12.2**) as well as two sheets of contoured perforated ADM (**Figure 12.3**). The authors'

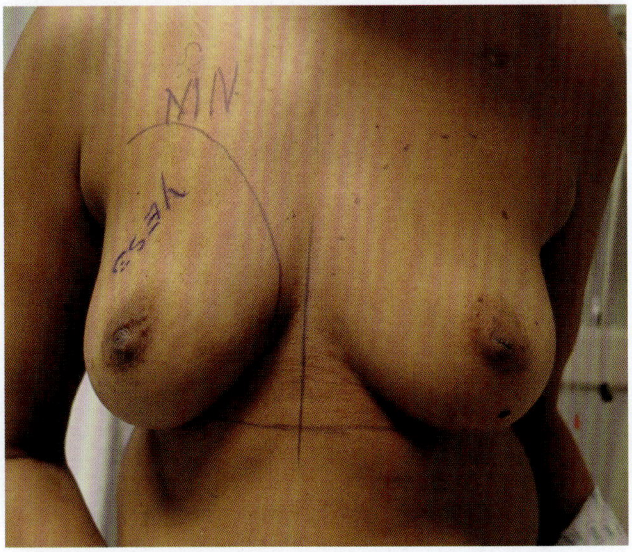

Figure 12.1 Preoperative markings include the sternal midline, inframammary folds, breast outline, and incision location.

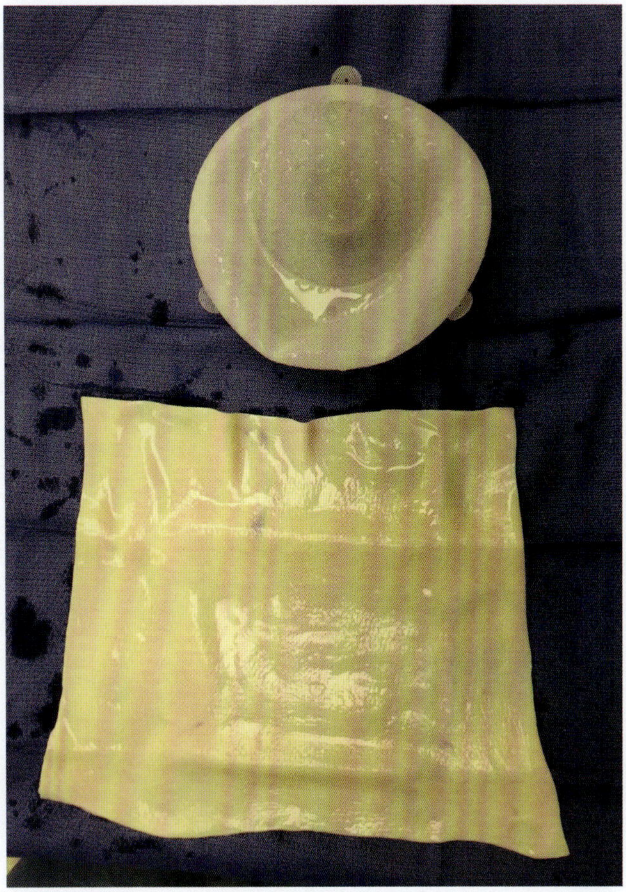

Figure 12.2 A 16 × 20 cm sheet of acellular dermal matrix for tissue expander coverage.

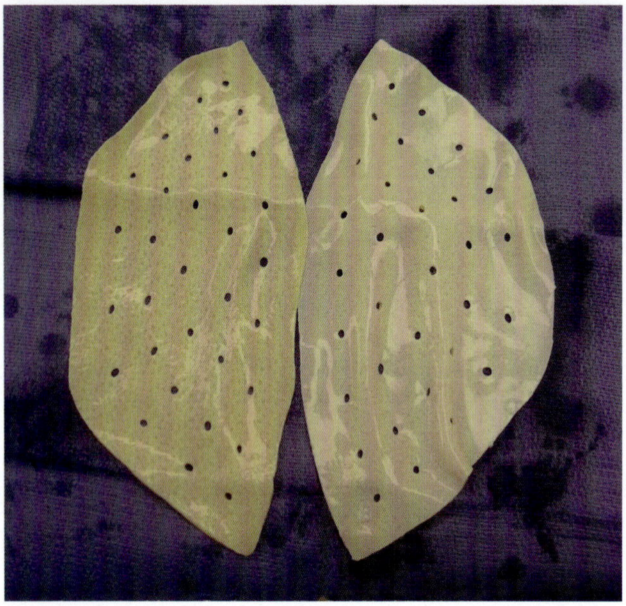

Figure 12.3 Two contour medium perforated sheets of acellular dermal matrix can be sewn together along the short axis.

algorithm for ADM size selection is based on tissue expander volume. For tissue expanders less than 350 mL, two small contoured sheets are appropriate; between 350 and 600 mL, two contour medium sheets are preferred: and over 600 mL, two large contoured sheets are used. While the mastectomy is in progress, two sheets of contoured perforated ADMs are sutured together along the short axis with a 3-0 Vicryl suture. The benefit of the two contoured sheets sewn together is that it creates a curved surface that drapes well over the tissue expander (**Figure 12.4**).

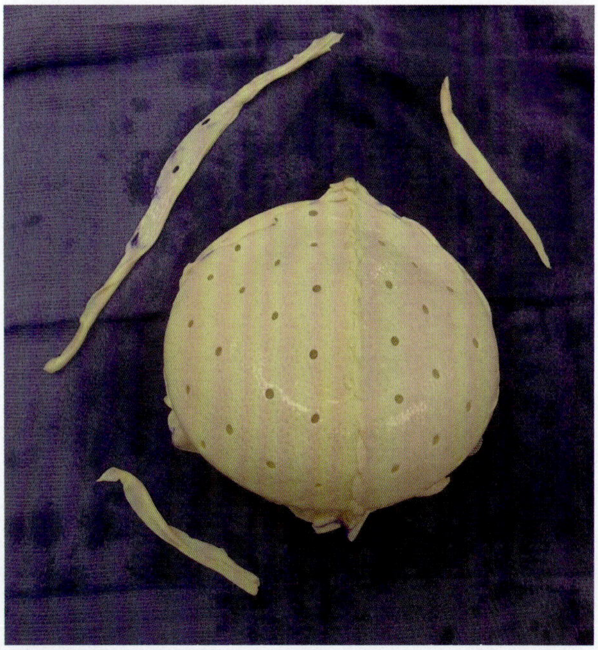

Figure 12.4 The acellular dermal matrix is placed around the tissue expander and the excess is trimmed.

The preferred thickness of the ADM ranges from 2 to 3 mm.

- All air is removed from the tissue expander and replaced with either air or saline to approximately 50% of capacity depending on the mastectomy skin flaps. The authors' preference is to use air because it is lightweight and offloads pressure on the mastectomy skin flaps, is evenly distributed within the tissue expander, and minimizes suture pull through from the pectoralis major muscle because of the effects of gravity when using saline.

Tissue Expander Insertion—The Off-Label Technique

- The tissue expander may be wrapped throughout its 360° surface or along its anterior surface only or 180° (**Figure 12.4**). The benefits of the off-label approach are that it reduces the amount of time in the operating room and is a simple procedure. The benefits and reasons for the 360° approach are that scar tissue formation is minimized throughout the entire surface of the device; whereas with the 180° approach, scar tissue formation anteriorly is minimized. However, the posterior surface of the tissue expander can still adhere to the underlying pectoralis major muscle (**Figure 12.5**).
- With the 360° approach, the ADM construct is draped over the tissue expander and sutured together along the posterior surface of the device with a 3-0 Vicryl. With the 180° approach, the ADM is redraped over the tissue expander and posterior spanning sutures (3-0 Vicryl) are used to secure the ADM on the anterior surface of the tissue expander (**Figure 12.5**).
- The suture tabs on the expander are exteriorized by making small slits in the ADM.

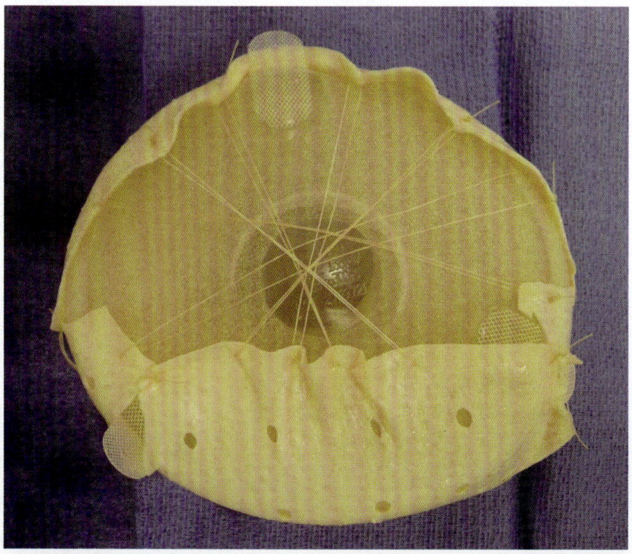

Figure 12.5 The acellular dermal matrix can be wrapped around the expander and secured with posterior spanning sutures.

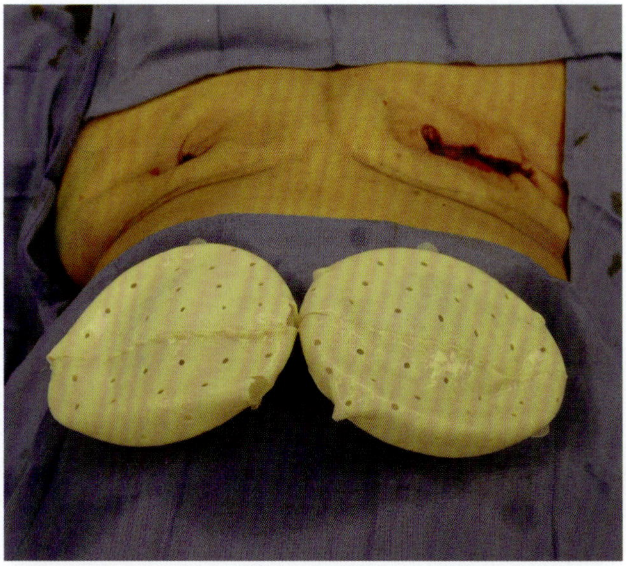

Figure 12.6 The two tissue expander/acellular dermal matrix constructs are ready to be inserted into the prepectoral space.

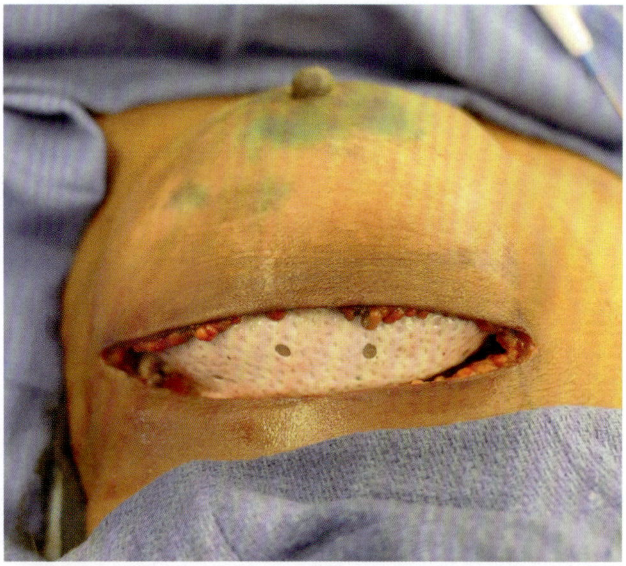

Figure 12.7 The tissue expander/acellular dermal matrix construct is inserted and the tabs are sutured to the pectoralis major muscle.

- The tissue expander–ADM construct is placed into the mastectomy space (**Figures 12.6 and 12.7**). The construct is positioned medially along the medial border of the breast and inferiorly along the IMF.

Tissue Expander Insertion—The On-Label Technique

- The ADM construct is placed in the mastectomy pocket to line and support the soft tissues. The dermal surface of the ADM is inset to abut the subcutaneous surface of the mastectomy.
- Following a nipple-sparing mastectomy through an IMF approach, the superior anchoring sutures are placed securing the superior edge of the ADM to the pectoralis major muscle. This is followed by medial and laterally based sutures, again securing the edge of the ADM to the pectoralis major muscle.
- Following a skin-sparing mastectomy, the ADM is typically anchored to the pectoralis major muscle superiorly, medially, and inferiorly using absorbable sutures.
- The tissue expander is inserted such that the medial and inferior aspects of the device abut the medial and inferior borders of the breast, respectively. The tabs are sutured to the pectoralis manor muscle with absorbable sutures.
- The final step is to tuck 3 to 4 cm of ADM under the tissue expander to serve as a gutter and assist in maintaining the position of the tissue expander and to minimize inferior descent of the device.

Technique—Preparing to Close

- The tissue expander tabs are sutured to the pectoralis major muscle with absorbable sutures. Air-filled tissue expanders are less likely to result in superior tab suture pull through when the patient is standing due to less weight or downward force. It is important to obtain three-point tab fixation with prepectoral placement to minimize edge palpability of the tissue expander.
- One or two closed suction drains are inserted. The authors' preference is to use a single drain unless the patient has a BMI > 30 or if extensive axillary surgery has been performed.
- The wound is irrigated with an antibiotic solution. The authors' preference is to first irrigate with a 50% povidone-iodine solution followed by a triple antibiotic solution.
- The incision is closed in layers using absorbable sutures.
- Options for incisional dressings include steri-strips, xeroform, and gauze as well as incisional vacuum-assisted devices. Following nipple-sparing mastectomy, Tegaderm is placed over the entire surface of the breast to assist with stabilizing the position of the nipple–areolar complex (**Figure 12.8**).

PREPECTORAL RECONSTRUCTION WITHOUT BIOPROSTHETIC MESH (STAGE 1)

Prepectoral prosthetic breast reconstruction without bioprosthetic mesh has demonstrated success.[13] The surgical technique described with is that of Salibian et al following nipple-sparing mastectomy.

- Important aspects of the mastectomy include placing the incision 2 mm above the IMF to preserve the ligamentous support and minimize the risk

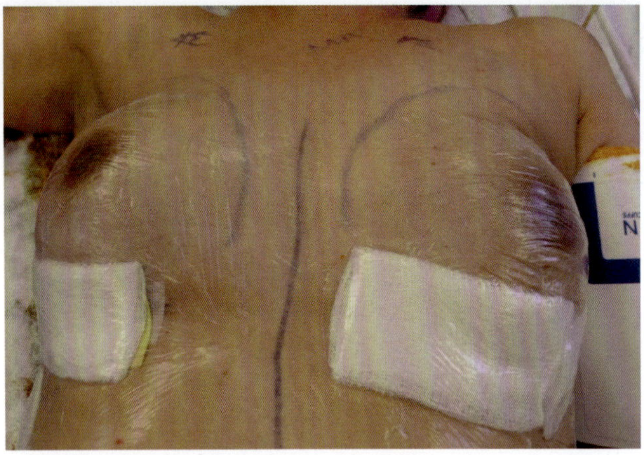

Figure 12.8 The postoperative dressings include a Tegaderm splint around the breast to maintain the position of the nipple–areolar complex.

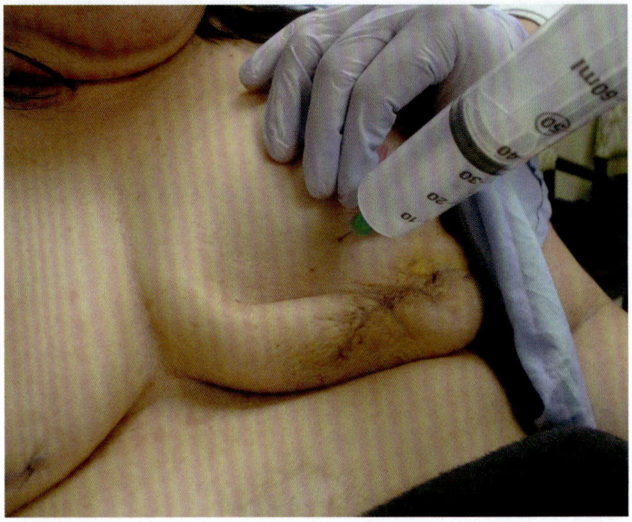

Figure 12.9 Two or 3 weeks postoperatively, the air is removed from the tissue expander and replaced with saline.

of inferior descent. It is also important to ensure adequate thickness of the mastectomy skin flaps and preserve as much normal subcutaneous tissue as possible.

- The mastectomy and tissue expander technique is the same following therapeutic and prophylactic mastectomy. Tabbed tissue expanders are highly recommended to minimize the risk of device malposition. Fixation of the tissue expander is usually 5 mm above the IMF.
- The tissue expander is minimally filled with saline to prevent undue pressure on the mastectomy skin flaps.

POSTOPERATIVE MANAGEMENT OF THE PREPECTORAL TISSUE EXPANDER

- Drain removal typically occurs 1 to 2 weeks following device placement. Antibiotics are typically delivered postoperatively for 3 to 5 days postoperatively.
- In patients with air-filled tissue expanders, the air is usually evacuated and replaced with saline 2 weeks postoperatively (**Figure 12.9**). In patients who continue with air expansion, it is important to recognize that air will diffuse from the device and more frequent expansions may be necessary. Postoperative expansion occurs in the office in small increments (50 mL). In patients with ADM, final expansion volumes are less than the desired volume to avoid overstretching of the skin. In patients without ADM who may or may not require radiation, the breast is expanded 50 to 100 mL more to account for skin and capsular contracture.

PREPECTORAL RECONSTRUCTION WITH THE IMPLANT (STAGE 2)

The second stage is usually performed 2 to 3 months later when no radiation is delivered and 4 to 9 months later when radiation is delivered. Permanent implant selection is based on tissue characteristics and patient expectations. Round or shaped devices can be used. If preoperative rippling and wrinkling is present, autologous fat grafting can be considered.

- Preoperative markings include the sternal midline, the IMFs bilaterally to assess any positional discrepancy, and the superior position of the tissue expander.
- The prior incision is opened and the dissection progresses through the ADM. The tissue expander is removed.
- The periprosthetic space is inspected for ADM adherence and the need for capsulotomy or capsulorrhaphy is assessed.
- When no ADM has been used, capsulotomy is usually necessary and is performed laterally, superiorly, and medially. When ADM has been used, capsulotomy is rarely necessary.
- Capsulorrhaphy is considered when the footprint needs to be tightened and is usually performed using electrocautery (popcorn technique) as well as a two-layer suture repair.[14]
- The permanent implant can be round or shaped and is usually slightly larger in volume than the tissue expander. The goal is to maintain a mild-to-moderate degree of tension on the skin envelope to minimize the incidence of rippling and wrinkling. With larger devices (> 500 mL), an inferior capsulorrhaphy is often considered to strengthen the position of the IMF and minimize the risk of inferior malposition or descent.

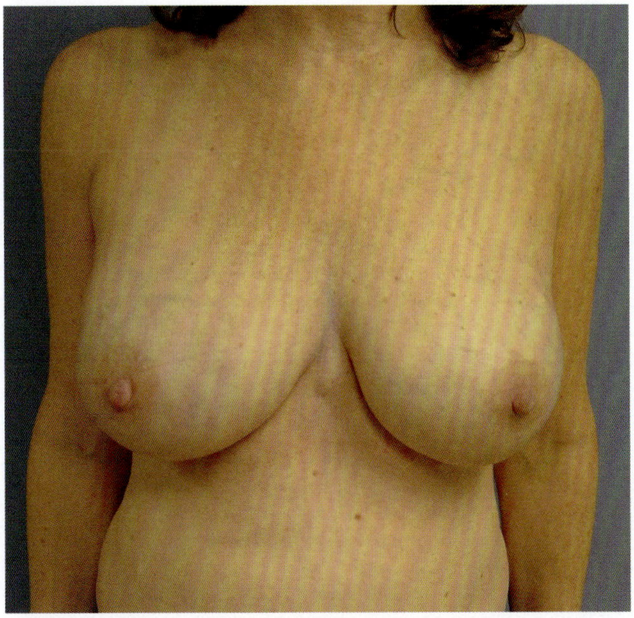

Figure 12.10 Preoperative photograph of a patient scheduled to have bilateral nipple-sparing mastectomy.

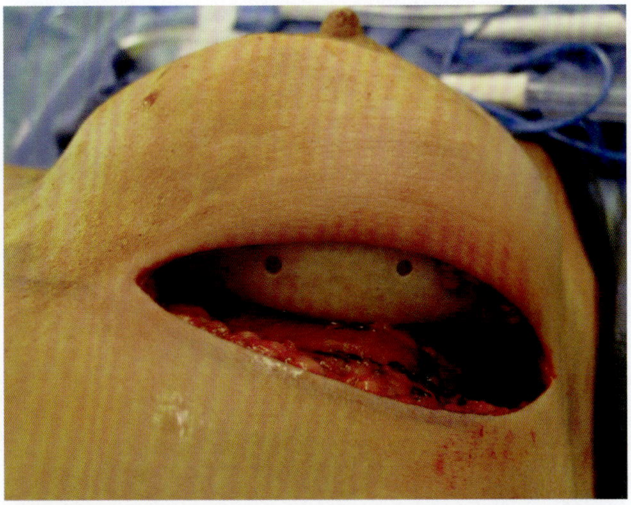

Figure 12.11 The 400-mL tissue expander and acellular dermal matrix are placed in the prepectoral space through the inframammary incision.

- When fat grafting is necessary, the regions to be grafted are delineated and the fat is injected via the incision between the ADM and the skin.
- **Figures 12.10 to 12.14** illustrate a prepectoral reconstruction in a patient from start to completion.

OUTCOMES

Reported outcomes following prepectoral reconstruction without any bioprosthetic material have been generally favorable. Salibian et al retrospectively reviewed 155 women and 250 breasts over a 10-year period following

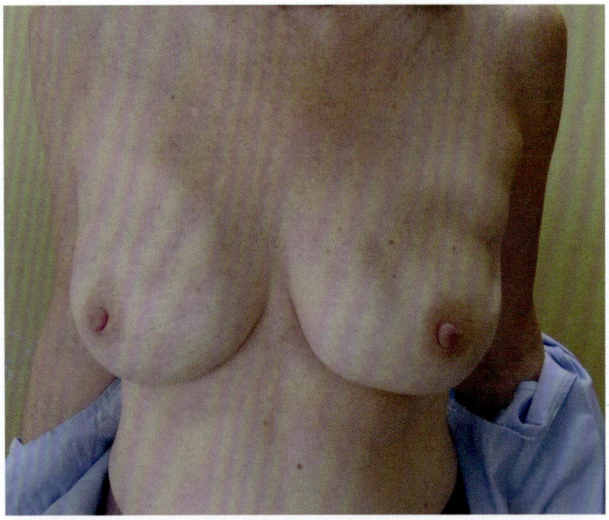

Figure 12.12 The tissue expander is gradually filled with saline during the postoperative phase.

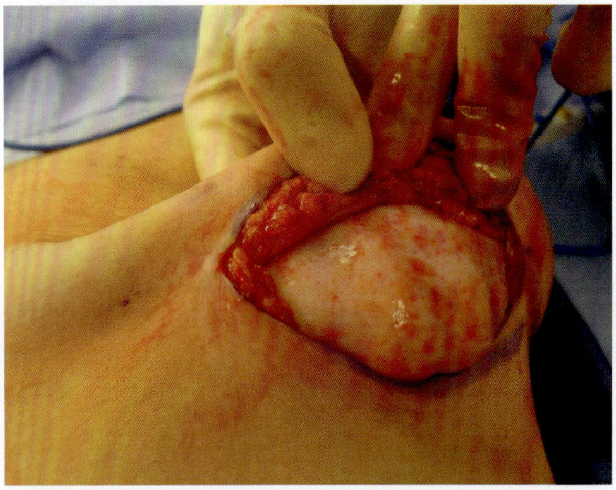

Figure 12.13 The acellular dermal matrix is pictured at time of the exchange demonstrating excellent incorporation and revascularization.

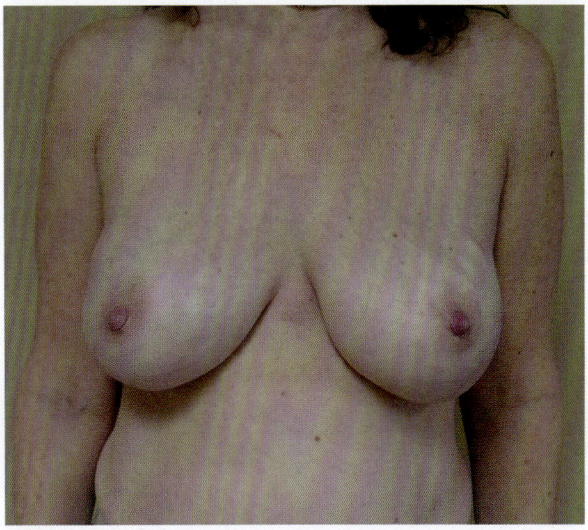

Figure 12.14 Postoperative photograph at 6 months following insertion of a 500-mL SCX silicone gel implant.

nipple-sparing mastectomy and two-stage prosthetic reconstruction without bioprosthetic soft-tissue support.[13] Mean follow-up was 55 months (range, 23.6-138.1). The range for tissue expander size was 275 to 450 mL. Fill volumes varied widely with an intraoperative tissue expander fill volume that ranged from 30 to 540 mL (mean, 248 mL) and a final implant volume that ranged from 275 to 800 mL (mean, 515 mL). Adverse events included tissue expander explantation in 6.8%, capsular contracture in 7.6%, and mild to moderate rippling in 3.6%. The overall aesthetic evaluation was graded as good to very good in 85.2% of women.

Reported outcomes for prepectoral reconstruction with bioprosthetic materials have also been favorable. Vidya et al reported on a prospective multicenter study of 100 prepectoral breast reconstructions using a porcine ADM and demonstrated 2% implant loss due to nipple necrosis or wound break down at 18 months follow-up.[15] Sigalove et al performed a retrospective review of 353 prepectoral reconstructions using human ADM in 207 patients demonstrating an infection rate of 4%, seroma rate of 2%, and a skin flap necrosis rate of 2.5%.[12] Woo et al performed a retrospective review of 135 prepectoral reconstructions using human ADM demonstrating successful reconstruction in 96% with minor surgical complications in 14% of patients. Comparative studies between prepectoral and total muscle coverage following the first stage of tissue expander breast reconstruction have demonstrated similar morbidities with regard to infection (0% vs 3%) and seroma (1% vs 1%); however, when combining all complications, they were increased with submuscular (18% vs 8%).[16]

SUMMARY

Prepectoral placement of devices using the two-stage prosthetic breast reconstruction appears to be safe and effective in properly selected patients. Proper patient selection includes ensuring viability and perfusion of the mastectomy skin flaps and accurate assessment of patient expectations. Bioprosthetic materials appear to be used in the majority of cases and provide benefits by adding to the thickness of the mastectomy skin flaps, reducing the inflammatory response around an implant, and compartmentalizing the device.

KEY REFERENCES

1. Woo A, Harless C, Jacobson SR. Revisiting an old place: single surgeon experience on post-mastectomy subcutaneous implant-based breast reconstruction. *Breast J*. 2017;23(5):545-553.
2. Sigalove S, Maxwell GP, Sigalove NM, et al. Prepectoral implant-based breast reconstruction: rationale, indications, and preliminary results. *Plast Reconstr Surg*. 2017;139(2):287-294.
3. Reitsamer R, Peintinger F. Prepectoral implant placement and complete coverage with porcine acellular dermal matrix: a new technique for direct to implant breast reconstruction after nipple-sparing mastectomy. *J Plast Reconstr Aesthet Surg*. 2015;68:162-167.
4. Bernini M, Calabrese C, Cecconi L, et al. Subcutaneous direct-to-implant breast reconstruction: surgical, functional, and aesthetic results after long-term follow-up. *Plast Reconstr Surg Glob Open*. 2016;3(12):e574.
5. Kobraei EM, Cauley R, Gadd M, Austen WG Jr, Liao EC. Avoiding breast animation deformity with pectoralis-sparing subcutaneous direct-to-implant breast reconstruction. *Plast Reconstr Surg Glob Open*. 2016;4(5):e708.
6. Sbitany H, Piper M, Lentz R. Prepectoral breast reconstruction: a safe alternative to submuscular prosthetic reconstruction following nipple-sparing mastectomy. *Plast Reconstr Surg*. 2017;140:432.
7. Thorarinsson A, Frojd V, Kolby L, Lidén M, Elander A, Mark H. Patient determinants as independent risk factors for postoperative complications of breast reconstruction. *Gland Surg*. 2017;6(4):355-367.
8. Nahabedian MY, Tsangaris TE, Momen B, Manson PN. Infectious complications following breast reconstructions with expanders and implants. *Plast Reconstr Surg*. 2003;112:467.
9. Disa JJ, Ad-El DD, Cohen, SM, Cordeiro PG, Hidalgo DA. The premature removal of tissue expanders in breast reconstruction. *Plast Reconstr Surg*. 1999;104:1662.
10. Blondeel PN, Hijawi J, Depypre H, Roche N, Van Landuyt K. Shaping the breast in aesthetic and reconstructive breast surgery: an easy three-step principle. Part IV—aesthetic breast surgery. *Plast Reconstr Surg*. 2009;124:372.
11. Bernini M, Calabrese C, Cecconi L, et al. Subcutaneous direct-to-implant breast Reconstruction: Surgical, functional, and aesthetic results after long-term follow-up. *Plast Reconstr Surg Glob Open*. 2016;3(12):e574.
12. Zenn MR. Staged immediate breast reconstruction. *Plast Reconstr Surg*. 2015;135(4):976-979.
13. Salibian AH, Harness JK, Mowlds DS. Staged suprapectoral expander/implant reconstruction without acellular dermal matrix following nipple-sparing mastectomy. *Plast Reconstr Surg*. 2017;139:30-39.
14. Harris R, Raphael P, Harris SW. Thermal capsulorrhaphy: a modified technique for breast pocket revision. *Aesthet Surg J*. 2014;34(7):1041-1049.
15. Vidya R, Masià J, Cawthorn S, et al. Evaluation of the effectiveness of the prepectoral breast reconstruction with Braxon dermal matrix: first multicenter European report on 100 cases. *Breast J*. 2017;23(6):670-676.
16. Zhu L, Mohan AT, Abdelsattar JM, et al. Comparison of subcutaneous versus submuscular expander placement in the first stage of immediate breast reconstruction. *J Plast Reconstr Aesthet Surg*. 2016;69(4):e77-e86.

CHAPTER 13

DIRECT-TO-IMPLANT PREPECTORAL RECONSTRUCTION WITH ROUND IMPLANTS

Michelle C. Roughton and Rafi Fredman

KEY POINTS

- DTI breast reconstruction with smooth round silicone implants following mastectomy provides high-quality aesthetic results in appropriately selected candidates.
- Surgical and technologic advances have allowed for successful prepectoral implant placement, which may eliminate several complications of subpectoral implant placement.

INTRODUCTION

In the 1960s, breast reconstruction was performed with implants in the subcutaneous space. Complications were common, including implant rippling and visibility, skin necrosis, implant exposure, and capsular contracture. To mitigate these complications, the reconstructive technique was modified to provide additional soft-tissue coverage and the implant was moved to a submuscular position.

Submuscular implant placement is performed with either total muscular coverage or a dual-plane approach. In the latter, the pectoralis major was allowed to window shade up and the inferior border was secured to the mastectomy skin flap. Both techniques have limitations. Total submuscular coverage did not frequently result in a natural-appearing breast, and sole reliance on the mastectomy flap in the inferior pole risked many of the complications that submuscular placement sought to avoid, namely, mastectomy skin necrosis and capsular contracture.

A turning point in implant-based reconstruction came with the introduction of acellular dermal matrices (ADMs) to the market. By utilizing ADM for lower pole coverage, total submuscular coverage could be avoided, a larger implant could be placed, and an additional layer of tissue would exist between the implant and mastectomy flap at the lower pole. This technique allowed for safe and successful direct-to-implant (DTI) breast reconstruction and has arguably become the standard of care for DTI reconstruction.

DTI breast reconstruction in the subpectoral dual plane has been shown to provide excellent aesthetic results; however, animation and pain continue to be problematic. In addition, implant size may be limited to the inherent subpectoral space. Although not a limiting factor for smaller breasted women, larger breasted women may not be able to return to their premastectomy size, despite having an adequate skin envelope.

The sine qua non of subcutaneous implant reconstruction is that its success is reliant on the viability of the overlying mastectomy skin flap. These flaps are often thin, which puts the skin at risk for ischemia, breakdown, and subsequent implant-related infection. Thin skin provides little camouflage over the structure of the implant that can result in unacceptable implant visibility and rippling. Over the past decade, advances in surgical techniques and technologies have allowed for each of these issues to be addressed and reconsideration of the benefits of prepectoral implant placement.[1-5]

Consistently well-perfused mastectomy skin flaps are a crucial factor in enabling successful placement of implants in the prepectoral space. The mastectomy skin flap is always carefully assessed clinically, before selection of reconstructive technique. We do not routinely use tissue perfusion technology. We apply topical nitroglycerin to the nipple–areolar complex (NAC) and surrounding skin and frequently to the peri-incisional area of skin-sparing mastectomies (SSMs) as well. We use one package of nitropaste per patient (let us figure out how much this is). Nevertheless, full-thickness mastectomy skin necrosis remains the most common complication in our experience.

Over the past decade, implant manufactures have developed more highly cohesive silicone implants that cause less rippling and feel more natural than earlier generation implants. With these attributes, they require less soft-tissue coverage to mask their inherent deficiencies. Nevertheless, thinner patients and thin flaps will still have some rippling with prepectoral implant placement. This is easily addressed with fat grafting to the upper pole of the mastectomy skin. In addition to masking rippling, fat grafting also improves the transition from chest wall to implant, creating a more natural slope, and increasing upper pole fullness. We have found that with highly cohesive implants, rippling is less of a problem and patients require fat grafting less frequently than with earlier generations of silicone implants. Rarely do we fat graft more than once with the highly cohesive devices.

By placing the implant above the pectoralis major muscle, the skin envelope can be filled without any volume restriction by overlying muscle. With subpectoral DTI, a smaller implant may need to be placed to fit under the muscle despite a voluminous skin envelope. In prepectoral DTI reconstructions, the skin envelope can be fully filled and the breast size can often be augmented without additional stretch on the skin. This is especially true in women with involutional ptosis.

We believe ADM to be essential to the success of prepectoral DTI. ADM provides an additional layer of tissue between implant and skin, which may reduce many of the complications seen when implants were placed directly under the skin. We believe the ADM to function as a barrier between the mastectomy skin and the implant. In some cases where we have seen ADM exposure from either mastectomy skin necrosis or incisional dehiscence, we have been able to close the mastectomy skin secondarily without changing the underlying device. We have yet to see any Baker grade three or four capsular contracture in these patients. We hypothesize that placing an implant under ADM is protective against capsular contracture, a finding that is supported in several previously published studies.[6] However, we have not attempted prepectoral implant placement without use of ADM and cannot comment on the success rate of this technique.

Postmastectomy radiation therapy (PMRT) is an integral part of the oncologic management of breast cancer and more patients are receiving PMRT than previously. PMRT has an adverse effect on the outcomes of implant-based reconstruction with studies showing a higher incidence of capsular contracture and need for unplanned revisions. In our experience, radiating a prepectoral placed implant does not significantly increase the risk of capsular contracture or need for major revision. This may be a result of not placing the implant under a radiated and fibrotic muscle as well as the presence of ADM, which may protect against the development of capsular contracture.

Early in our experience with prepectoral techniques, we observed that patients have less postoperative pain than do patients with subpectoral implant or expander placement. Our patients who underwent prepectoral DTI require less narcotics than did patients who underwent either subpectoral DTI or expander reconstruction. In the current US opioid epidemic, the ability to perform breast reconstruction in a manner that reduces the need for narcotic medication is significant. Many of our immediate prepectoral DTI reconstructions are now performed on an outpatient basis with discharge the same day as surgery.

In an era of soaring health care costs, it is essential to consider the cost-effectiveness of different breast reconstruction techniques. A recent cost–utility analysis showed that subpectoral DTI was more cost-effective than expander-based reconstruction, with a margin of \$44 336.59.[7] Factors in the prepectoral technique used in this series (I have friends who use no ADM) that could result in additional costs include the cost of a larger, 16 × 20 cm piece of ADM, as well additional fat grafting procedures. Nevertheless, given that the prepectoral technique has outcomes and complication rates similar to those of subpectoral reconstruction, and considering the large cost margin by which subpectoral DTI remains cost-effective over expander-based reconstruction, prepectoral DTI would likely remain cost-effective when compared to expander-based reconstruction. A thorough cost–utility analysis will need to be performed to quantify this and assess whether prepectoral DTI is cost-effective compared to subpectoral DTI.

PREOPERATIVE PLANNING

Our initial consultation in a patient planning to undergo SSM or nipple-sparing mastectomy for breast cancer or breast cancer prophylaxis involves an in-depth discussion of the various methods of reconstruction, both autologous and implant based. In situ or invasive breast cancer patients, or patients undergoing prophylactic mastectomy are considered for prepectoral implant placement. Patient-specific goals are discussed and standard measurements are taken to determine the optimal implant width and projection. Given the potential for implant contour visibility and rippling, we use smooth round highly cohesive silicone implants for our reconstructions. In our experience, the round implant is more mobile and favored by patients relative to anatomic devices. Furthermore, in a prepectoral approach, the anatomic devices, in our hands, are more likely to rotate, because the textured surfaces do not adhere to the ADM.

In our experience, a relative contraindication to prepectoral DTI has been the lack of a fat grafting donor site. We tend to reconstruct these very thin women as a dual plane with ADM. However, these same patients who are typically the most active may not tolerate visible animation deformity and thus it remains ever important to review the trade-offs

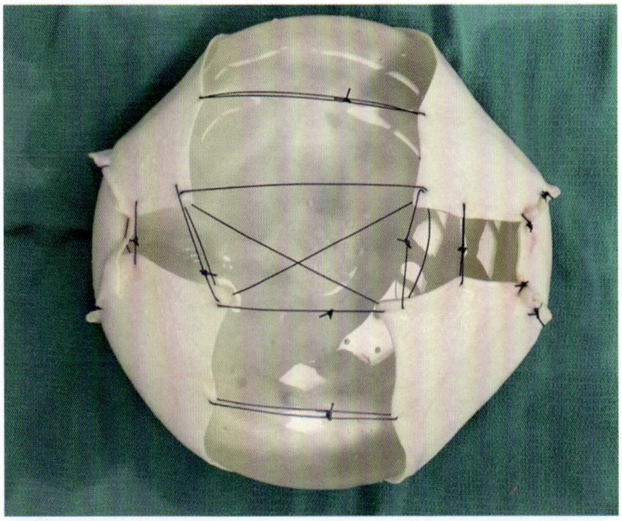

Figure 13.1 Smooth round silicone implant wrapped with a single 16 × 20 cm piece of acellular dermal matrix. Photograph showing posterior aspect of implant.

of the two planes with the patient. Furthermore, if there is a preexisting subpectoral augmentation, we utilize the space available and commonly stay subpectoral with the reconstruction.

SURGICAL MANAGEMENT

The most crucial point in the decision-making process occurs in the operating room, when the mastectomy skin flaps are assessed. If the flaps are found to be too thin, or poorly perfused, either a tissue expander is placed or, more commonly, a delayed approach is utilized with a 2-week delay before expander or implant placement. Once they have demarcated, if the skin flaps are adequate in surface area, we proceed with prepectoral implant placement. If not, we elect for prepectoral tissue expander.

TECHNIQUE: PREPECTORAL DIRECT-TO-IMPLANT RECONSTRUCTION WITH ROUND IMPLANTS

Implant sizers are placed into the pocket following mastectomy and the optimal implant volume and profile are chosen. The lateral breast border of mastectomy skin is secured to the chest wall with sutures to prevent lateral displacement of the implant. A 16 × 20 cm piece of ADM is prepared and placed on the implant to cover the entire anterior surface and as much of the posterior surface as possible with a single piece of ADM. The posterior edges are secured to each other with spanning sutures (**Figure 13.1**). The ADM-covered implant is then placed into the pocket. A single drain is placed in the pocket and the incision is closed in layers. Nitroglycerine paste is placed on the NAC and/or mastectomy skin. Several large pieces of Tegaderm (3M, Minneapolis, MN) are placed over the breast and used to secure the nipple (when present) in its ideal location on the implant. This also assists with immobilization to allow the ADM to adhere to the mastectomy flaps. Preoperative and postoperative photographs are shown in **Figures 13.2 to 13.4**.

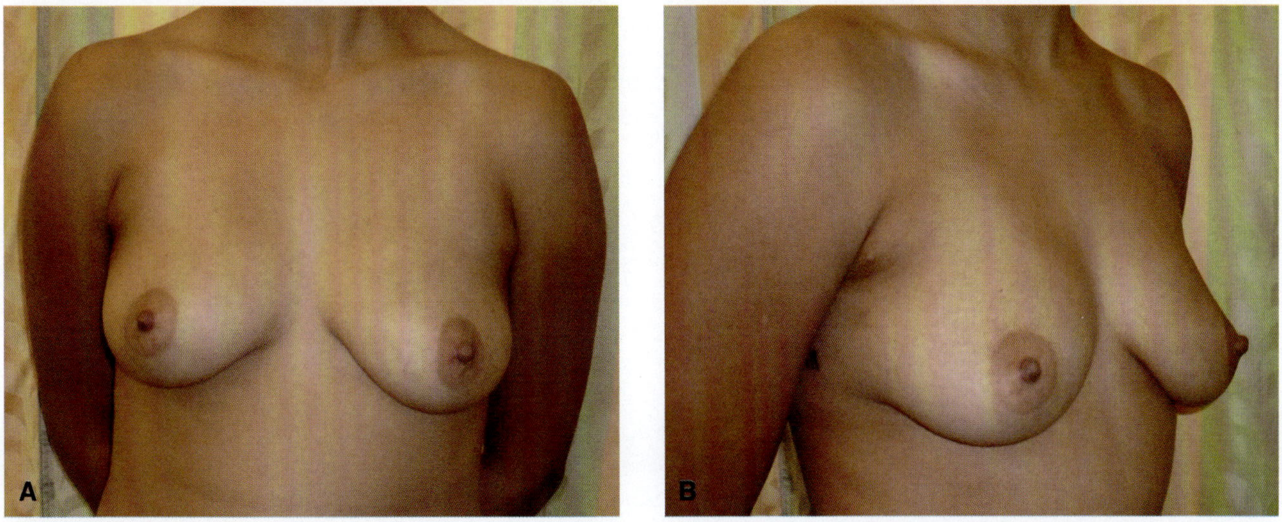

Figure 13.2 **A 25-year-old woman (body mass index 23.87 kg/m^2), *BRCA2* gene mutation, underwent bilateral prophylactic nipple-sparing mastectomy and immediate bilateral prepectoral direct-to-implant breast reconstruction.** She has Natrelle Inspira SCX 700cc implant (Allergan, Inc., Irvine, CA) in the right breast, SCX 580-mL implant in the right breast, and underwent fat grafting. (A-C) Preoperative and (D-F) postoperative views 13 months after surgery.

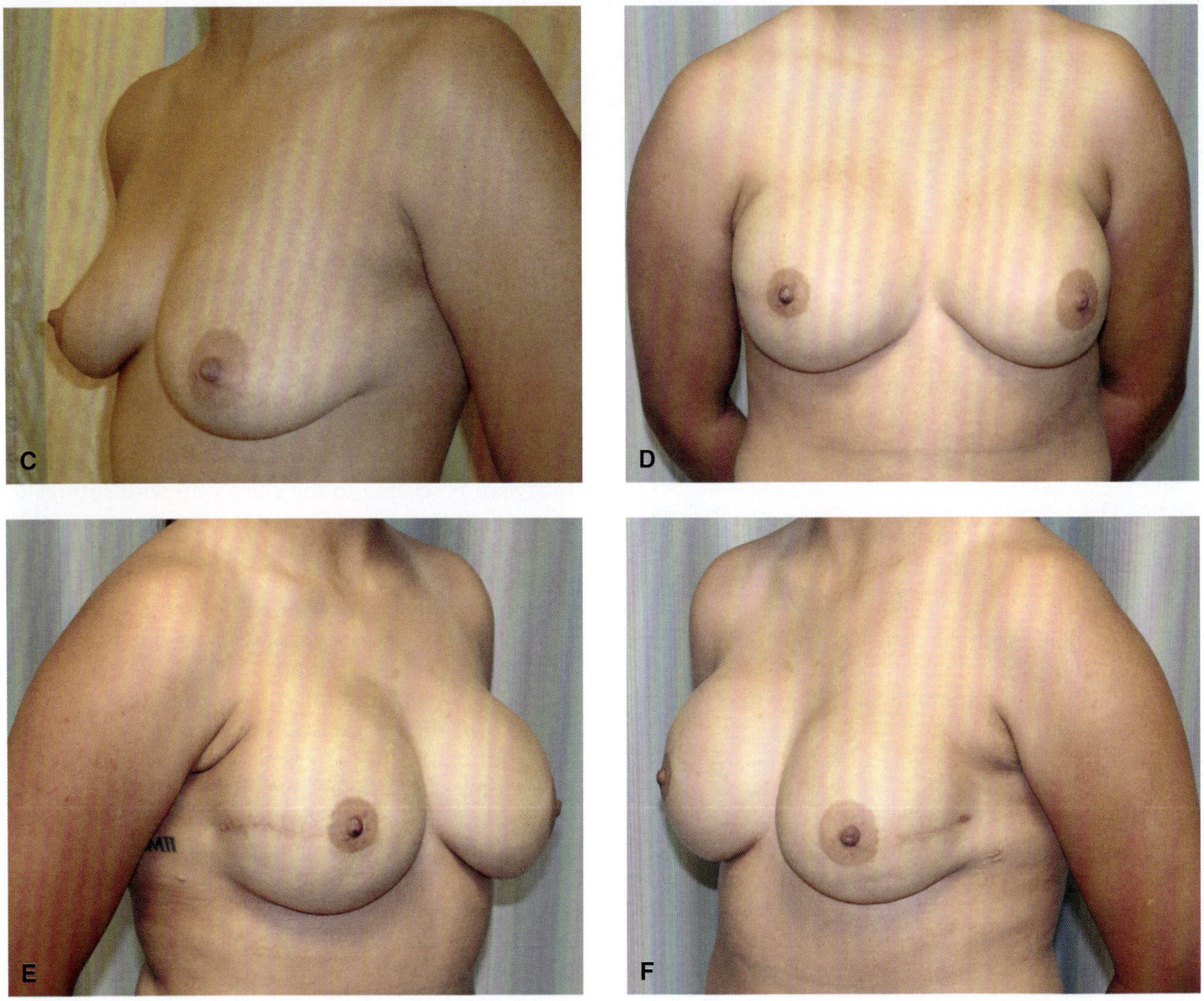

Figure 13.2 (*continued*)

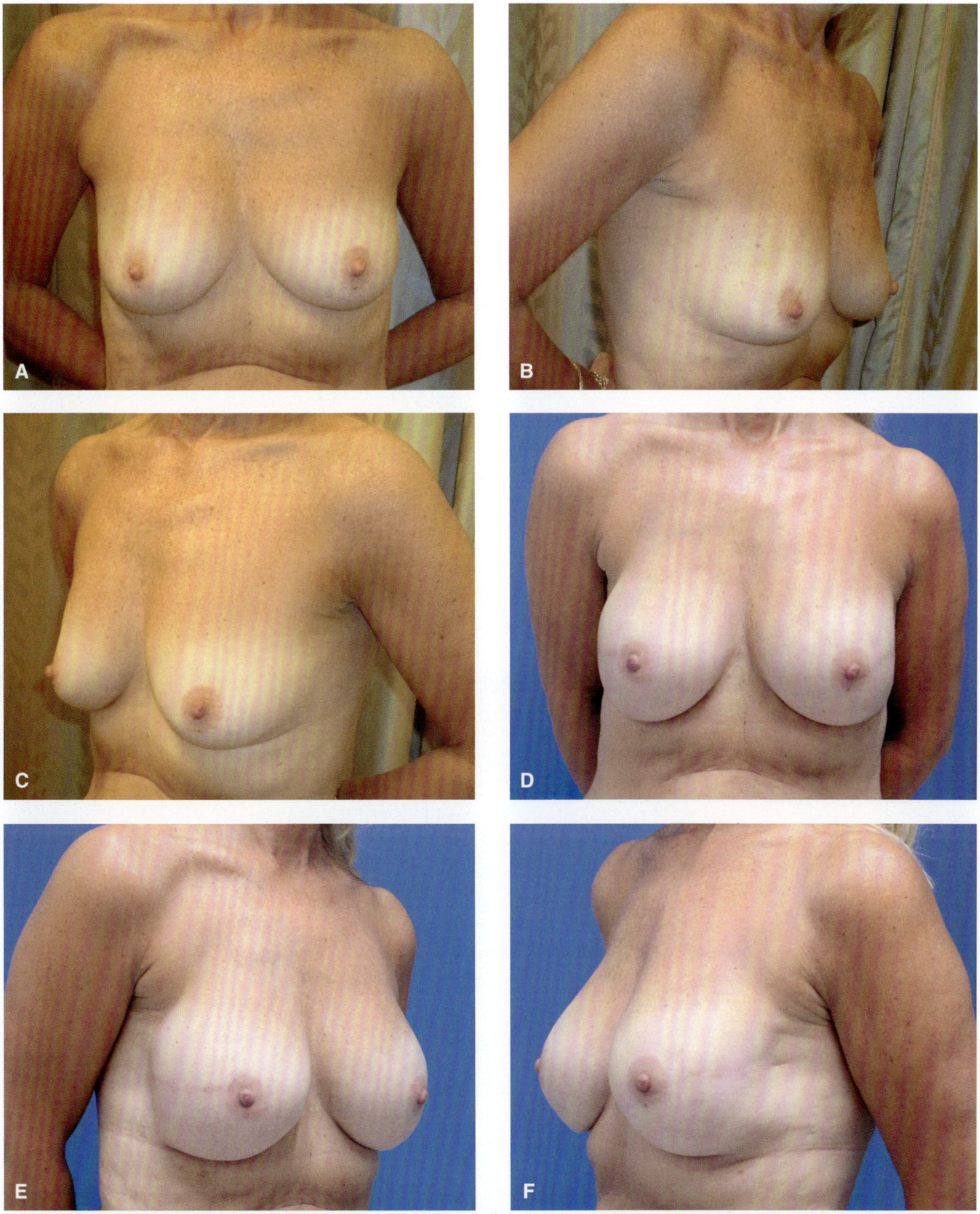

Figure 13.3 **A 56-year-old woman (body mass index 21.58 kg/m^2), right breast cancer, underwent bilateral nipple-sparing mastectomy and immediate bilateral prepectoral direct-to-implant breast reconstruction.** She has Natrelle Inspira SRF 385-cc implants (Allergan, Inc., Irvine, CA) and underwent fat grafting. (A-C) Preoperative and (D-F) postoperative views 16 months after surgery.

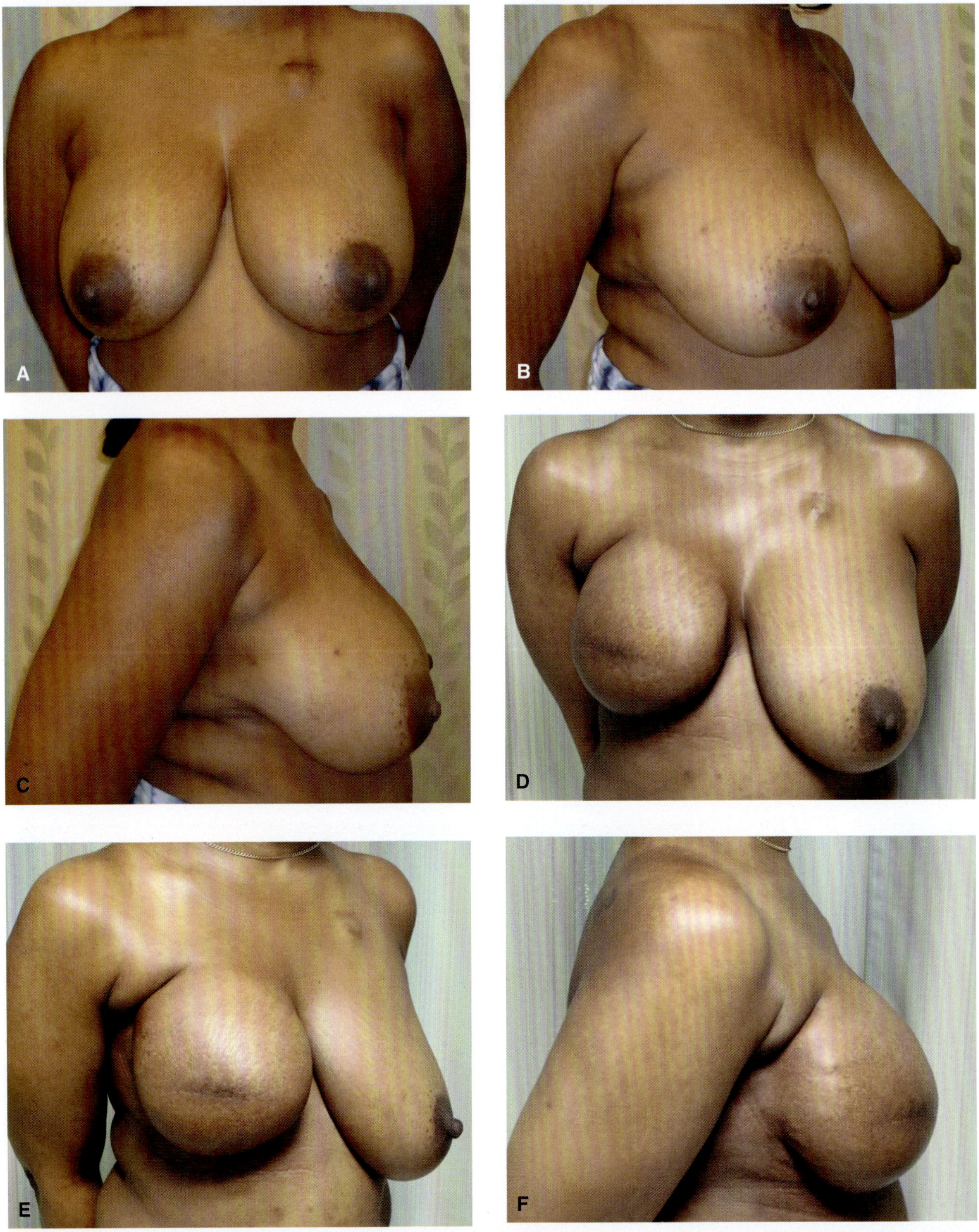

Figure 13.4. **A 42-year-old woman (body mass index 25.96 kg/m^2), right breast cancer, underwent right skin-sparing mastectomy and immediate prepectoral direct-to-implant breast reconstruction.** She received post mastectomy radiation therapy. She has Natrelle Inspira SCX 800-cc implants (Allergan, Inc., Irvine, CA). (A-C) Preoperative and (D-F) postoperative views 8 months after surgery without further surgery or evidence of capsular contracture.

SUMMARY

Prepectoral DTI with round silicone implants provides reliable results with a similar safety profile to other implant-based reconstructive techniques. Prepectoral DTI eliminates implant animation and results in patients requiring fewer narcotics after surgery.

KEY REFERENCES

1. Sbitany H, Piper M, Lentz R. Prepectoral breast reconstruction: a safe alternative to submuscular prosthetic reconstruction following nipple sparing mastectomy. *Plast Reconstr Surg*. 2017;140(3):432-443.
2. Vidya R, Iqbal FM. A guide to prepectoral breast reconstruction: a new dimension to implant-based breast reconstruction. *Clin Breast Cancer*. 2017;17:266-271.
3. Sigalove S, Maxwell GP, Sigalove NM, et al. Prepectoral implant-based breast reconstruction: rationale, indications, and preliminary results. *Plast Reconstr Surg*. 2017;139:287-294.
4. Caputo GG, Marchetti A, Dalla Pozza E, et al. Skin-reduction breast reconstructions with prepectoral implant. *Plast Reconstr Surg*. 2016;137:1702-1705.
5. Woo A, Harless C, Jacobson SR. Revisiting an old place: single-surgeon experience on post-mastectomy subcutaneous implant-based breast reconstruction. *Breast J*. 2017;23(5):545-553.
6. Salzberg CA, Ashikari AY, Berry C, Hunsicker LM. Acellular dermal matrix-assisted direct-to-implant breast reconstruction and capsular contracture: a 13-year experience. *Plast Reconstr Surg*. 2016;138:329-337.
7. Krishnan NM, Fischer JP, Basta MN, Nahabedian MY. Is single-stage prosthetic reconstruction cost effective? A cost-utility analysis for the use of direct-to-implant breast reconstruction relative to expander-implant reconstruction in postmastectomy patients. *Plast Reconstr Surg*. 2016;138:537-547.

CHAPTER 14

PREPECTORAL IMMEDIATE DIRECT-TO-IMPLANT BREAST RECONSTRUCTION WITH ANTERIOR ALLODERM COVERAGE

Glyn Jones, Victor King, and Aran Yoo

KEY POINTS

- If skin flap perfusion is acceptable with a sizer in place, reconstruction is performed as single stage.
- On the basis of the mastectomy weight and the patient's desire for final bra cup size, a temporary sterile implant sizer is selected and placed beneath the mastectomy skin anterior to the pectoralis major muscle.
- If the vascularity of a larger skin area is found to be compromised, inadequate to cover even an expander, the procedure is aborted and skin closure is performed with a plan to perform delayed reconstruction.

INTRODUCTION

Breast reconstruction has been performed with a two-stage approach using expanders placed in the subpectoral plane since the 1970s when Radovan introduced the tissue expander concept. At that time, mastectomy techniques involved major breast skin resection, leaving little domain for an implant to be placed. Tissue expansion played a major role in creating new skin surface area, resulting in the creation of more aesthetically pleasing implant-based breast mounds. The subpectoral plane was associated with improved outcomes in terms of capsular contracture and, to a lesser extent, soft-tissue coverage. In the interim during the 1990s to early 2000s, mastectomy techniques evolved into both skin-sparing and nipple-sparing approaches. This resulted in a dramatically increased amount of available skin and domain into which an implant could be placed, negating much of the original conceptual basis for tissue expansion. More recently, expansion was often coupled with lower pole acellular dermal matrix (ADM) coverage,[1-5] which provided greater pocket control and potentially reduced capsular contracture rates.

Over the past 10 to 15 years, interest has turned to the benefits of single-stage subpectoral direct-to-implant (DTI) reconstruction using lower pole coverage with ADM.[6-12] The results from this procedure often surpassed those of traditional two-stage expander-implant reconstruction and the safety profile appeared to be excellent. However, the subpectoral plane remains an area of controversy because of the negative effects resulting from animation of the muscle.

PROBLEMS WITH THE SUBPECTORAL PLANE

1. The breast is a subcutaneous structure and prevents adhesion between the pectoralis major muscle and the skin. Following a mastectomy, it is an inevitable consequence of submuscular reconstruction that the pectoralis major muscle becomes adherent to the overlying mastectomy skin flap. With muscle contraction, the adherent skin is distorted and animates in an embarrassing manner, often causing severe distortion of the breast. The encapsulated implant beneath the muscle follows suit and is pulled upward with the contracting muscle, further exacerbating the tendency to abnormal shape and motion.

2. Subpectoral implant placement causes significant loss of power of approximately 15% to 20% as evidenced by recent studies, which also confirm thinning of the muscle by about 50%. This functional deficit has only been quantified recently and confirms anecdotal patient reports of relative weakness following both reconstruction and augmentation in the submuscular plane.
3. Submuscular implant insertion results in bowstringing of the muscle across the domed surface of the implant resulting in tightness and discomfort, both of which accompany activities of daily living.
4. Although subpectoral placement has been advocated as a means of reducing capsular contracture, recent work has supported the belief that contracture is primarily a function of biofilm formation and not of implant position in relation to the muscle. Although there may be a slight advantage to subpectoral placement because of the massaging pressure and forces generated by the pectoralis major muscle, it is appearing less and less likely to be a major factor in reducing contracture.
5. Implant rippling has always been a problem in breast reconstruction, and subpectoral implant positioning has been cited as helping to reduce the problem by providing soft-tissue padding over the implant. Although this may appear to be true at surface value, the pectoralis major muscle may actually be partially responsible for causing rippling. Ripples always lie vertically or slightly obliquely in the implant (never horizontally) and are almost always at right angles to the line of pull of the pectoralis major muscle. This is remarkably similar to the rhytids seen around the mouth and in the crows' feet area, which exist as a direct consequence of the action of the underlying orbicularis muscles pulling at right angles to the skin. A similar mechanism may be at work in creating implant rippling where the pectoralis major muscle may contract across the encapsulated implant, decreasing the implant's diameter resulting in heaped up ripples in the gel. In this scenario, the pectoralis major may actually be a causative factor in creating rippling rather than alleviating the problem. It is remarkable how little serious rippling is being seen in prepectoral reconstruction when the reverse was once thought to be likely.

Given all of these concerns about subpectoral implant positioning, together with the availability of ADMs, the prepectoral location became an area of considerable interest for breast reconstruction.

Recent work has focused on two-stage prepectoral expander-implant reconstruction with ADM coverage.[12-15] Given the successful results achieved with this approach, the senior author transitioned to single-stage prepectoral reconstruction with total anterior ADM coverage. Although over 150 breasts have been operated upon using this approach, the data reported on later in this chapter pertains to our study on 2.5-year follow-up data of a series of 73 breasts reconstructed in 50 patients using prepectoral DTI reconstruction.

SURGICAL TECHNIQUE

Following completion of the mastectomy, the plastic surgery team reprepped the mastectomy skin with ChloraPrep (Becton Dickinson, Franklin Lakes, NJ) before applying fresh sterile drapes. Skin flaps were then assessed for quality and thickness and hemostasis was checked and secured.

DECISION MAKING WITH PERFUSION ASSESSMENT

The decision to proceed with prepectoral immediate reconstruction was made if the tumor was located more than 5 mm from the posterior aspect of the breast so as to reduce concerns about monitoring for recurrence on the pectoral muscle surface.

In this study, the decision to perform single-stage prepectoral DTI reconstruction was predicated only on the basis of perfusion device assessment using Indocyanine green (ICG) laser fluorescence with an appropriate breast sizer positioned beneath the mastectomy skin envelope.

If skin flap perfusion was acceptable with a sizer in place, reconstruction was performed irrespective of risk factors such as body mass index (BMI), breast size, or smoking history. This decision had been reached when our prior experience with subpectoral DTI indicated very limited correlation between the usual stated risk factors and breast outcomes *if skin perfusion viability with a sizer in place was preselected as being adequate on fluorescence imaging.*

On the basis of the mastectomy weight and the patient's desire for final bra cup size, a temporary sterile implant sizer was selected and placed beneath the mastectomy skin anterior to the pectoralis major muscle. The mastectomy skin was then draped over the sizer and temporarily stapled closed. Laser fluorescence angiography was performed with 3cc of ICG, using the SPY Elite imaging system (Novadaq Inc., Mississauga, Canada). If areas of concern were noted on fluorescence imaging, SPY-Q analysis was performed and questionable areas were debrided to healthy skin edge bleeding. Adequacy of perfusion was assessed to determine whether the selected implant volume could be accommodated safely beneath the resulting overlying skin envelope. A decision was made to proceed with DTI prepectoral reconstruction when perfusion was deemed acceptable on perfusion imaging. If perfusion was poor and skin surface area had to be sacrificed, reconstruction reverted to a more traditional two-stage approach with an expander placed in the prepectoral position at the index operation. This study reports only those patients with adequate skin perfusion on ICG fluorescence imaging. If the vascularity of a larger skin area was found to be compromised, inadequate to cover an expander, the procedure was aborted and skin closure was performed with a plan to perform delayed reconstruction.

The sizer was removed and the mastectomy pocket was irrigated first with 50% povidone-iodine solution, then with triple antibiotic solution consisting of 1 L of Ringers lactate containing 1 g cefazolin, 80 mg gentamicin, and 50 000 units of bacitracin. A sheet of 16 × 20 cm thick AlloDerm RTU (ready to use) (Allergan/LifeCell, Irvine, CA) was washed for at least 10 minutes with sterile saline. The sheet was perforated repeatedly with a 3-mm dermatologic punch to allow for improved fluid drainage. The AlloDerm was then trimmed at its uppermost corners to shape it to the tapering profile of the underlying anatomic implant's base contour. This technical caveat is deemed extremely important because it controls the position of the anatomic implant without allowing for any rotation of the device. The narrower upper pole of the pocket blocks any attempted movement of the implant's broader base into this narrow upper space, limiting the risk of rotation deformity developing.

ANTERIOR TENTING TECHNIQUE OF ACELLULAR DERMAL MATRIX FIXATION

AlloDerm is sutured to the anterior surface of the pectoralis major muscle with running 2-0 PDS sutures. Suturing commences at 12 o'clock and runs down either side of the allograft leaving an open access window laterally or inferiorly depending on the location of the mastectomy incision, to facilitate ease of implant insertion. For nipple-sparing mastectomies with lateral approaches, a lateral access window is used, whereas with the inferolateral approach, an inferior window is utilized. For skin-sparing mastectomies incorporating a central transverse incision, an inferior window is used (**Figure 14.1A and B**).

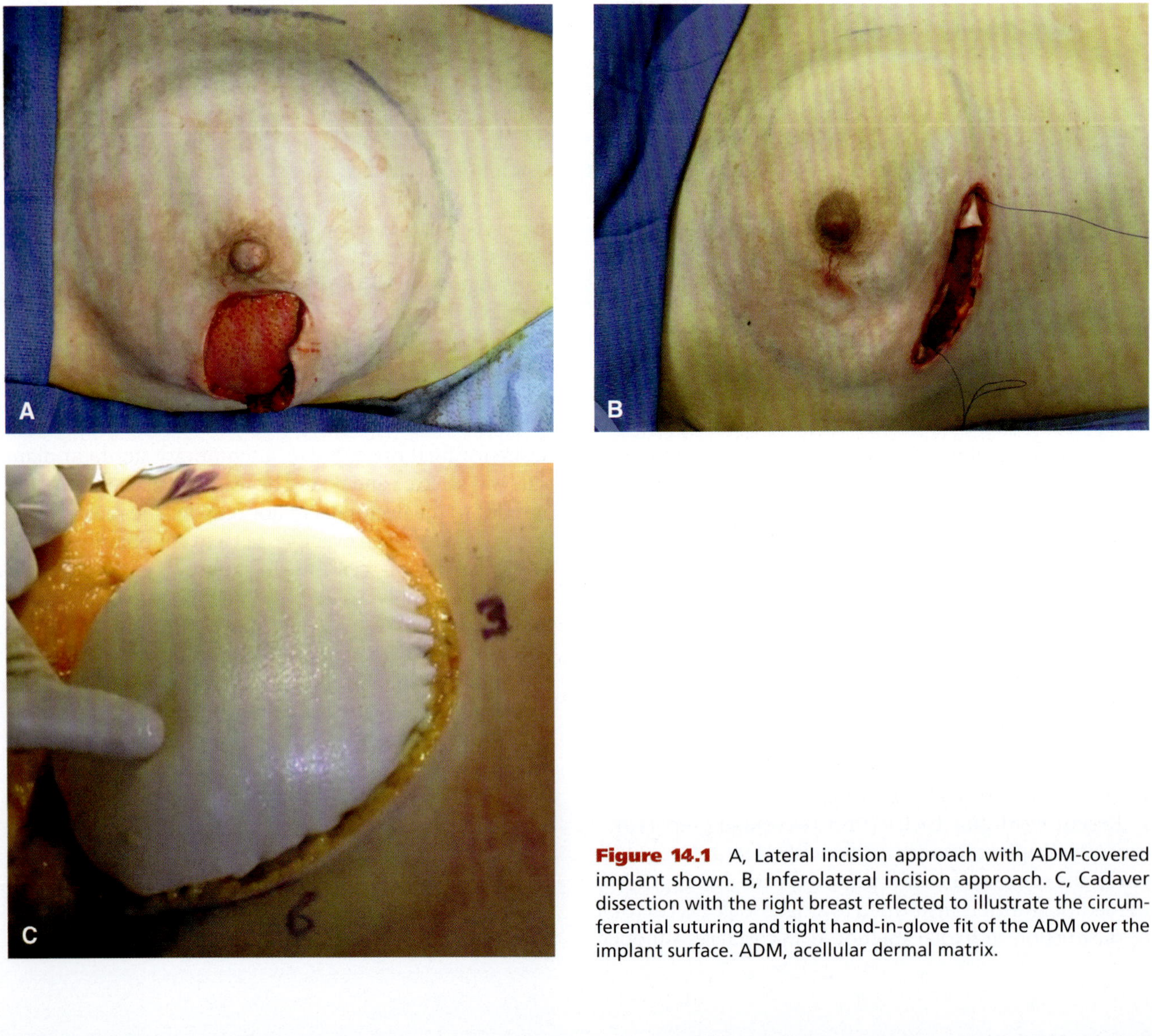

Figure 14.1 A, Lateral incision approach with ADM-covered implant shown. B, Inferolateral incision approach. C, Cadaver dissection with the right breast reflected to illustrate the circumferential suturing and tight hand-in-glove fit of the ADM over the implant surface. ADM, acellular dermal matrix.

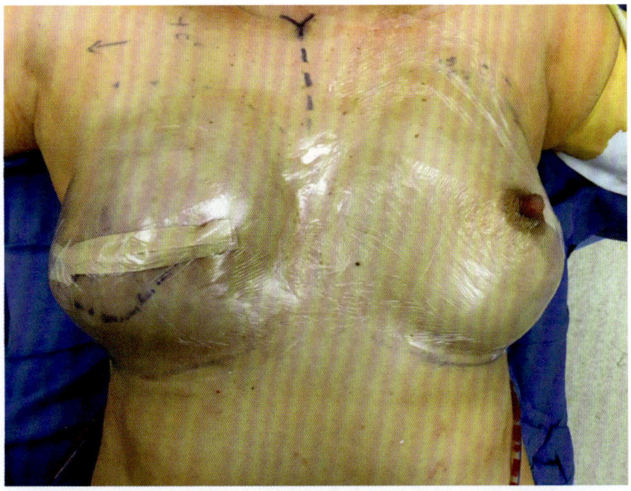

Figure 14.2 A completed prepectoral direct-to-implant reconstruction with skin-sparing mastectomy on the right and nipple-sparing mastectomy on the left indicating the Tegaderm bra dressing.

Adherence to Adams' 14-point biofilm reduction protocol[16] is central to this procedure, the key points of which are as follows:

- The pocket is irrigated with povidone-iodine followed by a triple antibiotic solution.
- The surgeon changes gloves and is the only individual to touch the device at any time.
- Insertion is facilitated with a Keller funnel (Keller Medical Inc., Stuart, FL) in all patients, allowing for no contact between the implant and skin.

All patients in this series were reconstructed with full height and full or extra full profile anatomic cohesive gel implants (Allergan), depending on their original breast shape and projection. The AlloDerm was pulled taut over the surface of the implant and sutured to the chest wall with the remaining tails of 2-0 PDS. Care was taken to ensure a tight "hand-in-glove" fit of the AlloDerm over the anterior surface of the implant to reduce risk of rotation (**Figure14.1C**). The pocket was again washed with antibiotic solution and the subcutaneous space was drained with a 15-French fully fluted, hubless channel drain. If full axillary dissection had been performed, an additional drain was placed to the axilla. Closure was performed in two layers with 3-0 Monocryl (Ethicon) and the entire reconstruction was covered with a gently applied Tegaderm "bra" to preserve the correct orientation of skin and nipple in relation to the underlying implant shape. Antibiotics were given perioperatively and then orally for 5 days postoperatively (**Figure 14.2**).

CLINICAL STUDY DATA ON PREPECTORAL DTI RECONSTRUCTION

Our study reported on a cohort of patients treated over a 30-month period; 73 breast reconstructions were performed in 50 consecutive patients using single-stage prepectoral implant placement with total anterior AlloDerm coverage (Allergan/LifeCell, Irvine, CA). All reconstructions were performed using anatomic cohesive gel full height and full or extra full profile textured surface implants (Allergan). All patients had either active breast cancer (stage <T2N-1M0pN1a) or were oncogene positive. Mastectomies were performed by two independent breast surgeons dedicated to practicing surgery of the breast only. Nipple-sparing and skin-sparing mastectomies were almost equally represented in this series. The senior author performed all of the reconstructions (**Tables 14.1 and 14.2**).

RESULTS

Seventy-three breasts in 50 patients were operated upon with an average BMI of 28.4 and average mastectomy weight of 551 g (range 184-1350 g). Nipple-sparing mastectomy was performed in 53% and skin sparing in 47%. Dedicated breast surgeons performed all mastectomies. Reconstruction was considered successful if patients achieved complete healing with a stable result at 8 weeks post mastectomy. Ninety-seven percent of all patients achieved stable breast reconstructions in one stage within these parameters. Minor delayed wound healing with superficial blistering occurred in six patients (8%) with no full-thickness losses, some of which were related to Steri-strip shear blisters. Treatment involved topical wound care. Delayed healing was not significantly associated with any of the usual risk factors in this study,

TABLE 14.1 PATIENT CHARACTERISTICS (*N* BREASTS = 73)

Variable	Average	Min	Max
Age	47	26	67
BMI	27	18	44
Mastectomy weight	551	184	1350
Days for drain removal	14	4	37
Follow-up weeks	48	13	103
Nipple to notch	25	17	39
IMF to nipple	9	5	19
Variable	**N**	**%**	
Nipple-sparing mastectomy	39	53	
Skin-sparing mastectomy	34	47	
Smoking history	23	32	
Preoperative radiation	1	1	
Postoperative radiation	7	10	
FX profile implant	48	66	
FF profile implant	23	32	

Abbreviations: BMI, body mass index; IMF, inframammary fold.

TABLE 14.2 POSTOPERATIVE COMPLICATIONS (*N* BREASTS = 73)

Complication	N	%
Minor upper pole contour deformity	35	47.9
Minor seroma	8	10.9
Rippling	9	12.3
Blistering requiring local wound care	6	8.2
Infection with implant loss	2	2.7
Cellulitis requiring PO antibiotics	2	2.7
Change in implant size	2	2.7
Explantation	2	2.7
Major seroma	1	1.3
Hematoma	1	1.3
Dehiscence with resuturing	1	1.3
Capsular contracture Grades III-IV	0	0
Necrosis requiring debridement	0	0
Animation deformity	0	0
Full-thickness necrosis	0	0

Abbreviation: PO, by mouth.

despite the fact that 32% of patients had a history of smoking, whereas 17% were active smokers just before mastectomy. All patients claimed to have stopped smoking postoperatively. One percent had preoperative radiation, whereas 10% underwent postoperative radiotherapy. There were two implant losses (2.7%), both related to infection. Two patients (2.7%) developed peri-incisional cellulitis treated with oral antibiotic therapy. One patient required in-office resuturing of a small central dehiscence after skin-sparing mastectomy and healed uneventfully.

Average drain duration to the subcutaneous plane was 13 days. One patient developed recurrent seroma requiring drain reinsertion by interventional radiology (1.2%). A further eight patients (10%) experienced early postoperative seromas occurring after drain removal, treated with aspiration in the office. There was only one hematoma (1.3%).

All nonradiated patients have maintained grade 1 capsules with a maximal follow-up of 32 months, with no signs of progressive capsular contracture (0%). One patient had undergone preoperative radiation therapy, whereas another eight patients underwent postoperative radiation therapy. All patients within the radiation category have maintained grades 1 to 2 capsular contracture, apart from one who has developed a grade 3 capsular contracture at 2 years (1.3%).

Fat grafting rates have been substantially reduced using this technique. When subpectoral round implant DTI reconstruction was performed, fat grafting was performed universally in all patients to reduce upper pole hollowing and rippling, as well as animation deformity. In this study, fat grafting was performed in 37% of patients for added upper pole volume or, to camouflage visible upper medial implant margins occurring in 47% of cases, a significantly reduced rate when compared with the author's almost 100% rate of upper pole fat grafting with round implants. Minimal rippling occurred in only nine patients (12%), which was much lower than expected, probably due to the stiffer consistency of the cohesive gel implants used. Bottoming out was predicted to be a problem by many skeptics, yet this has not been seen in any patients. There has been no animation deformity whatsoever. Patients noted very little discomfort or tightness and all returned to preoperative activity levels with full range of active shoulder motion. This is particularly noticeable in patients who have been converted to the prepectoral position from the subpectoral plane for animation deformity. Patient satisfaction has been high. There have been no breast cancer recurrences in any of the patients treated, irrespective of tumor location within the breast at 32 months longest follow-up (now almost 3 years at the time of writing), and no cases of implant-associated anaplastic large cell lymphoma. Malrotation occurred in one patient at 3 months, requiring reoperation. Two patients requested upsizing to a larger, higher profile implant at 12 to 15 months (**Figures 14.3 to 14.5**).

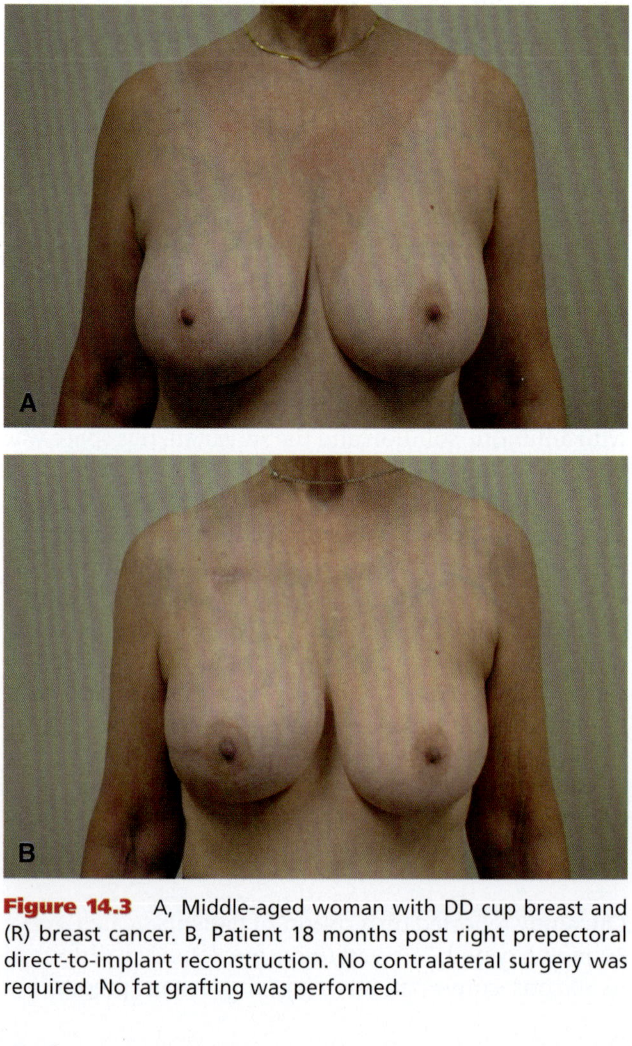

Figure 14.3 A, Middle-aged woman with DD cup breast and (R) breast cancer. B, Patient 18 months post right prepectoral direct-to-implant reconstruction. No contralateral surgery was required. No fat grafting was performed.

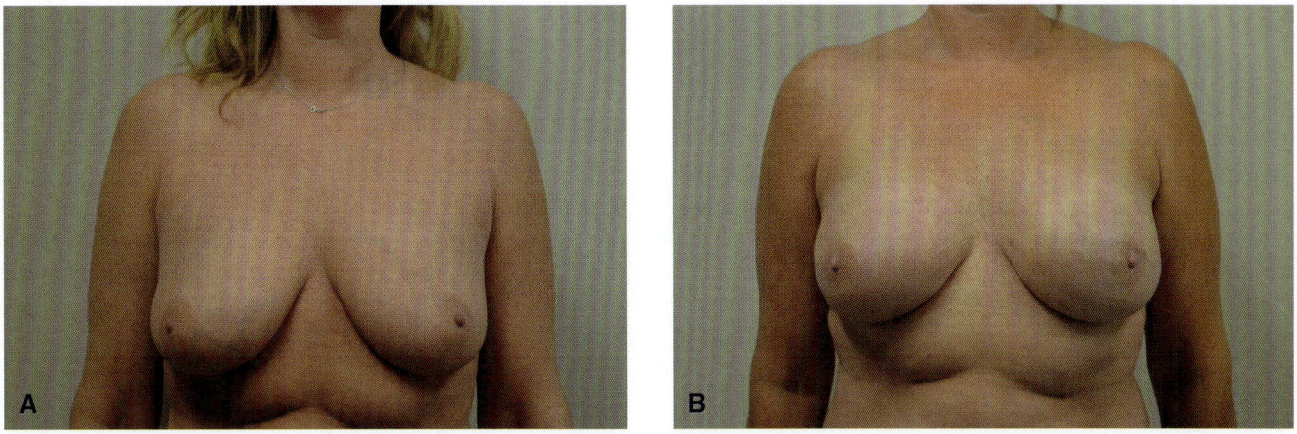

Figure 14.4 A, *BRCA*-positive young woman with C cup breasts. B, The patient 9 months after bilateral nipple-sparing mastectomies and immediate prepectoral direct-to-implant with cohesive gel implants.

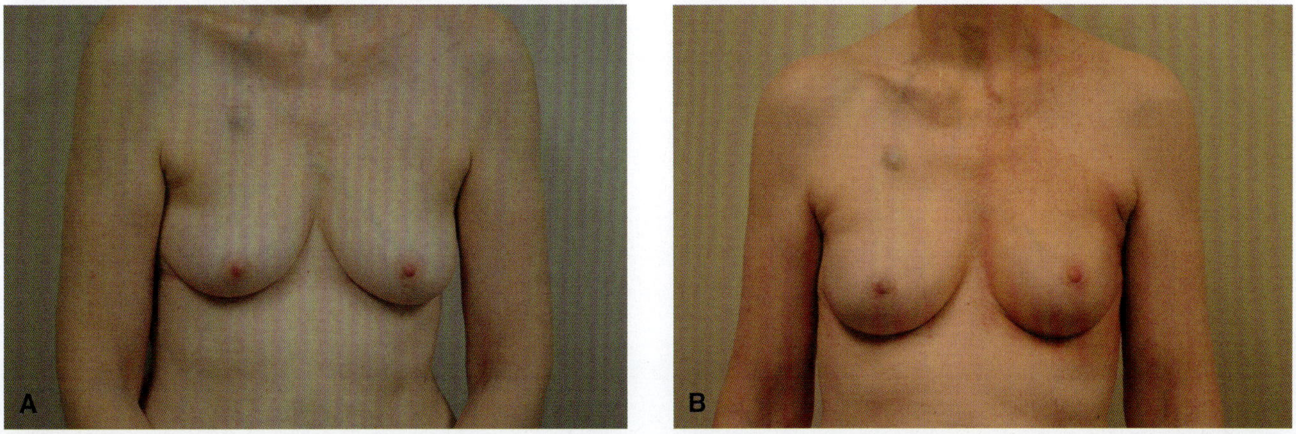

Figure 14.5 A, A 50-year-old woman with left breast cancer following neoadjuvant chemotherapy. B, The patient 6 months following left therapeutic and right prophylactic mastectomies with immediate prepectoral breast reconstruction with cohesive gel implants and postoperative radiation therapy to the left breast.

DISCUSSION

The first published report on prepectoral breast reconstruction with DTI insertion was by Snyderman[15] in 1971. Complications were unacceptably high in terms of poor shape, severe rippling due to the use of thin-shell, low-cohesivity gel implants and high capsular contracture rates. The procedure fell into disrepute as the subpectoral approach gained traction after Gruber's report in 1981.[17] In 1976, Radovan introduced the tissue expander, and since that time expander-based submuscular approaches have dominated implant-based reconstruction. In the interim, although skin- and nipple-sparing mastectomy techniques have almost eliminated the original purpose for which breast expansion was developed, tissue expansion continues to be widely used. With the skin domain issue resolved, surgeons have been left with attempting to improve aesthetic outcomes, capsular contracture rates, chest wall or shoulder discomfort, and animation deformity.[6,9,18-21]

Salzberg and Spear[1-3] introduced ADM use into dual-plane reconstruction, resulting in better shape, lower pole support, and reduced capsular contracture rates. Salzberg advocated single-stage submuscular DTI reconstruction and reported excellent outcomes with 2.3% contracture rates at 11 years.[3] It was this paper which triggered the senior author's interest in DTI prepectoral breast reconstruction. In addition, Maxwell's bioengineered prepectoral expander concept[22] and the data from Woo and Jacobson[13] prompted us to further investigate the possibility of performing single-stage prepectoral implant insertion with total anterior ADM coverage.

Why Anterior Acellular Dermal Matrix Coverage?

Many surgeons have asked why ADM is essential to this procedure. Given that we have newer implant technologies and understand biofilm formation better,[16] why not simply place an implant in the prepectoral space and save a considerable amount of money? The answer to this question lies in two major issues

1. ADM appears to play a role in lowering capsular contracture rates.

2. ADM controls implant position in an otherwise patulous mastectomy pocket, allowing for precise pocket shape control, which in turn shapes, the breast.

In a series of 19 breasts, Hammond[19] performed prepectoral conversion in an attempt to eliminate severe animation deformity by changing implants from a subpectoral to prepectoral position without routinely incorporating ADM. He reported successful elimination of animation, but 21% of patients developed capsular contracture within a relatively short time frame necessitating capsulectomy to achieve correction. Vardanian et al[23] reported 3.9% and 19.4% capsular contracture rates in patients undergoing reconstruction with and without ADM, respectively. Salibian et al[24] recently reported on prepectoral two-stage expander reconstruction without ADM, yielding 7.6% capsular contracture rates after 2 years. This supports the contention that despite the presumed use of biofilm reduction technique in these papers, the lack of full anterior ADM coverage may be crucial to successful longer-term outcomes.[25] The complete absence of capsular contracture in our series and that reported by Sigalove[12] supports this contention.

It goes without saying that the mastectomy pockets presented to us by breast surgeons are not precisely shaped to fit an implant. They extend far beyond the boundaries of our current implant profiles and breach the lateral mammary crease to access the axillary tail and approach sentinel nodes. When tabbed expanders are used, they can be sutured into position to control their place on the chest wall without ADM use if desired. Implants lack tabs and slide around inside the fresh mastectomy pocket if not constrained by some form of internal support such as ADM or deepithelialized "autoderm" flaps. ADM is therefore essential to allow controlled positioning of the implant within the fresh mastectomy pocket.

Seroma is a common occurrence following unreconstructed mastectomy, with rates varying between 15% and 45% being reported in the breast surgical literature. Seromas requiring aspiration occurred in 10% of our patients, one of which (1.3%) required reinsertion of a drain by interventional radiology. Longer drain retention to 3 weeks instead of the 2-week average we used may result in lower seroma rates.

In our series, we experienced a 2% implant loss rate secondary to true periprosthetic infection, which is similar to the 2% to 6% rates published in other series. We also saw an additional 4% incidence of cellulitis requiring oral antibiotic therapy with complete resolution. Two reports comparing retropectoral versus prepectoral DTI approaches using titanium mesh-wrapped implants found low complication rates in each group with comparable outcomes over 12 months, but found superior aesthetic outcomes in the prepectoral group. In their study, skin viability remained the primary determinant of initial success.[9,26] Recently, Vidya et al published a multicenter European study on 100 prepectoral breast reconstructions using total implant wrap with porcine ADM and also reported a 2% implant loss rate secondary to infection and 1% delayed healing with 17 month follow-up.[27,28]

Skin vascularity is a critical component of success in any breast reconstruction.[29] This is particularly true of the prepectoral single-stage approach. Skin necrosis is heavily dependent on gentle tissue handling and preservation of flap blood supply by the breast surgeon in addition to the impact of comorbid conditions.[29] We had observed, when performing dual-plane immediate DTI reconstruction in the past, that ICG imaging allowed us to perform the procedure in a wide range of patients exhibiting the typical risk factors associated with morbidity, namely, smoking, obesity, large-volume mastectomy, and prior radiation. In this study, we evaluated skin viability using ICG perfusion in the presence of a temporary prepectoral sizer. Although not foolproof, it represents the most accurate means for evaluating skin perfusion to date.[30-32] The decision to proceed with prepectoral DTI insertion was predicated entirely on the viability of the overlying skin covering an implant volume deemed adequate to achieve a good aesthetic outcome concordant with the patient's desire for breast size. Using this approach there were no full-thickness necrosis in our series, with an 8% incidence of minor delayed healing. Much to our surprise, there was no significant correlation with the presence of risk factors in most patients.

When we embarked on this study, many surgeons expressed concern that the stress imposed by a full volume implant pressing against the mastectomy skin envelope would result in increased skin necrosis. This has not been our experience when compared with our prior subpectoral expander or DTI experience. The weight of the implant beneath the skin is borne entirely by the ADM stretched over the device in a tight hand-in-glove fit and not by the skin. The skin is draped gently over the ADM, resulting in minimal stress from implant weight and gravity. By accounting for adequate skin perfusion for a given implant size, we have been able to proceed with this approach despite many patients falling into high-risk categories such as high BMI, smoking history, and large breast size.[6,29,33] This supports the contention that intraoperative skin perfusion assessment remains the most critical factor in determining success.

The claim that mastectomy skin thickness is a primary determinant of whether one should proceed with prepectoral reconstruction is invalid. Rather, it is cutaneous perfusion that determines outcome, not placing a numerical value on skin thickness alone. Skin thickness may be a concern for postoperative rippling, but even this has not been as common as we expected. The addition of ADM to thicken the soft-tissue cover is invaluable, and fat grafting can be performed as an additional adjunct.

The quality of aesthetic outcomes from this procedure has been excellent when compared with the senior author's personal experience of subpectoral reconstruction (whether two stage or single stage). This is due in part to the use of anatomic cohesive gel implants, which are less prone to rippling and provide excellent shape approaching that of the natural breast. The prepectoral location prevents muscle adherence to the skin, completely eliminating animation deformity and the compressive effect of the muscle on an underlying implant. The lack of animation deformity and minimal impact on upper extremity/shoulder function alone is extremely gratifying. In addition, prepectoral placement allows the surgeon complete control of the medial breast boundary, creating a softly contoured natural cleavage (see **Figure 14.3A and B**). One of the major aesthetic concerns of subpectoral implant placement, whether for reconstruction or cosmetic augmentation, has been the tendency to produce widely spaced breasts with poor cleavage definition. Natural cleavage and retention of lower pole fullness without skin retraction is a notable benefit of the prepectoral approach, creating superior aesthetic results in our hands. Bottoming out and pseudoptosis has not been seen in any patients after 3 years of careful follow-up. Long-term follow-up will be necessary to evaluate this further. Prepectoral reconstructions appear to tolerate radiation well and have better aesthetic and functional outcomes in our hands than did our radiated subpectoral implants (see **Figure 14.5A and B**).

Although this procedure is not for every patient, the outcomes suggest that in the face of adequate skin perfusion, immediate prepectoral DTI reconstruction provides outstanding results and spares patients the discomfort and inconvenience of expansion, as well as a mandatory second procedure. Although the cost of a larger sheet of ADM is an issue, paying for only one prosthetic device and one mandatory operation is more cost-effective in our institution than the two mandatory procedures and devices required of expander-implant reconstruction.

SUMMARY

Immediate prepectoral DTI reconstruction with intraoperative skin perfusion assessment appears to be a safe, reproducible procedure. It is applicable to a wider range of patient profiles than was previously anticipated. It eliminates animation deformity entirely, creating a comfortable, well-shaped reconstruction that appears to be maintained. Postoperative complication rates are low and similar to those of two-stage procedures. Prepectoral reconstructions tolerate postoperative radiation better in our hands than subpectoral reconstruction. Application of a 14-point biofilm reduction[16] protocol and the use of ADMs have rendered capsular contracture negligible. In our hands, subpectoral reconstruction has been completely replaced by prepectoral techniques. Data from multiple centers is increasingly supportive of prepectoral single-stage reconstruction becoming an established modality with excellent aesthetic as well as functional outcomes.

KEY REFERENCES

1. Spear SL, Parikh PM, Reisin E, Menon NG. Acellular dermis-assisted breast reconstruction. *Aesthetic Plast Surg.* 2008;32:418-425.
2. Salzburg CA, Ashikari AY, Koch RM, Chabner-Thompson E. An 8-year experience of direct-to-implant immediate breast reconstruction using human acellular dermal matrix (AlloDerm). *Plast Reconstr Surg.* 2011;127:514-524.
3. Salzberg CA, Ashikari AY, Berry C, Hunsicker LM. Acellular dermal matrix-assisted direct-to-implant breast reconstruction and capsular contracture: a 13-year experience. *Plast Reconstr Surg.* 2016;138(2):329-337.
4. Nahabedian MY. Acellular dermal matrices in primary breast reconstruction: principles, concepts and indications. *Plast Reconstr Surg.* 2012;130:44S-53S.
5. Namnoum JD. Expander/implant reconstructions with AlloDerm: recent experience. *Plast Reconstr Surg.* 2009;124(2):387-394.
6. Clarke-Pearson EM, Lin AM, Hertl C, Austen WG, Colwell AS. Revisions in implant-based breast reconstruction: how does direct-to-implant measure up? *Plast Reconstr Surg.* 2016;137(6):1690-1699.
7. Basta MN, Gerety PA, Serletti JM, Kovach SJ, Fischer JP. A systematic review and head-to-head meta-analysis of outcomes following direct-to-implant versus conventional two-stage implant reconstruction. *Plast Reconstr Surg.* 2015;136(6):1135-1144.
8. Berna G, Cawthorn SJ, Papaccio G, Balestrieri N. Evaluation of a novel breast reconstruction technique using the Braxon® acellular dermal matrix: a new muscle-sparing breast reconstruction. *ANZ J Surg.* 2014;87(6):493-498.
9. Bernini M, Calabrese C, Cecconi L, et al. Subcutaneous direct-to-implant breast reconstruction: surgical, functional, and aesthetic results after long-term follow-up. *Plast Reconstr Surg Glob Open.* 2016;3(12):e574.
10. Downs RK, Hedges K. An alternative technique for immediate direct-to-implant breast reconstruction—a case series. *Plast Reconstr Surg Glob Open.* 2016;4(7):e821.
11. Reitsamer R, Peintinger F. Prepectoral implant placement and complete coverage with porcine acellular dermal matrix: a new technique for direct-to-implant breast reconstruction after nipple-sparing mastectomy. *J Plast Reconstr Aesthet Surg.* 2015;68(2):162-167.
12. Sigalove S, Maxwell GP, Sigalove NM, et al. Prepectoral implant-based breast reconstruction: rationale, indications, and preliminary results. *Plast Reconstr Surg.* 2017;139(2):287-294.
13. Woo A, Harless C, Jacobson SR. Revisiting an old place: single surgeon experience on post-mastectomy subcutaneous implant based breast reconstruction. *Plast Reconstr Surg.* 2015;136(4 suppl):83.
14. Zhu L, Mohan AT, Abdelsattar JM, et al. Comparison of subcutaneous versus submuscular expander placement in the first stage of immediate breast reconstruction. *J Plast Reconstr Aesthet Surg.* 2016;69(4):e77-e86.
15. Snyderman RK, Guthrie RH. Reconstruction of the female breast following radical mastectomy. *Plast Reconstr Surg.* 1971;6:565-567.
16. Adams WP, Culbertson EJ, Deva, AK, et al. Macrotextured breast implants with defined steps to minimize bacterial contamination around the device: experience in 42,000 implants. *Plast Reconstr Surg.* 2017;140:427-431.
17. Gruber RP, Kahn RA, Lash H, Maser MR, Apfelberg DB, Laub DR. Breast reconstruction following mastectomy: a comparison of submuscular and subcutaneous techniques. *Plast Reconstr Surg.* 1981;67(3):312-317.
18. Scheflan M, Colwell AS. Tissue reinforcement in implant-based reconstruction. *Plast Reconstr Surg Glob Open.* 2014;2(8):e192.
19. Hammond DC, Schmitt WP, O'Connor EA. Treatment of breast animation deformity in implant-based reconstruction with pocket change to the subcutaneous position. *Plast Reconstr Surg.* 2015;135:1540-1544.
20. Hammond DC, O'Connor EA, Scheer JR. Total envelope fat grafting. a novel approach in breast reconstruction. *Plast Reconstr Surg.*2015;135:691-694.

21. Cheng A, Lakhiani C, Saint-Cyr M. Treatment of capsular contracture using complete implant coverage by acellular dermal matrix: a novel technique. *Plast Reconstr Surg*. 2013;132(3):519-529.
22. Maxwell PG, Gabriel A. Bioengineered breast: concept, technique, and preliminary results. *Plast Reconstr Surg*. 2010;126: 1842-1847.
23. Vardanian AJ, Clayton JL, Roostaeian J, et al. Comparison of implant-based immediate breast reconstruction with and without acellular dermal matrix. *Plast Reconstr Surg*. 2011;128:403e-410e.
24. Salibian AH, Harness JK, Mowlds DS. Staged suprapectoral expander/implant reconstruction without acellular dermal matrix following nipple-sparing mastectomy. *Plast Reconstr Surg*. 2017;139(1):30-39.
25. Basu CB, Leong M, Hicks MJ. Acellular cadaveric dermis decreases the inflammatory response in capsule formation in reconstructive breast surgery. *Plast Reconstr Surg*. 2010;126(6):1842-1847.
26. Casella D, Bernini M, Bencini L, et al. TiLoop® Bra mesh used for immediate breast reconstruction: comparison of retropectoral and subcutaneous implant placement in a prospective single institution series. *Eur J Plast Surg*. 2014;37(11):599-604.
27. Vidya R, Iqbal FM. A guide to prepectoral breast reconstruction: a new dimension to implant-based breast reconstruction. *Clin Breast Cancer*. 2017;17(4):266-271.
28. Vidya R, Masià J, Cawthorn S, et al. Evaluation of the effectiveness of the prepectoral breast reconstruction with Braxon dermal matrix: first multicenter European report on 100 cases. *Breast J*. 2017;23(6):670-676.
29. Qureshi AA, Broderick KP, Belz J, et al. Uneventful versus successful reconstruction and outcome pathways in implant-based breast reconstruction with acellular dermal matrices. *Plast Reconstr Surg*. 2016;138(2):173e-183e.
30. Phillips BT, Lanier ST, Conkling N, et al. Intraoperative perfusion techniques can accurately predict mastectomy skin flap necrosis in breast reconstruction: results of a prospective trial. *Plast Reconstr Surg*. 2012;129(5):778e-788e.
31. Munabi NC, Olorunnipa OB, Goltsman D, Rohde CH, Ascherman JA. The ability of intra-operative perfusion mapping with laser-assisted indocyanine green angiography to predict mastectomy flap necrosis in breast reconstruction: a prospective trial. *J Plast Reconstr Aesthet Surg*. 2014;67(4):449-455.
32. Duggal CS, Madni T, Losken A. An outcome analysis of intraoperative angiography for postmastectomy breast reconstruction. *Aesthet Surg J*. 2014;34(1):61-65.
33. Becker H, Lind JG II, Hopkins EG. Immediate implant-based prepectoral breast reconstruction using a vertical incision. *Plast Reconstr Surg Glob Open*. 2015;3(6):e412.

CHAPTER **15**

ANTERIOR/POSTERIOR ACELLULAR DERMAL MATRIX COVERAGE IN PREPECTORAL PROSTHETIC BREAST RECONSTRUCTION

Steven R. Sigalove, Maurice Y. Nahabedian, Steven R. Jacobson, G. Patrick Maxwell, and Allen Gabriel

KEY POINTS

- A variety of techniques are covered in this section, with some being on label and others off label.
- Covering both anterior and posterior surfaces with ADM does inhibit capsule formation and may have implications in formation of capsular contracture.
- Perforated ADM on the lower pole is critical for these cases.

INTRODUCTION

Prepectoral prosthetic breast reconstruction has seen an ever-growing revival during the past 5 to 10 years. What started off in the early 1970s as primitively placing a fixed volume silicone implant directly below thin mastectomy skin flaps that yielded high complication rates and failures has evolved into a highly successful and rewarding procedure for both surgeon and patient. Using the Bioengineered Breast Concept described by Dr. Patrick Maxwell, we have furthered the reconstructive process, using materials such as acellular dermal matrices (ADMs), form-stable silicone gel implants, and autologous fat grafting. These sophisticated materials, combined with improved mastectomy skin flaps, technology to objectively assess perfusion, and a true team approach connecting plastic surgeons, breast surgeons, medical oncologists, and radiation oncologists, have given our patients new and exciting hope regarding their aesthetic and functional outcomes following mastectomy with reconstruction. Prepectoral prosthetic reconstruction has become the workhorse of my prosthetic practice. Patients are generally extremely happy, their recoveries are shorter, and their aesthetic outcomes are routinely excellent. Issues that lead us to the rebirth of prepectoral reconstruction such as hyperanimation deformities, chronic pain, and muscle spasms, as well as aesthetic considerations such as lack of cleavage, diminished projection, and breast "tightness" are no longer problems associated with prosthetic-based breast reconstruction. By not involving the pectoralis major muscle in our reconstruction, we are eliminating significant surgical morbidity, minimizing distracting forces on the implant, which, over time, manifest as soft-tissue displacement, and are minimizing functional impairment.

RATIONALE FOR PREPECTORAL PLACEMENT

Subpectoral prosthesis placement with partial muscle coverage, with or without ADM, is currently the standard technique for implant-based breast reconstruction. Many of the disadvantages/complications of subcutaneous implant placement (implant visibility, palpability, and exposure; and capsular contracture) are mitigated with the subpectoral technique because of the thicker coverage provided by the muscle. The elevation of the muscle, however, has introduced its own set of problems. A major concern is functional impairment of the muscle, particularly the adduction, anteversion, and inward rotation of the upper limb. In addition, animation deformities caused by muscle contraction, chest tightness, pain, and muscle spasm are other significant concerns. Furthermore, subpectoral placement creates an unnatural state because the natural breast is anterior to the muscle. Despite these concerns, patients who have had dual-plane reconstruction with ADM can have aesthetically pleasing results; but with any contraction of the pectoralis major, animation deformity on the chest can immediately be noted. Fat grafting is utilized as a means of establishing a natural gliding surface between the thin mastectomy flap and the pectoralis/ADM interface, which decreases the pain and the visual deformities associated with the scarred mastectomy flap being pulled by the pectoralis major. This ameliorates, but does not eliminate animation deformity, and some degree of animation remains.

As a further means to alleviate muscle-related issues, surgeons have resorted to moving the implant from the subpectoral back to the prepectoral (subcutaneous) position in certain revision cases. Using the bioengineered breast concept has overcome the original limitations of subcutaneous placement and has greatly improved the aesthetic outcomes. Using form-stable implants and reinforcing the entire breast pocket with ADM to mimic muscle coverage and use of fat grafting to enhance the thickness and the gliding ability of the subcutaneous pocket has produced consistent outcomes with resolution of animation deformity and implant-related complications in appropriately selected patients.

Prepectoral Device Placement

Prepectoral breast reconstruction offers the patient several short and relatively painless outpatient procedures with minimal recovery time. By not dividing and elevating the pectoralis major muscle (**Figure 15.1**), primary prepectoral reconstruction can be performed as an outpatient procedure, particularly with the addition of regional anesthetic nerve blockade. Patients have minimal pain postoperatively, and use of opioids for analgesia has been reduced considerably. Many patients are placed on nonsteroidal anti-inflammatory medications and do quite well. Owing to the relatively painless recovery, patient satisfaction is quite high.

Patients who have undergone prepectoral reconstruction also do not complain of chest tightness, chronic pain, pectoralis major muscle spasms, or hyperanimation deformities. Hyperanimation deformities were challenging to correct, and patients were dissatisfied with the appearance and even the pain associated with it. These findings were often present in women who have undergone dual-plane or full muscle coverage breast reconstruction; and before the rebirth of prepectoral breast reconstruction, these patients would be either salvaged with autologous reconstruction or they would opt to have their devices removed and would forego any reconstruction due to persistent pain and discomfort.

With prepectoral breast reconstruction, aesthetic outcomes are, on the whole, quite impressive. Without the distracting forces of the pectoralis major muscle negatively acting on the implant, the device is truly shaping the reconstructed breast. In addition, over long periods of time, the pectoralis major muscle does not exert a force on the device, which historically has led to inframammary fold

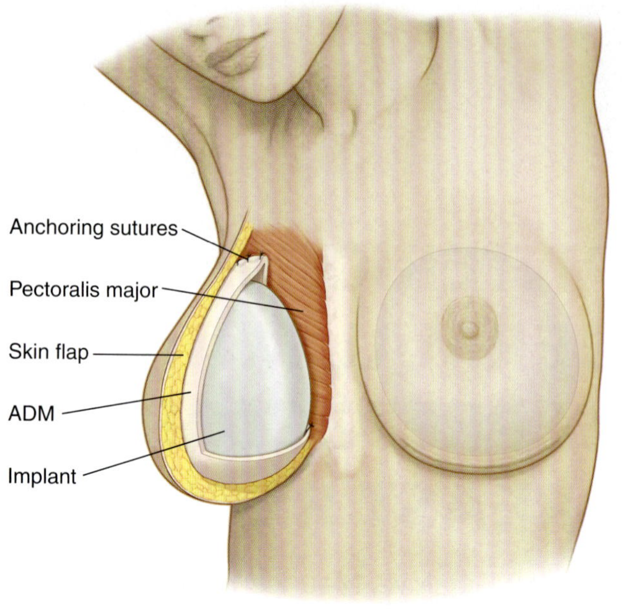

Figure 15.1 Prepectoral reconstruction with anterior acellular dermal matrix coverage.

(IMF) malposition, bottoming out, or lateral migration. The cleavage lines of the reconstructed breast are more predictable, because the medial insertion of the pectoralis major muscle on the sternum does not limit the medial extent of the device. This, combined with autologous fat grafting, has enabled the reconstructive breast surgeon to create beautiful and highly predictable aesthetic outcomes.

The concept of prepectoral prosthetic breast reconstruction centers on placement of a device (tissue expander or implant) directly onto the pectoralis major muscle following mastectomy. The device is placed into the prepectoral space, which has been inset with ADM, or it is placed as a prefabricated ADM–device construct. This chapter focuses on the various techniques of ADM–device assembly.

OPTIONS IN ADM–DEVICE ASSEMBLY

Lower Pole Gutter with Anterior Reinforcement (On Label)

This is the classic on-label use of ADM in prepectoral breast reconstruction. In this application, the ADM is used both to create a gutter at the IMF and to support the overlying anterior mastectomy skin flaps. This technique is straightforward and is easily performed during either single- or two-stage prosthetic reconstruction, particularly when the mastectomy has been performed through a skin-sparing, breast-splitting incision, because the exposure is excellent.

This on-label technique is often used, because it only requires one piece of ADM per side, minimizing product costs. Once the decision has been made to proceed with prepectoral reconstruction, the ADM is first rinsed in normal saline and is then fenestrated with a #11 blade (some

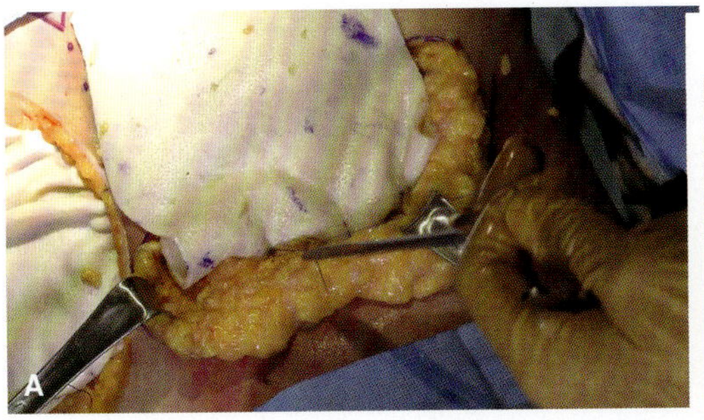

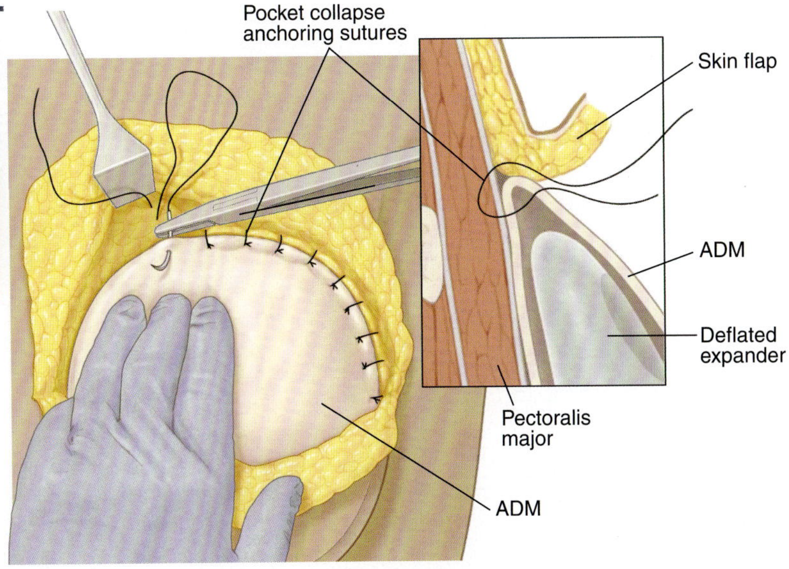

Figure 15.2 A and B, Securing the ADM with posterior ADM cuff. ADM, acellular dermal matrix.

institutions have preperforated ADM already). The ADM is then cut to size, depending on the device measurements—an extra 3 cm is added for device height to allow for a 3-cm cuff, which will be created at the IMF. The last 3 cm of ADM is placed directly onto the pectoralis major muscle at the IMF, with the dermal side down, because the remaining portion is folded and brought superiorly, creating a fold or gutter at the IMF. Using a 2-0 PDS suture, interrupted bites are taken on the back of this fold in a full-thickness through and through manner, extending from the ADM to the IMF. Care is taken to ensure the suture passes through the surfaces of both the ADM and the chest wall (muscle, periosteum, or fascia) at the fold. Once the gutter has been created, the tissue expander or implant is placed directly onto the pectoralis major muscle (tissue expander is sutured to the muscle via suture tabs and is filled with 120 cc of air). The ADM is then draped superiorly over the device, and the 12 o'clock suture is placed first, insetting the ADM directly to the pectoralis muscle. Care is taken to ensure that the ADM is affixed just distal to the superior aspect of the device. There should be little to no space between the edge of the device and the ADM. The remainder of the ADM is trimmed if needed and is inset to the pectoralis muscle with interrupted 2-0 PDS suture. Two 15 French hubless Blake drains are then inserted into the pocket, one in the upper and one in the lower pole, both between the ADM and the skin flaps. The incision is closed in two layers. In two-staged reconstruction, air is then injected into the expander to obliterate dead space and to maximize ADM-skin flap adherence. The end point of intraoperative air expansion is skin tension. After this, the skin flaps are reassessed with the skin perfusion assessment device (Indocyanine green [ICG] in my practice) to ensure that no ischemia has been created. The incisions are dressed with negative pressure wound management devices.

In **Figure 15.2**, a 16 × 20 cm piece of ADM has been trimmed to fit the dimensions of the pocket and has been inset to the pectoralis major muscle at the IMF, leaving a 3-cm cuff of ADM that will adhere to the muscle. This 3-cm cuff will prevent dehiscence at the fold as expansion progresses. An end-to-end inset of the ADM to the fold leads to dehiscence and thus loss of lower pole support. By maintaining the cuff, dehiscence is prevented, and lower pole support is thus maintained (**Figures 15.2A and B, 15.3**).

After this, the tissue expander is sutured directly to the pectoralis major muscle via the suture tabs (**Figure 15.4**). The ADM is draped superiorly and is trimmed and inset to the pectoralis major muscle with absorbable sutures (**Figure 15.5**).

Advantages of On-Label Techniques

This technique is an on-label method of insetting the ADM during prepectoral breast reconstruction. It requires only one piece of ADM per side; thus, costs are minimized when

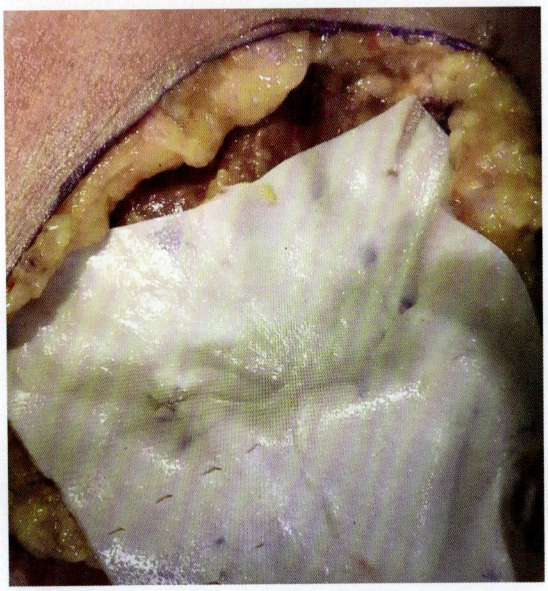

Figure 15.3 Through and through bites along the back of the acellular dermal matrix create a 3- to 4-cm cuff at the inframammary fold.

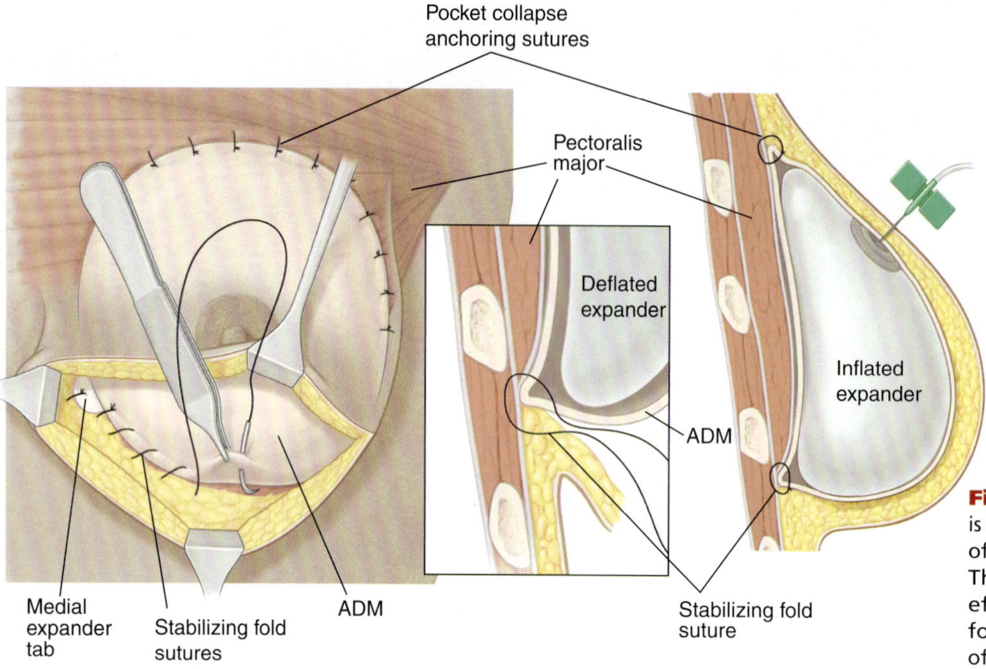

Figure 15.4 A 3- to 4-cm cuff is seen along the anterior surface of the pectoralis major muscle. The cuff will create a gutter effect at the inframammary fold, which reduces incidence of bottoming out.

compared to other types of inset, which is discussed later. This technique is straightforward, and the novice prepectoral reconstructive breast surgeon will quickly gain comfort with this technique. This technique is particularly useful during skin-sparing mastectomies or Wise-pattern mastectomies because the exposure is excellent, which facilitates inset. The gutter created at the IMF reduces the risks of fold malposition, and, thus, fold malposition with this technique is rare.

Disadvantages of On-Label Techniques

This technique (unlike others which are discussed) requires completion of the mastectomy before beginning and can take longer to perform than some of the other techniques. In addition, only the anterior surface of the device is covered by ADM; therefore, having no posterior coverage can lead to capsule formation. This fact, in and of itself, may not necessarily be a disadvantage, but there may be negative implications because of lack of capsule that are discussed in the final section of this chapter.

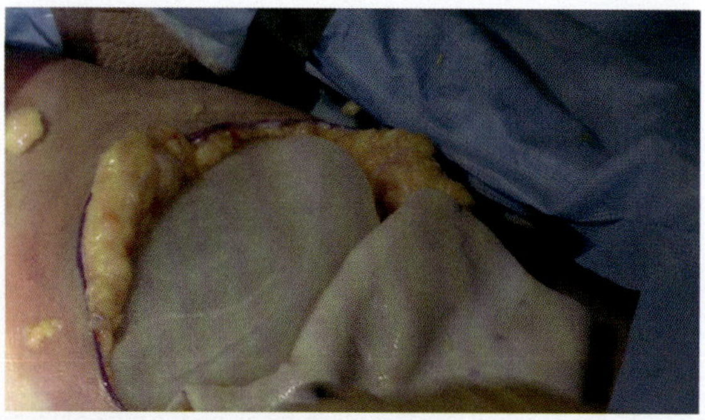

Figure 15.5 Tissue expander placed into pocket and tabs are sewn to the pectoralis major or acellular dermal matrix.

Prefabricated ADM–Device Construct (Off Label)

Another method of utilizing the ADM in prepectoral reconstruction is by creating an ex vivo prefabricated construct on the back table. This technique has gained popularity because of its ease of use as well as its efficient use of time; besides, this can be performed simultaneously with the mastectomy. On the basis of the size of the device, either one or two pieces of ADM can be used to "wrap" the expander (or implant). With a single piece of ADM, a "wonton" method is used; and if two pieces are used, a "ravioli" method is used.

When using devices up to 500 mL, typically a single sheet of 16 × 20 cm extra-thick ADM can be used to wrap the device easily. This technique is known as a "wonton" technique because the final construct resembles a wonton. With this technique, the ADM is first fenestrated with a #11 scalpel blade or preperforated sheets are utilized. The ADM is placed on the back table with the dermal side down. The device is then injected with 120 mL of air (if an expander is used) and is placed onto the center of the ADM facing down. The four corners are then brought together with a 4-0 chromic suture on FS-2 needle, creating four new corners. These new corners are then brought toward the center and are secured to the ADM with 4-0 chromic suture, creating eight dog-ears. The dog-ears are then trimmed, and the ADM is closed to itself. The suture tabs are then exteriorized and the device is inset to the pectoralis muscle via the exposed suture tabs with 2-0 PDS suture. Two 15 French Blake drains are then placed, one in the upper pole and one in the lower pole, and the incision is closed in layers. Air is then inflated into the expander to the point of mild tension. The flaps are reassessed for perfusion to ensure that no ischemia was created. Negative pressure is used to dress the incisions followed by compression foam in the upper outer quadrant.

Ravioli Technique (Off Label)

When devices of greater than 500 mL are used, a ravioli two-piece technique is often used. Once again, this ADM–device construct is prefabricated on the back table while the mastectomy is being performed. Once the device has been selected, two 16 × 20 cm pieces of extra-thick ADM are fenestrated. In situations where skin flap perfusion is modest, a thinner piece of ADM will be used anteriorly. The posterior sheet is placed with the dermal side down on the back table. The device is then placed directly in the center of the ADM and if an expander is used, it is inflated with 120 mL of air. The ADM is trimmed around the periphery with curved Mayo scissors. The second piece of ADM is placed directly on top of the device and is similarly trimmed peripherally. The two pieces are then sewn together using a 4-0 chromic FS-2 needle in a running manner, creating a seam around the periphery of the construct. The construct is then placed directly onto the pectoralis major muscle and is affixed directly to the underlying muscle with interrupted 2-0 PDS suture, anchoring the seam directly to the muscle. Care is taken to precisely inset the ADM at the IMF. If done through an inframammary incision, the construct is inset from the 4 o'clock to 8 o'clock position. Two drains are then placed, both between the ADM and the skin flaps, one in the upper pole and one in the lower pole. The incision is closed in layers, and the expander (if used) is inflated with air until mild skin tension is noted. The skin flaps are reassessed with ICG to ensure that no ischemia has been created. Negative pressure is used to dress the incisions followed by compression foam in the upper outer quadrant (**Figures 15.6** and **15.7A-E**).

Advantages of Off-Label Techniques

Prefabricated ADM–device constructs are beneficial because they are straightforward to prepare, and, most importantly, they can be devised on the back table while the mastectomy is being performed. This maximizes operative efficiency and reduces operating room time for both the patient and the surgeon significantly. These constructs can be easily inserted through any incision; and particularly when used in conjunction with a Keller funnel, even an inframammary incision is relatively straightforward.

In addition, by covering both the anterior and posterior surfaces of the device, there is no capsule formed. The

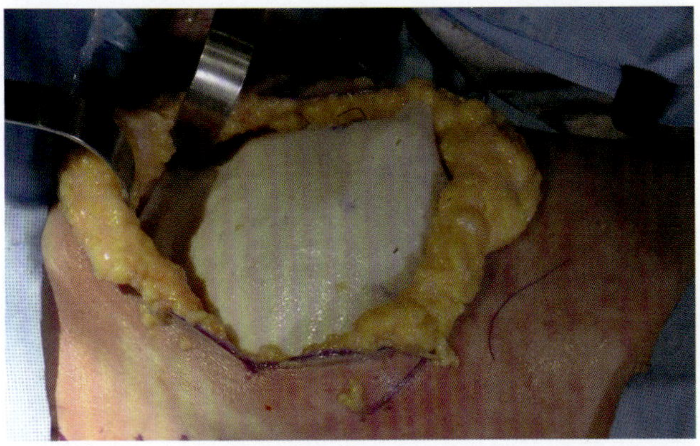

Figure 15.6 Acellular dermal matrix is draped over the expander and secured.

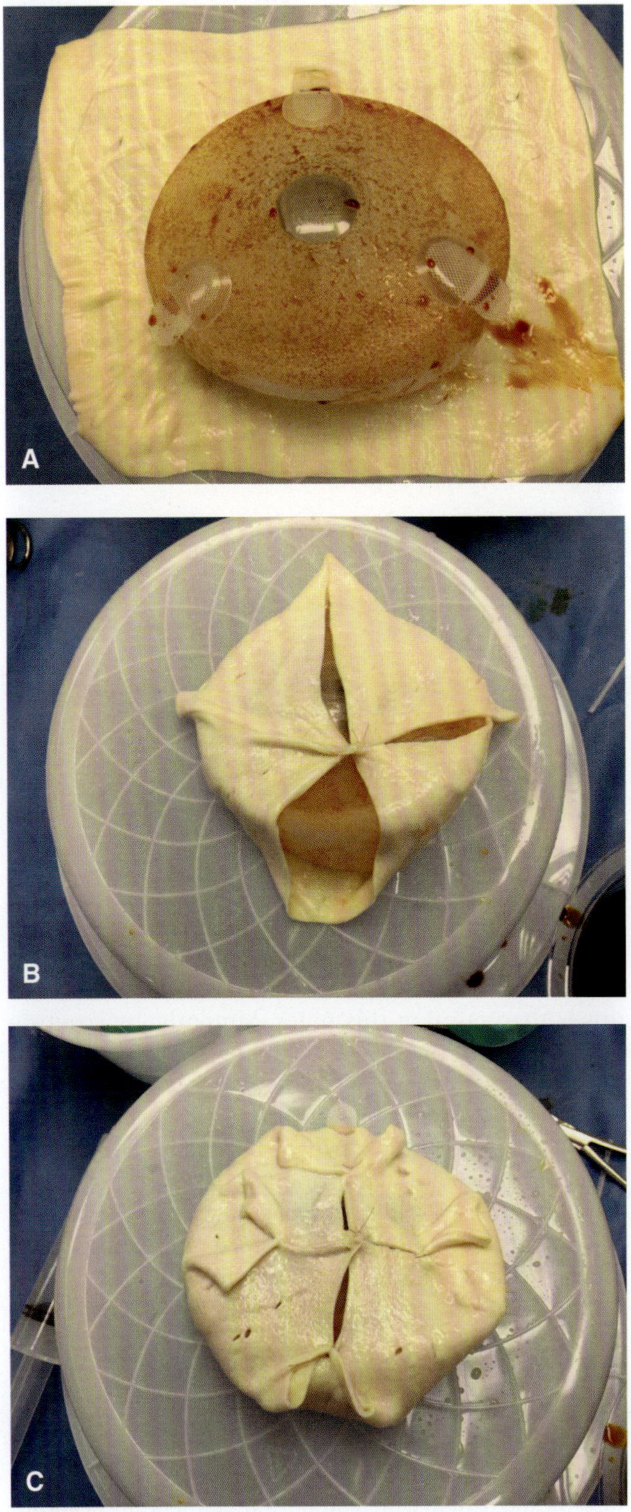

Figure 15.7 A-E, Complete wrap of acellular dermal matrix on the back table before insertion into the mastectomy pocket. This is an off-label technique.

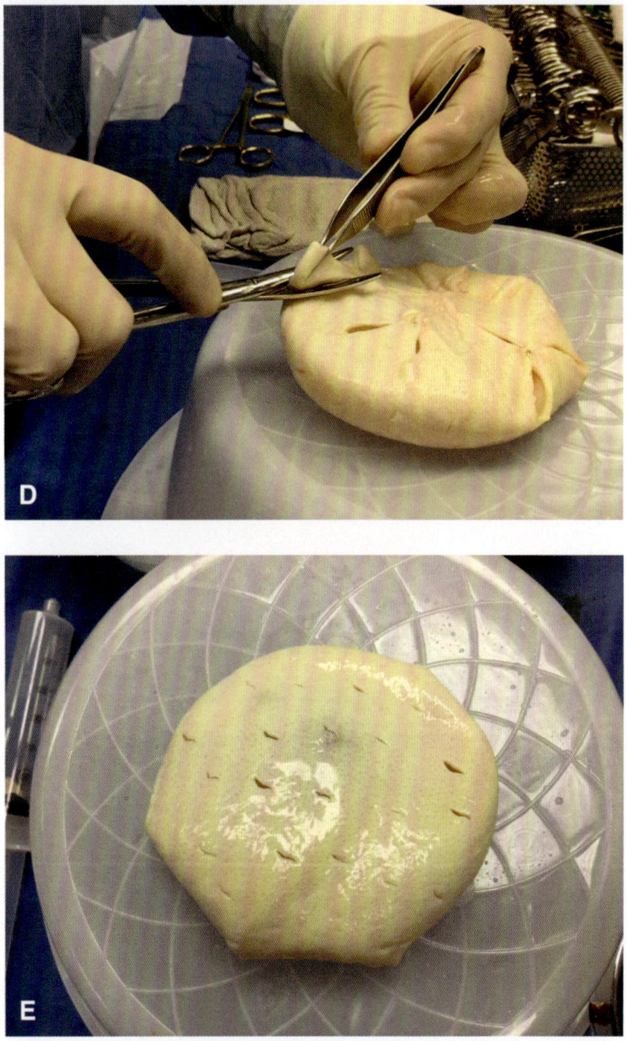

Figure 15.7 *(continued)*

lack of capsule has potential implications such as reduced capsular contracture as well as theoretically mitigating chances for developing capsular lymphoma; however, this is theoretical at this point. Similarly, by covering both aspects of the device, in the presence of infection or contamination, we feel quite comfortable salvaging many such cases by removing the ADM and device, and leaving a new device on top of the pectoralis major muscle to prevent skin contraction and to minimize autologous salvage in these settings. We have titled this the "naked expander" technique in the presence of contamination and it is elucidated in another chapter.

DISADVANTAGES OF OFF-LABEL TECHNIQUES

These off-label techniques, although efficient and provide surgeon and patient with reproducible aesthetically beautiful outcomes, are also more costly, because two pieces may be utilized per side, increasing overall case costs significantly. We believe that although increased, these additional costs are outweighed by the procedure's inherent value, which is described in great detail in another chapter.

Both the wonton and the ravioli techniques facilitate prepectoral reconstruction through any type of incision. These ex vivo techniques are considered "off label" because they are not truly supporting the native tissue and are being used in conjunction with a device (**Figures 15.8-15.11**).

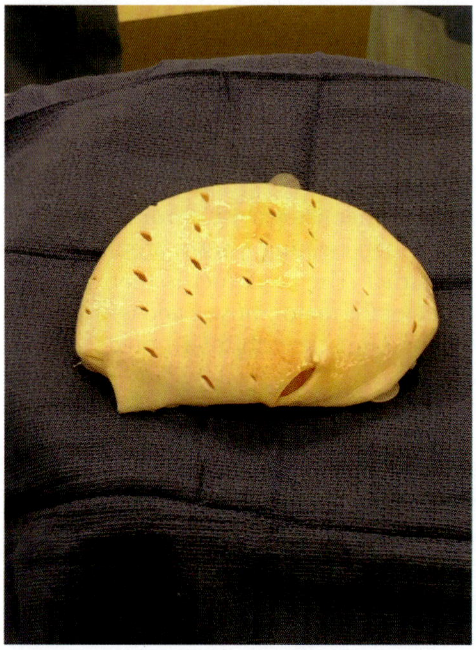

Figure 15.8 Complete wrap of acellular dermal matrix on the back table before insertion into the mastectomy pocket. This is an off-label technique.

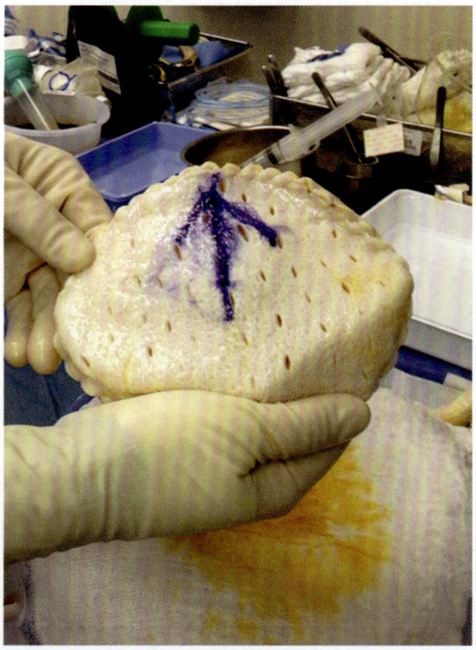

Figure 15.9 Complete wrap of tissue expander with acellular dermal matrix using "wonton" technique, anterior surface.

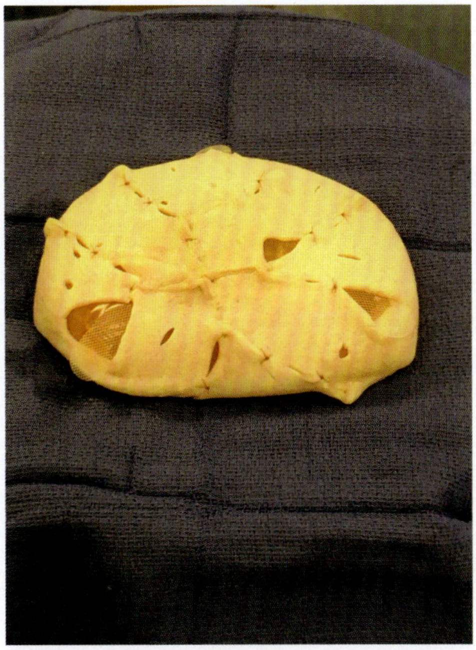

Figure 15.10 Posterior surface of completely wrapped expander with perforated acellular dermal matrix; see exteriorized suture tabs.

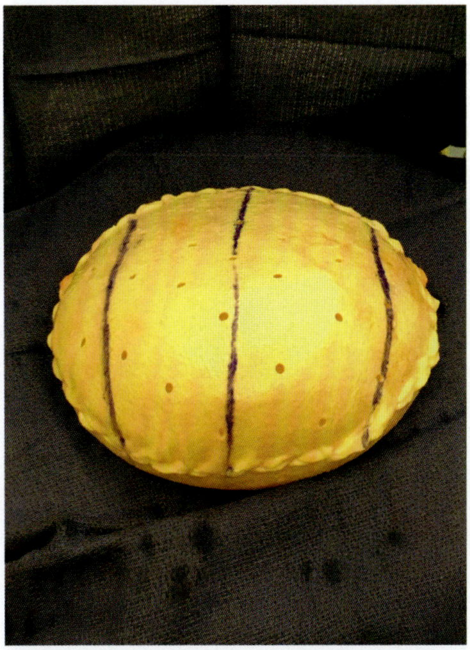

Figure 15.11 Anterior surface of wrapped expander with perforated acellular dermal matrix.

Once the prefabricated construct has been properly inset, the device is filled with air. Air has been used in the immediate setting of the mastectomy to reduce the weight and trauma on the fresh mastectomy skin flaps. In my practice, I use air throughout the entire expansion process, because it is simpler, more efficient, and more comfortable for the patients. The only time air is exchanged for saline is for patients undergoing postmastectomy external beam radiotherapy or if they are traveling by air (**Figure 15.12**).

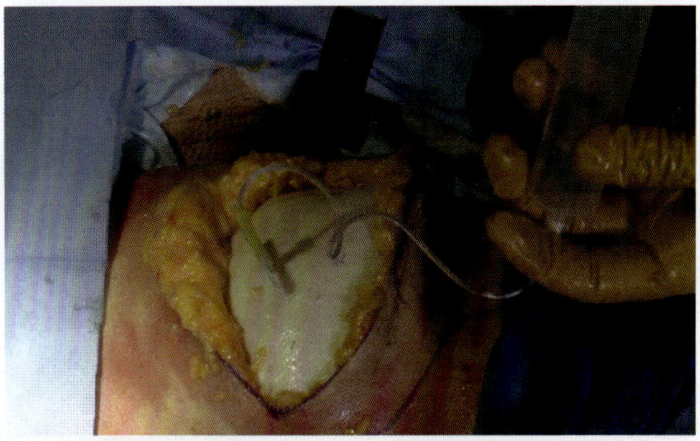

Figure 15.12 Air being placed into the tissue expander.

CASE EXAMPLES

CASE 1

This 33-year-old woman underwent a right nipple-sparing mastectomy with sentinel lymph node biopsy. She requested immediate reconstruction. Owing to her ptosis, prepectoral reconstruction with tissue expander and ADM was performed. Three months later, she underwent second-stage reconstruction with a right capsulotomy, tissue expander removal, placement of a highly cohesive anatomic silicone gel implant, and autologous fat grafting. The patient did not wish to undergo any form of symmetry procedure on the contralateral breast. This case illustrates the power of prepectoral reconstruction—particularly in a unilateral reconstruction—to mimic the natural ptosis of the native breast. The patient is seen 12 months following her mastectomy. She is overall quite pleased with her natural result, particularly without having to undergo a symmetry procedure on the left breast (**Figures 15.13-15.17**).

CASE 2

This 25-year-old woman underwent bilateral nipple-sparing mastectomies for left-sided invasive breast cancer. The patient carried the genetic mutation for breast cancer (*BrCA*-1) and underwent prophylactic right mastectomy with a left sentinel lymph node biopsy. She underwent two-stage reconstruction with placement of moderate-height/extra-projection tissue expanders with ADM. She underwent second-stage bilateral reconstruction

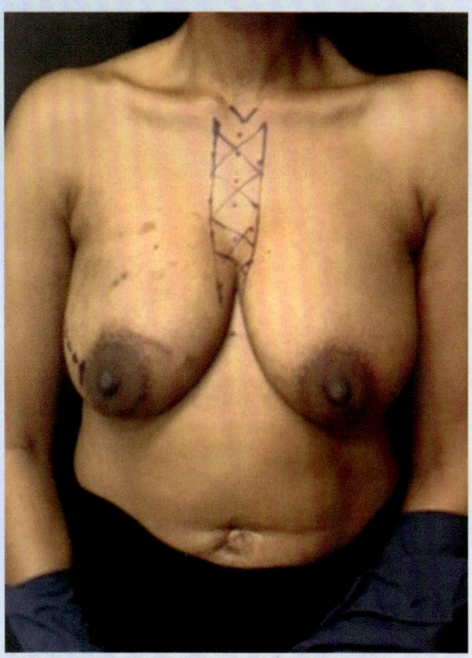

Figure 15.13 Anterior view of preoperative markings.

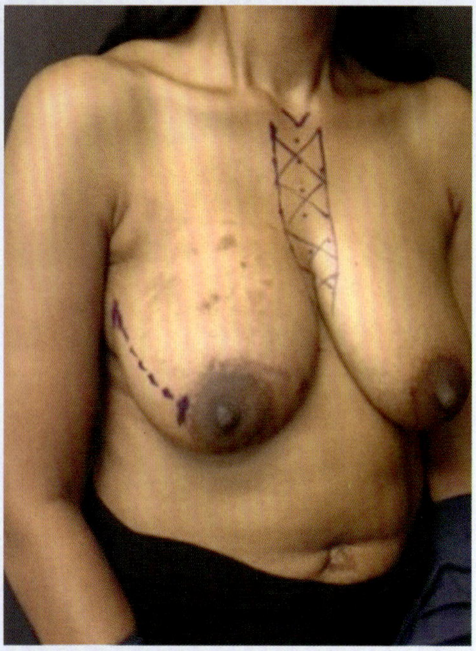

Figure 15.14 Antero-Lateral view of preoperative markings demonstrating a lateral incisional approach.

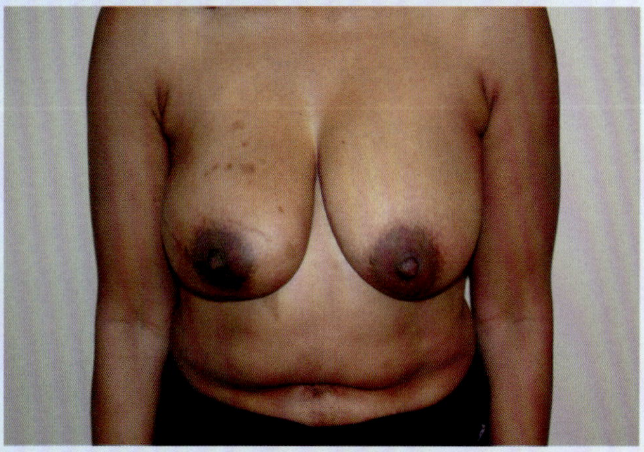

Figure 15.15

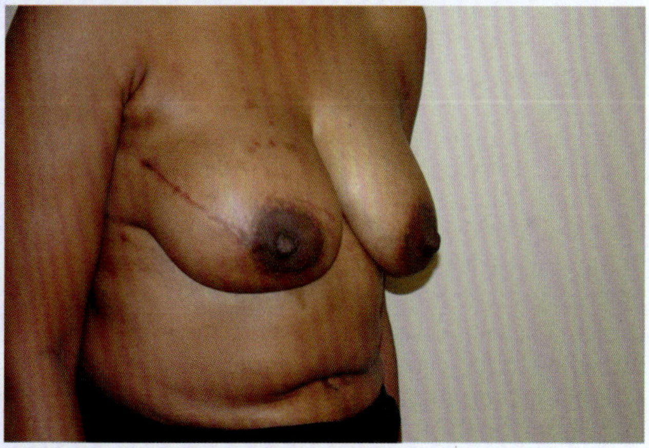

Figure 15.16

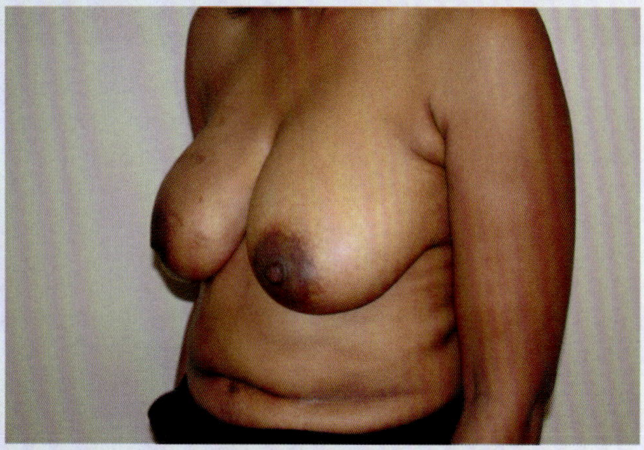

Figure 15.17

with exchange of tissue expanders for anatomically shaped highly cohesive silicone gel implants and autologous fat grafting. She is seen here 36 months following her mastectomies with a stable and overall natural result. She requested an overall augmented result and this was achieved because the anatomic implants truly shape the reconstructed breasts without the distracting forces of the pectoralis major muscle acting on the implant. An off-label "wrap" was used to complete the first stage of her reconstruction as the inframammary incision was utilized to perform the mastectomies (**Figures 15.18-15.21**).

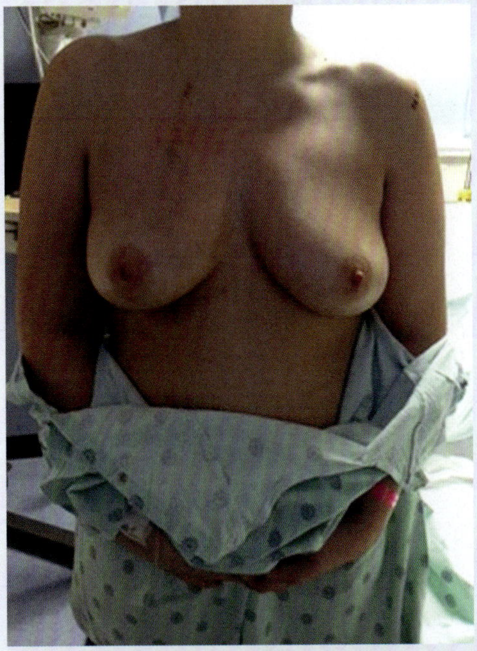

Figure 15.18

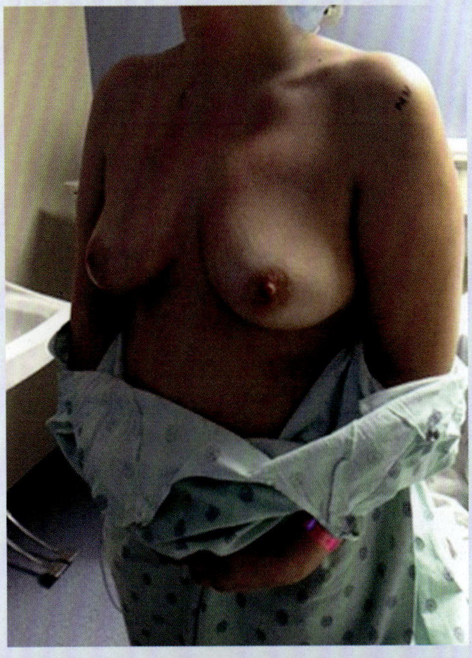

Figure 15.19

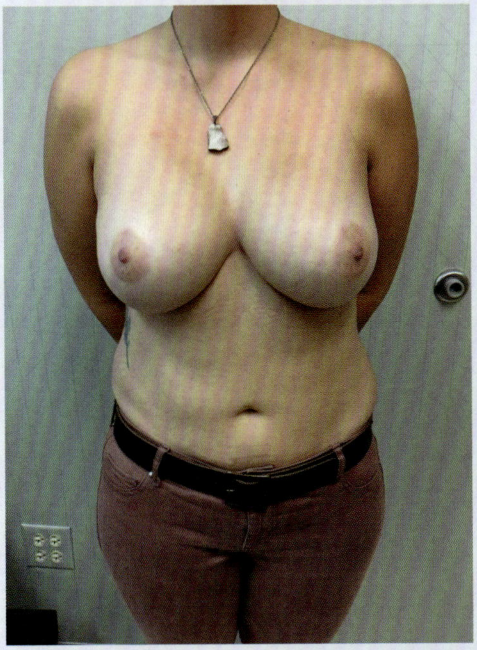

Figure 15.20

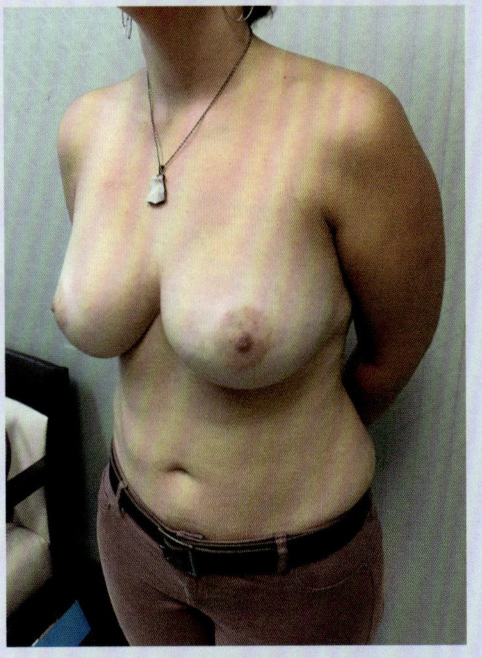

Figure 15.21

CASE 3

This 42-year-old woman underwent bilateral nipple-sparing mastectomies for left breast ductal carcinoma in situ. She underwent immediate placement of moderate-height extra-projection tissue expanders followed by second-stage reconstruction with anatomic gel implants. She is shown 12 months following her mastectomies. The psychological impact that reconstruction can offer is illustrated here, because this patient felt so pleased with her aesthetic outcome following nipple-sparing mastectomies and two-stage reconstruction that she went on to undergo abdominoplasty with concurrent autologous fat grafting to superomedial breasts (**Figures 15.22-15.26**).

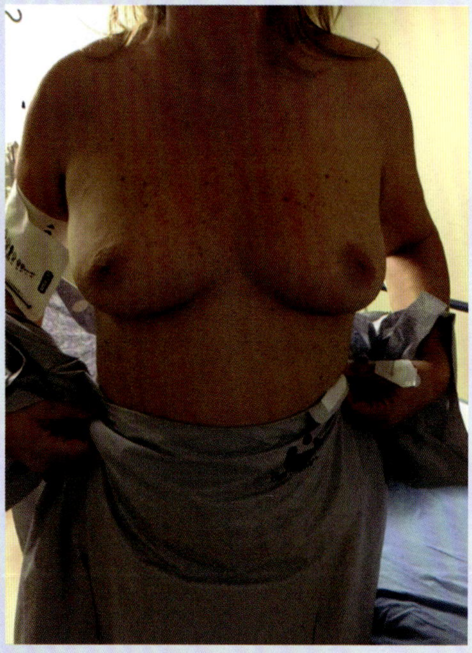

Figure 15.22

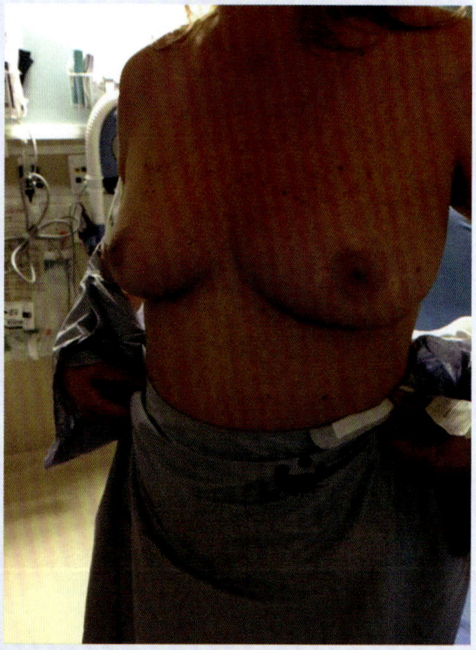

Figure 15.23

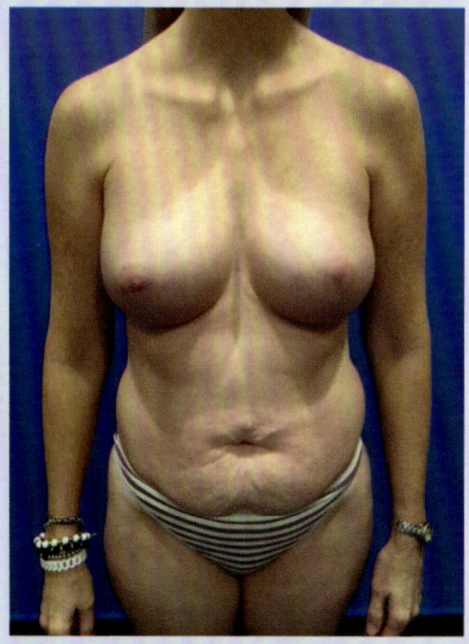

Figure 15.24

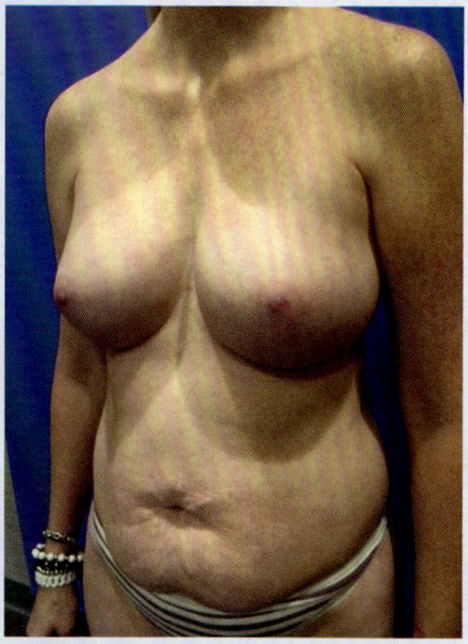

Figure 15.25

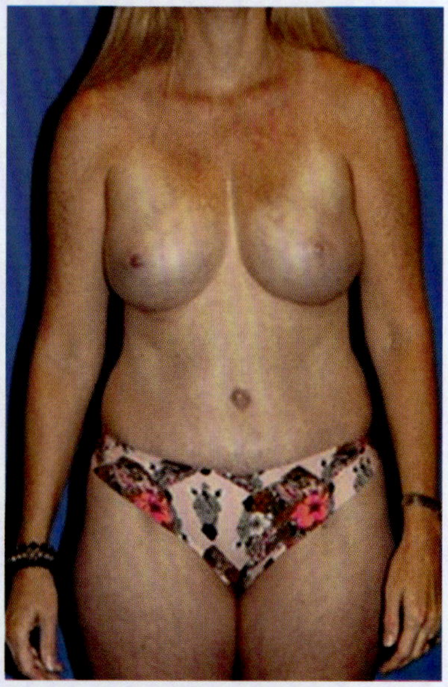

Figure 15.26

CASE 4

This 46-year-old obese hypermastic female underwent bilateral mastectomies for left breast cancer. I used a modified Goldilocks technique because the deepithelialized lower mastectomy skin flap was used as soft-tissue coverage for the expander/ADM construct. The upper skin flap is brought down to the IMF. She is seen on the table with 300 mL of air in each of the expanders (**Figures 15.27-15.31**).

Here she is shown with her expanders completely inflated with 650 mL of air before second-stage reconstruction.

She is shown 1 year following her mastectomies with full height anatomic gel implants and nipple reconstruction with areolar tattooing. Notice the lack of inverted "T," which I believe reduces incidence of wound breakdown (**Figure 15.32**).

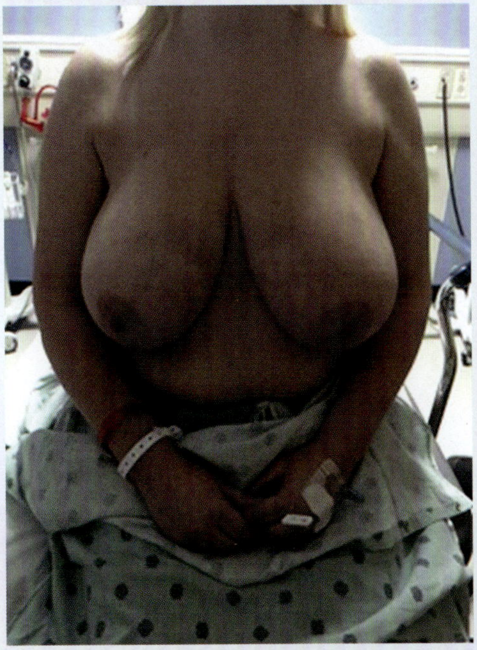

Figure 15.27

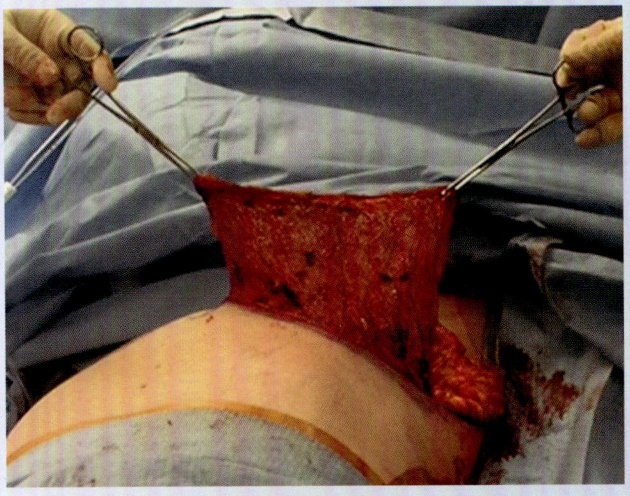

Figure 15.28

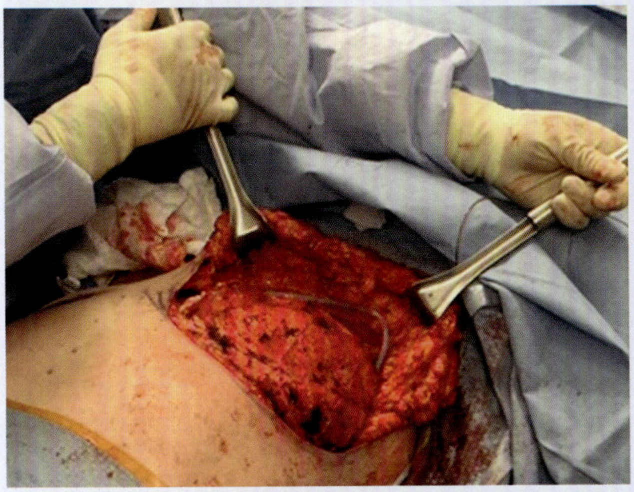

Figure 15.29

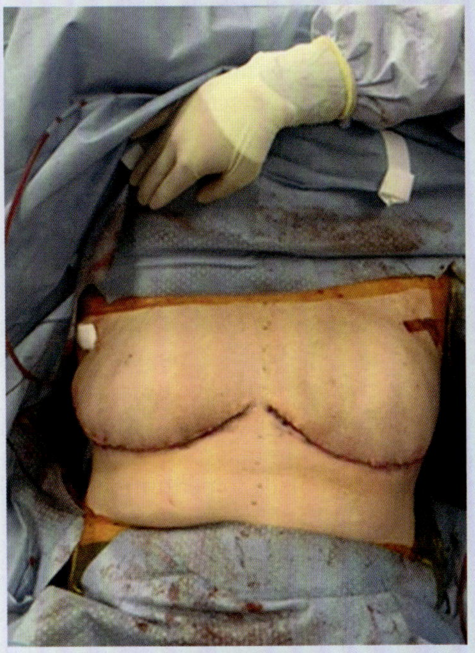

Figure 15.30

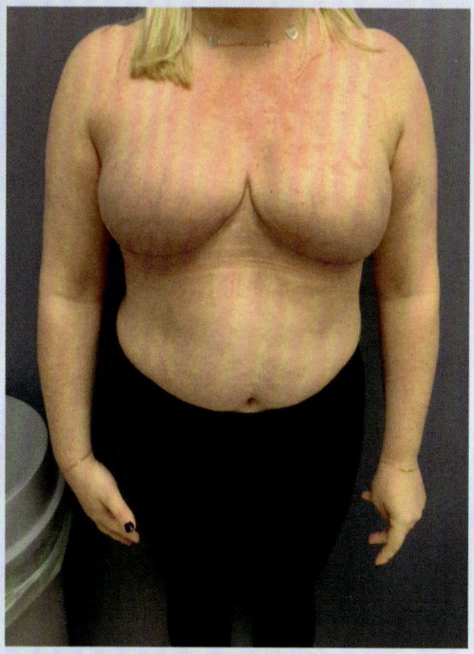

Figure 15.31

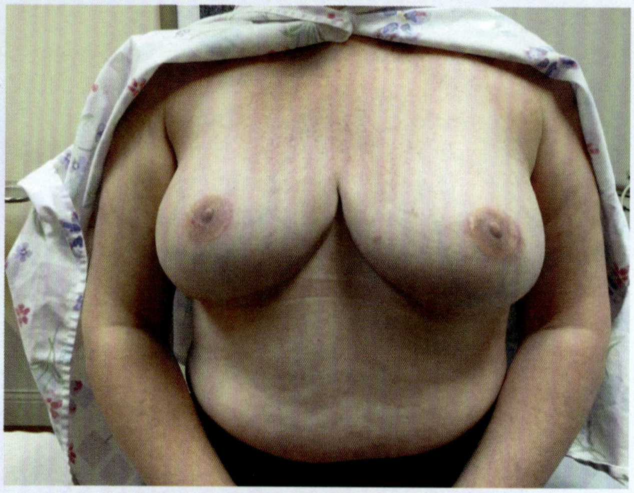

Figure 15.32

SUMMARY

In conclusion, there are many variables that can all have an effect on the final reconstructive outcome in prepectoral breast reconstruction. The technique that is used to inset the ADM, however, does not affect the final outcome. In my practice, I employ several different techniques on a regular basis, and the outcomes do not vary. What is important is to master all of the techniques and to utilize a specific technique depending on the situation. For example, I try to do mainly on-label ADM placement in the setting of two-stage reconstruction through a breast-splitting incision because it is straightforward and costs less. For the majority of the single-stage direct-to-implant reconstructions, particularly through an IMF incision, I routinely use the off-label technique with a Keller funnel because it is technically far easier to do with minimal traumatizing retraction of the already traumatized skin flaps. Whether the decision has been made to perform on- or off label, it is imperative to be precise in preoperative planning as well as being open and honest with the patient regarding potential risks as well as the likelihood of a perfect outcome and potential need for secondary surgeries in the future such as fat grafting. Prepectoral breast reconstruction has had an incredible awakening since its early inception in the 1970s; and because of improved techniques and technology, we are able to offer our patients extremely safe and reproducibly excellent aesthetic breast reconstructions on a routine basis.

BIBLIOGRAPHY

1. Sigalove S, Maxwell GP, Sigalove NM, et al. Prepectoral implant-based breast reconstruction: rationale, indications, and preliminary results. *Plast Reconstr Surg*. 2017139(2):287-294.
2. Sbitany H, Piper M, Lentz R. Prepectoral breast reconstruction: a safe alternative to submuscular prosthetic reconstruction following nipple-sparing mastectomy. *Plast Reconstr Surg*. 2017140(3): 432-443.
3. de Haan A, Toor A, Hage JJ, Veeger HE, Woerdeman LA. Function of the pectoralis major muscle after combined skin-sparing mastectomy and immediate reconstruction by subpectoral implantation of a prosthesis. *Ann Plast Surg*. 2007;59:605-610.
4. Breuing KH, Warren SM. Immediate bilateral breast reconstruction with implants and inferolateral AlloDerm slings. *Ann Plast Surg*. 2005;55:232-239.
5. Salzberg, CA. Nonexpansive immediate breast reconstruction using human acellular tissue matrix graft (AlloDerm). *Ann Plast Surg*. 2006;57:1-5.
6. Maxwell GP, Gabriel A. Bioengineered breast: concept, technique, and preliminary results. *Plast Reconstr Surg*. 2016;137:415-421.
7. Woo A, Harless C, Jacobson SR. Revisiting an old place: single-surgeon experience on post-mastectomy subcutaneous implant-based breast reconstruction. *Breast J*. 2017;23(5):545-553.
8. Vidya R, Iqbal FM. A guide to prepectoral breast reconstruction: a new dimension to implant-based breast reconstruction. *Clin Breast Cancer*. 2017;17:266-271.

CHAPTER 16

PREPECTORAL CONVERSION

Maurice Y. Nahabedian, G. Patrick Maxwell, and Allen Gabriel

Key Points

- Most patients with a subpectoral device will demonstrate some degree of device movement with pectoral muscle contraction.
- Prepectoral conversion involves the separation of the pectoral muscle from the mastectomy skin flap and returning the muscle back to its normal anatomic position.
- Acellular dermal matrices are commonly used to provide tissue support to the new prepectoral pocket.
- Anatomic or round implants can be used for prepectoral conversion procedures.
- Animation deformity is resolved with prepectoral conversion.

INTRODUCTION

Animation deformity following prosthetic breast reconstruction in the subpectoral position is an underreported problem.[1-3] Although there are various degrees of animation, most patients with a subpectoral device will demonstrate some degree of device movement with pectoral muscle contraction. Animation, on the other hand, is defined as distortion of the breast and chest with pectoral muscle contraction. The reason for this is that the periprosthetic capsule is adherent to the overlying pectoralis major muscle; and with contraction, the capsule-implant unit will move with the muscle causing visible distortion of the breast and overlying skin. This can occur following breast augmentation as well as breast reconstruction. However, it is much more common with reconstruction because there is no parenchymal buffer between the pectoralis major muscle and skin following a mastectomy; whereas, with augmentation, the breast parenchyma will minimize the degree of animation.

From a historical perspective, animation deformities have been difficult to manage. Contraction of the pectoralis major muscle is a natural event. Options for correction are varied. Denervation of the motor nerves resulting in paralysis is not practical given the importance of pectoral muscle function. Chemo paralytic agents such as botulinum toxin A can be considered, but it requires serial injections into the pectoralis major muscle to place the implant at risk for rupture.[4,5] Another option is to convert the location of the implant from the subpectoral space to the prepectoral space. This procedure is referred to as prepectoral conversion. Before the era of the bioengineered breast, this was not considered a viable option because of the increased incidence of capsular contracture, rippling and wrinkling, and skin erosion due to the aggressive nature of the mastectomies.[6] Only recently has it been recognized that adjunct procedures such as the use of acellular dermal matrices (ADMs) and autologous fat grafting can enhance outcomes and minimize untoward events in the setting of prepectoral implant placement.[1,7] This chapter reviews the preoperative planning and execution of converting implant position from the subpectoral to prepectoral position.

PREOPERATIVE PLANNING

Following prosthetic breast reconstruction, patients are followed up at regular intervals to assess surgical and aesthetic outcomes as well as patient satisfaction. From a historical perspective, plastic surgeons rarely assessed animation deformities because a viable solution was not available. Animation, however, was a common occurrence and a complaint among patients. Current practice includes an assessment of animation in all patients having subpectoral implants. Factors to consider include the degree of animation, thickness of the subcutaneous layer, history of radiation, and tobacco use. For patients with a mild degree of animation, surgical correction may not be necessary. **Table 16.1** provides a classification of animation deformities following prosthetic breast reconstruction.[3] For patients with moderate-to-severe

TABLE 16.1 CLASSIFICATION OF ANIMATION DEFORMITY

Breast Distortion	Lateral Displacement	Skin Rippling
Minimal	Minimal	None to minimal
Moderate	Moderate	Minimal
Moderate-severe	Moderate-severe	Moderate
Severe	Severe	Severe

animation deformity, surgical correction may be desired. Ideal candidates are those with reasonable mastectomy skin flap thickness. In general, it is recommended that at least 5 mm of subcutaneous fat be present. This is usually determined by pinching the upper and lower pole mastectomy skin. In patients with very thin mastectomy skin and a paucity of subcutaneous fat, prepectoral placement may not be possible because of the risk of severe rippling, wrinkling, and implant visibility. In patients who have been previously radiated or who are actively using tobacco products, prepectoral conversion may result in delayed healing or skin necrosis and should be avoided.

SURGICAL MANAGEMENT OF ANIMATION DEFORMITY

Preoperative photographs are obtained with the patient standing at rest and with animation (**Figures 16.1 and 16.2**). Patients are marked in the holding area in the standing position (**Figure 16.3**). Relevant landmarks include the

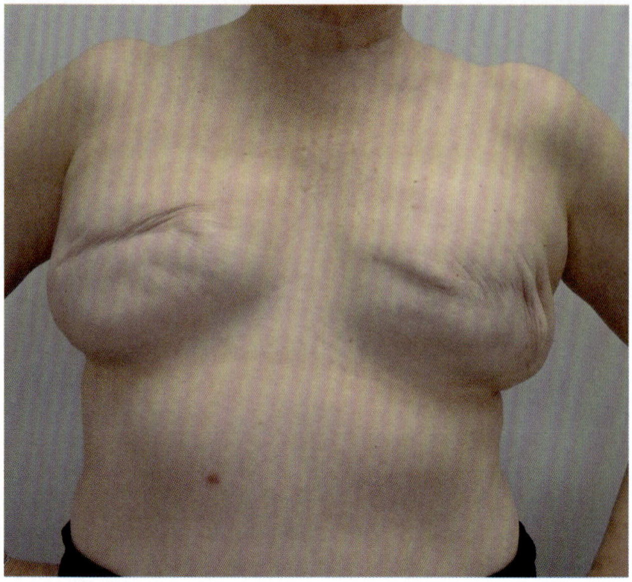

Figure 16.2 The degree of animation with pectoral contraction is illustrated.

sternal midline, inframammary fold, as well as the upper and lateral borders of the breast. The initial mastectomy incision is delineated and is the usual approach for prepectoral conversions. Prepectoral conversion can be performed following skin-sparing mastectomy or nipple-sparing mastectomy (NSM).

Patient Positioning and Anesthesia

Patients are placed on the operating table in the supine position with the arms abducted approximately 75°. The operation is usually performed under general anesthesia

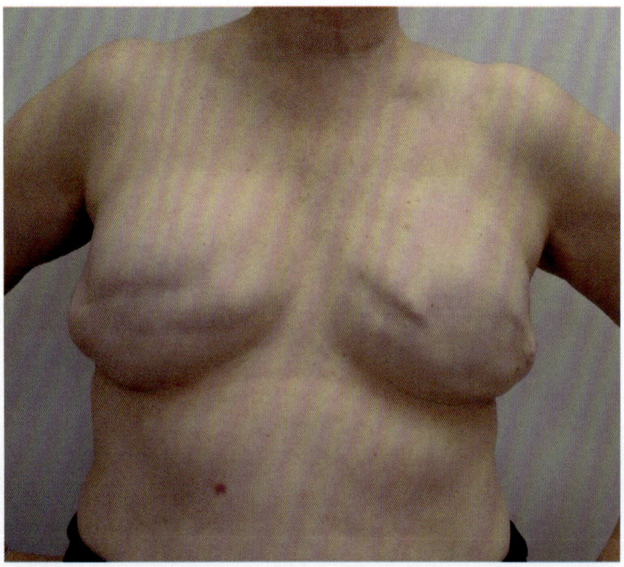

Figure 16.1 Image of a woman following bilateral skin-sparing mastectomy and subpectoral implants.

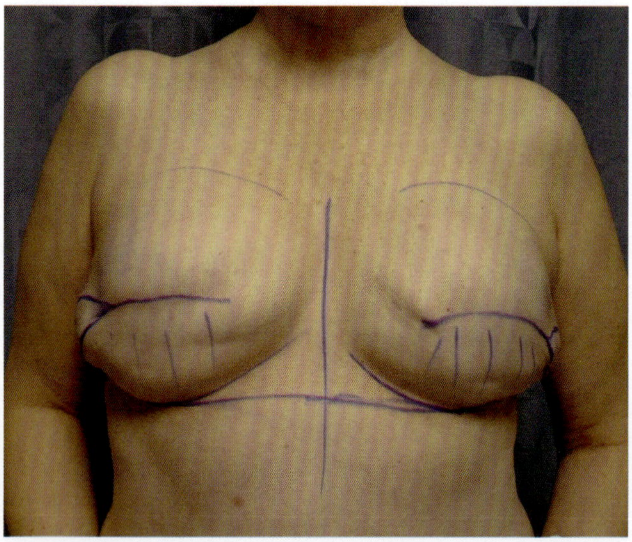

Figure 16.3 Preoperative marking delineating the sternal midline, inframammary folds, and the breast footprint.

with or without paralysis. Preoperative intravenous antibiotics are administered before the incision.

Surgical Technique—Skin-Sparing Mastectomy, Apical Incision

- The apical incision is delineated and incised. The dissection extends through the subcutaneous fat and stops at the level of the pectoralis major muscle.
- The dissection then proceeds in the direction of the inferior edge of the pectoralis major muscle. If ADM was used during the initial reconstruction, the ADM-pectoralis major muscle interface is incised to expose the periprosthetic space. The implant is removed.
- The pectoralis major muscle is then separated from the overlying mastectomy skin flap using low-set electrocautery, taking care not to cause thermal injury to the mastectomy skin flap. The muscle is freed medially, superiorly, and laterally from the mastectomy skin.
- The undersurface of the muscle is scored, repositioned onto the chest wall, and sutured to the chest wall using absorbable suture (**Figures 16.4 and 16.5**).

Surgical Technique—Nipple-Sparing Mastectomy, Inframammary Incision

- The patient is photographed while standing in repose and with animation (**Figures 16.6 and 16.7**). On the operating room table, photographs can document the amount of displacement (**Figure 16.8**). The inframammary incision site is delineated. The length of the incision is typically 8 to 12 cm depending on the breast volume. The dissection proceeds to the implant pocket and the implant is removed.
- The periprosthetic capsule is carefully examined and the inferior border of the pectoralis major muscle is identified. If ADM was used during the initial operation, it is retained along the lower pole. Electrocautery is used to incise the capsule approximately 5 mm from its distal edge of the pectoralis major muscle. The edge of the pectoralis major muscle is grasped with

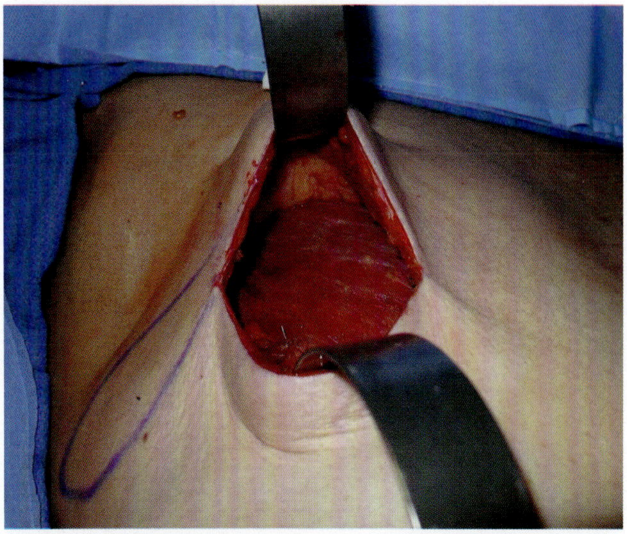

Figure 16.5 The pectoralis major muscle is sutured to the chest wall in its normal anatomic position.

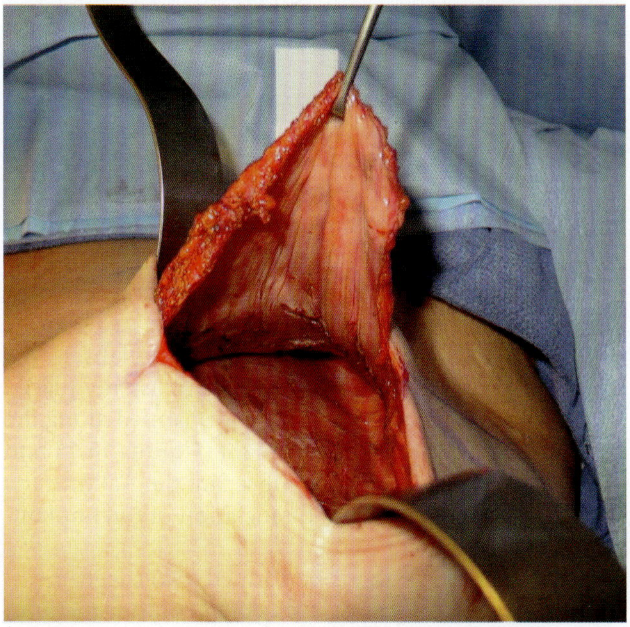

Figure 16.4 The implant is removed, the pectoralis major muscle is freed from the overlying mastectomy flap, and the undersurface of the pectoralis major muscle and the chest wall is scored.

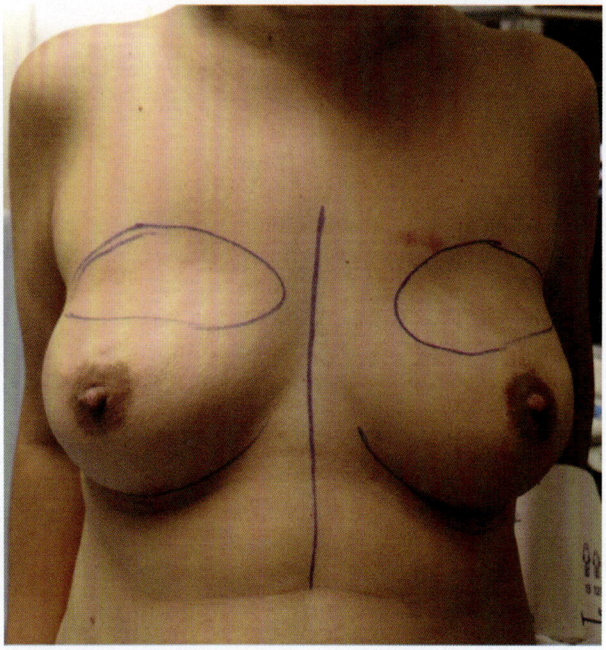

Figure 16.6 Preoperative markings of a patient following bilateral nipple-sparing mastectomy and subpectoral breast implants.

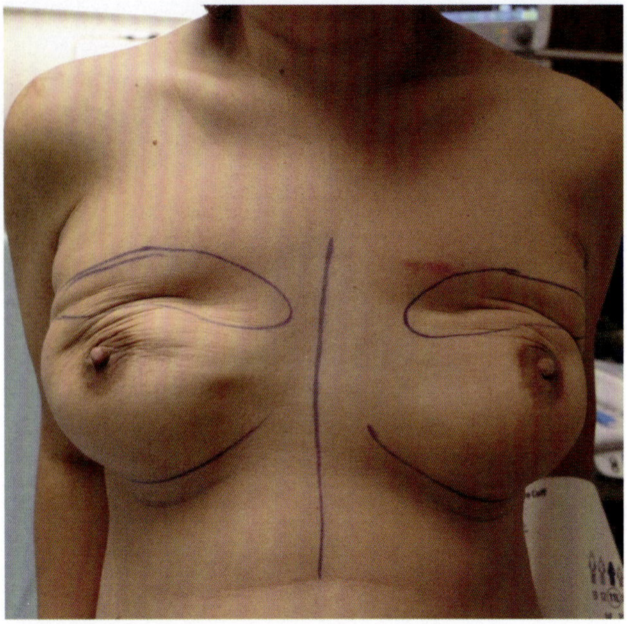

Figure 16.7 The degree of animation is depicted demonstrating severe distortion with pectoralis major contraction.

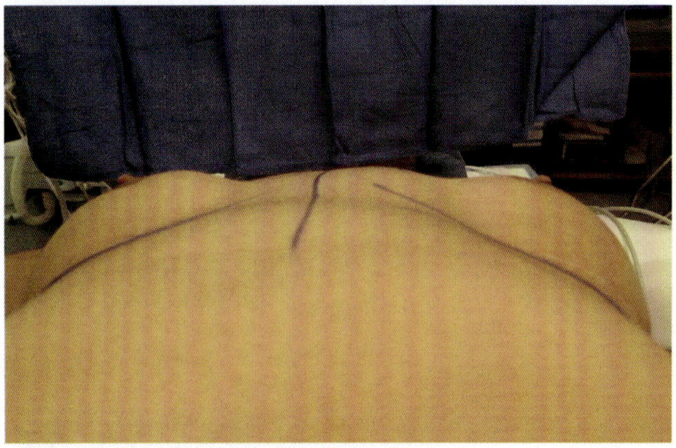

Figure 16.8 Supine preoperative photograph depicting lateral displacement bilaterally and a lack of projection.

atraumatic clamps and the dissection then proceeds between the pectoralis major and the mastectomy skin flap, ensuring that the subcutaneous fat remains on the skin flap. The muscle is freed throughout the entire periprosthetic space superiorly, medially, and laterally.

- The capsular surface of the pectoralis major and the posterior chest wall surface are scored using electrocautery to disrupt the capsule and to create two raw surfaces that will adhere to and minimize the risk of a seroma.
- The pectoralis major muscle is repositioned onto the chest wall and the periphery is sutured to the chest wall using absorbable sutures (**Figure 16.9**).

Surgical Technique—Implant Selection

- Implant selection is performed using biodimensional planning as well as understanding the desired goals

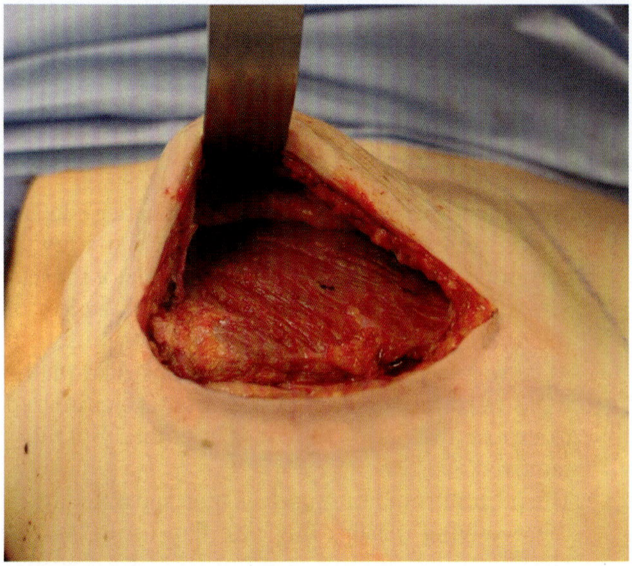

Figure 16.9 The pectoralis major muscle is separated from the mastectomy skin flap and sutured to the chest wall in its normal anatomic position.

and expectations of the patient.[8] Round or shaped breast implants can be used depending on surgeons' preference and patient desire. Patient input in this decision is critical because of the variability in implant cohesivity, visibility, degree or projection, upper pole contour, and likelihood of rotational artifact. A breast implant sizer is typically used to confirm the optimal size.

- If no ADM is used, a permanent implant is inserted into the prepectoral space.

Surgical Technique—Acellular xDermal Matrix

- ADMs can be used for partial (180°) or total coverage (360°) of the selected prosthetic device. When a 180° ADM wrap is performed, a single sheet measuring 16 × 20 cm or two contoured sheets can be used. The two contoured sheets are sutured together along the short axis using a soft absorbable suture (**Figure 16.10**). The ADM can be sutured along the perimeter of the periprosthetic space or it can be redraped directly over the selected implant. In the setting of a 180° wrap, sutures are usually placed along the edge of the ADM and spanned along the posterior surface of the implant (**Figures 16.11 and 16.12**). This maneuver will secure the ADM to the implant and prevent a dissociation of the implant-ADM construct.
- When a 360° wrap is performed, two sheets measuring 16 × 20 cm or 3 sheets of contour medium perforated ADM are usually required. The sheets of ADM are sutured together in a spherical manner around the implant using absorbable sutures.

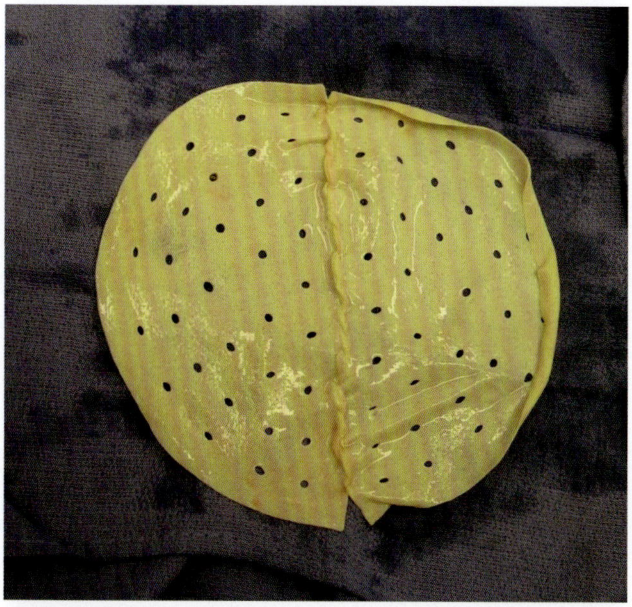

Figure 16.10 Two sheets of contour perforated acellular dermal matrix are sutured together.

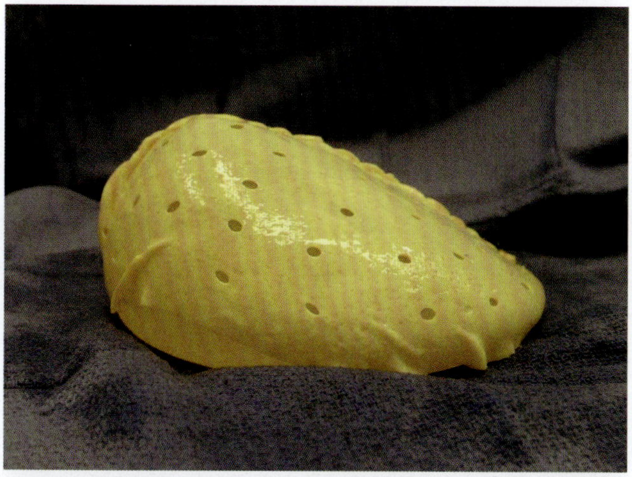

Figure 16.11 The acellular dermal matrix construct can be placed over a shaped silicone gel implant demonstrating complete anterior coverage.

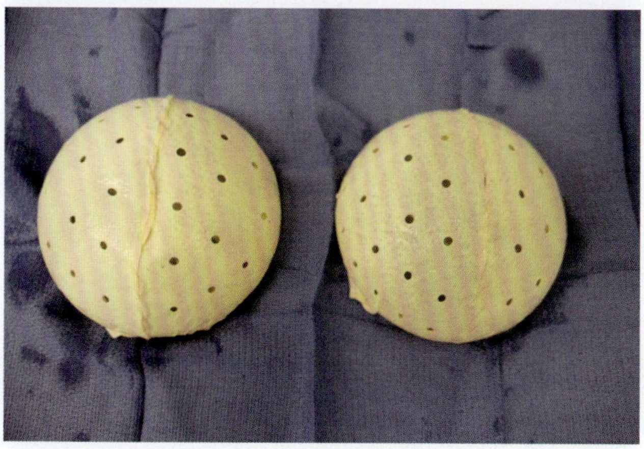

Figure 16.12 The acellular dermal matrix construct can be placed over a round silicone gel implant demonstrating complete anterior coverage.

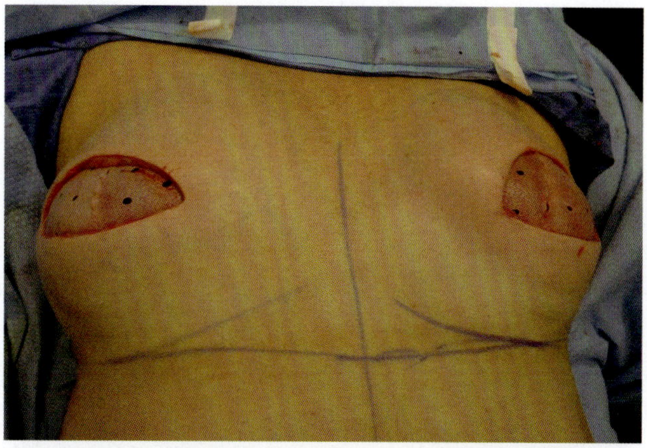

Figure 16.13 Intraoperative photograph demonstrating the implant and acellular dermal matrix in the prepectoral space through an apical (skin-sparing mastectomy) approach.

Surgical Technique—Implant Insertion

- The dimensions of the prepectoral space are assessed. The ideal inframammary fold position is confirmed and the lateral mammary fold position is defined.
- A closed suction drain is inserted into the prepectoral space.
- The implant with or without an ADM construct is inserted. It is important that hand-in-glove fit be obtained to minimize the risk of device malposition. This is especially important if a shaped implant is used. **Figure 16.13** illustrates implant insertion in the setting of skin-sparing mastectomy and **Figure 16.14** illustrates implant insertion following NSM.
- The entire space with the implant and ADM is irrigated with a 50% povidone-iodine solution. This is followed with a triple antibiotic or single antibiotic irrigation per U.S. Food and Drug Administration recommendations.
- The operating table is adjusted such that the patient is flexed approximately 45° at the waist. With NSM,

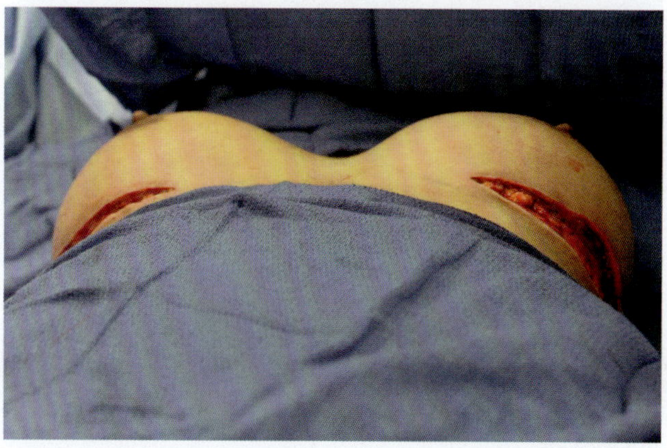

Figure 16.14 Intraoperative photograph demonstrating the implant and acellular dermal matrix in the prepectoral space through an inframammary (nipple-sparing mastectomy) approach.

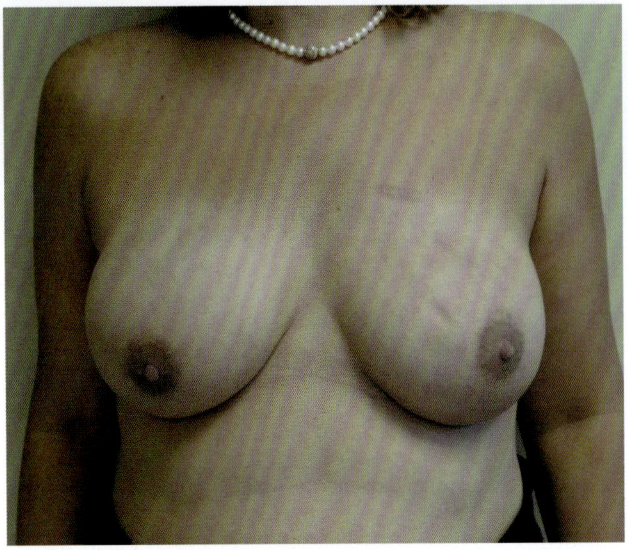

Figure 16.15 Postoperative photograph following prepectoral conversion using a round silicone gel implant and acellular dermal matrix (follow-up from Figure 16.6).

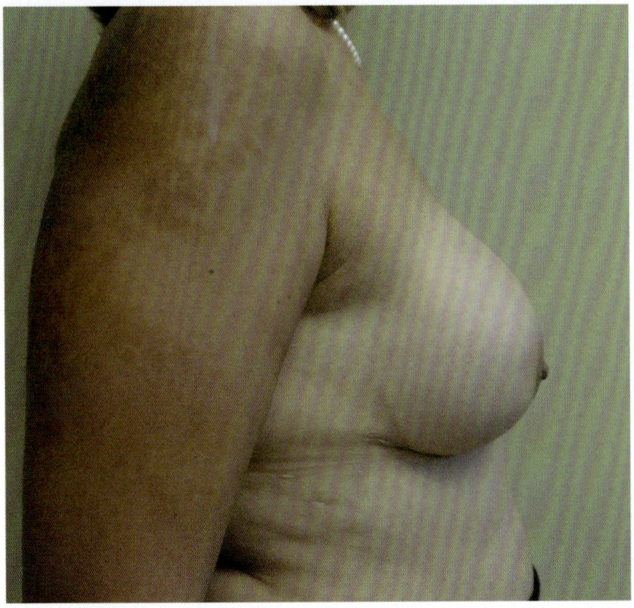

Figure 16.17 Right lateral view demonstrating no rippling and excellent contour.

the nipple-areolar complex is positioned in its ideal location and symmetry is confirmed.

- The skin is closed in the standard manner using absorbable monofilament sutures. Surgical dressings can include an incisional negative pressure wound therapy device or steri-strips, xeroform, and dry gauze. A soft compression bra is applied and the drains are placed on suction.

- **Figures 16.15 to 16.17** illustrate the final outcome following prepectoral conversion using a round silicone gel implant and ADM in the setting of NSM. **Figures 16.18 to 16.20** illustrate the final outcome following prepectoral conversion using a shaped silicone gel implant and ADM in the setting of skin-sparing mastectomy.

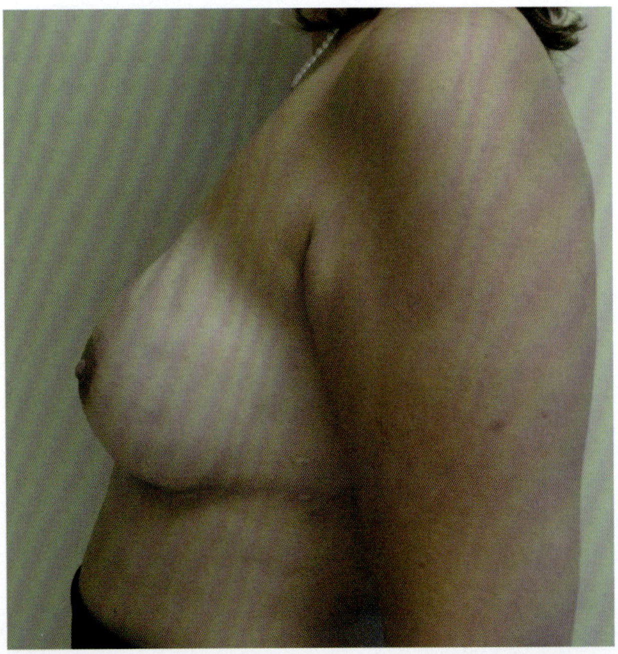

Figure 16.16 Left lateral view demonstrating slight rippling but excellent contour.

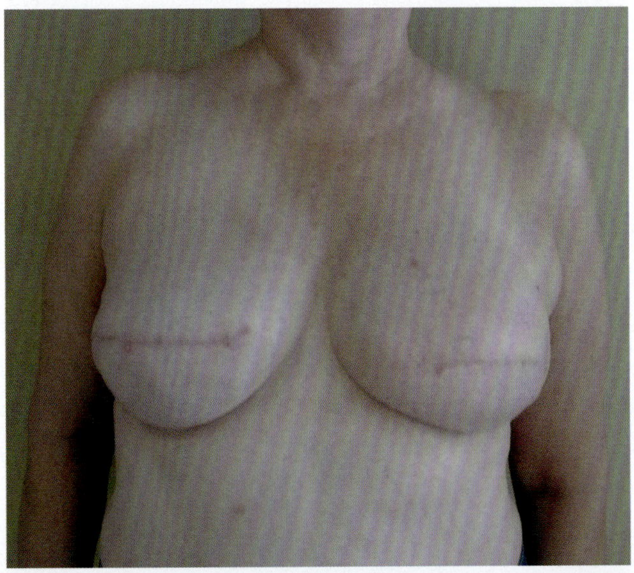

Figure 16.18 Postoperative image demonstrating excellent volume and contour (follow-up from Figure 16.1)

OUTCOMES

There are few studies in the literature that have adequately examined the incidence and treatment of animation deformity. Spear et al performed a review of 40 patients following subpectoral breast augmentation and demonstrated no distortion in 22%, minimal distortion in 62.5%, moderate distortion in 10%, and severe distortion in 5%.[9] Becker et al, in a review of 25 patients following subpectoral breast reconstruction, demonstrated that 80% of patients questioned had some degree of bothersome animation.[3] A classification of animation was created to facilitate the categorization and treatment of these patients (**Table 16.1**). Of those patients with animation, 20% had grade 1 distortion (minimal), 44% had grade 2 (moderate), 24% had grade 3 (moderate-severe), and 12% had grade 4 (severe). Correction of this animation had occurred or was planned in 7/25 patients (28%). Hammond et al evaluated 19 breasts with severe animation deformity and corrected them with prepectoral conversion without using ADM. All patients experienced complete resolution of animation. Complications occurred in five breasts (26.3%) and included Baker three-fourth capsular contracture in four (21.1%) and a seroma in one (5.3%). No breast had a visible implant deformity infection, or required device removal.

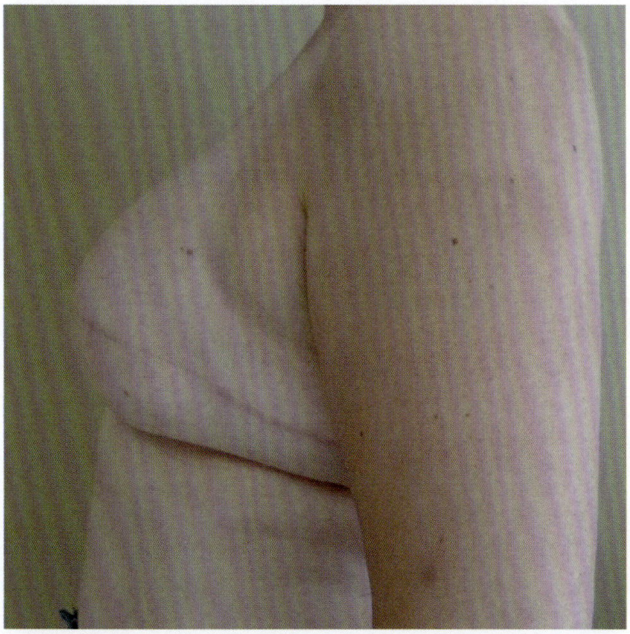

Figure 16.19 Left lateral view demonstrating no rippling and excellent contour.

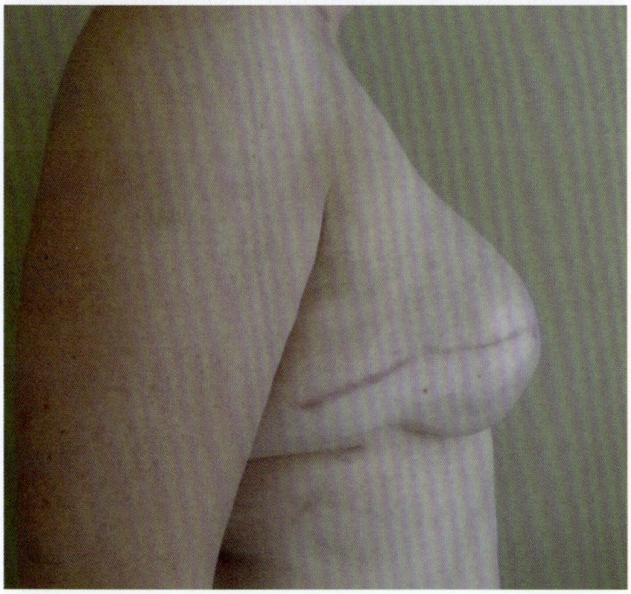

Figure 16.20 Right lateral view demonstrating no rippling and excellent contour.

KEY REFERENCES

1. Sbitany H, Piper M, Lentz R. Prepectoral breast reconstruction: a safe alternative to submuscular prosthetic reconstruction following nipple-sparing mastectomy. *Plast Reconstr Surg*. 2017;140: 432-443.
2. Hammond DC, Schmit WP, O'Connor EA. Treatment of breast animation deformity in implant-based reconstruction with pocket change to the subcutaneous position. *Plast Reconstr Surg*. 2015; 135:1540.
3. Becker H, Fregosi N. The impact of animation deformity on quality of life in post-mastectomy reconstruction patients. *Aesth Surg J*. 2017;37(5):531-536.
4. Gabriel A, Champaneria MC, Maxwell GP. The efficacy of Botulinum Toxin A in post-mastectomy breast reconstruction: a pilot study. *Aesth Surg J*. 2015;35(4):402-409.
5. Figus A, Mazzocchi M, Dessy LA, Curinga G, Scuderi N. Treatment of muscular contraction deformities with botulinum toxin type A after latissimus dorsi flap and sub-pectoral implant breast reconstruction. *J Plast Reconstr Aesthet Surg*. 2009;62:869-875.
6. Schlenker JD, Bueno RA, Ricketson G, Lynch JB. Loss of silicone implants after subcutaneous mastectomy and reconstruction. *Plast Reconstr Surg*. 1978;62(6):853-861.
7. Sigalove S, Maxwell GP, Sigalove NM, et al. Prepectoral implant-based breast reconstruction: rationale, indications, and results. *Plast Reconstr Surg*. 2017;139(2):287-294.
8. Tebbetts, JB. A system for breast implant selection based on patient tissue characteristics and implant-soft tissue dynamics. *Plast Reconstr Surg*. 2002 1; 109 (4):1396-1409.
9. Spear SL, Schwartz J, Dayan JH, Clemens MW. Outcome assessment of breast distortion following submuscular breast augmentation. *Aesthetic Plast Surg*. 2009;33:44-48.

CHAPTER **17**

DELAYED PREPECTORAL BREAST RECONSTRUCTION

Allen Gabriel, Maurice Y. Nahabedian, and G. Patrick Maxwell

KEY POINTS

- Delayed prepectoral breast reconstruction can be performed in all patients who are not candidates for immediate prepectoral reconstruction.
- In patients with prior breast irradiation, prepectoral reconstruction is performed as a latissimus-based procedure.
- In all cases, reconstruction is performed as an expander/implant procedure.
- Most patients would require fat grafting as an additional procedure.
- In patients with mastectomy incision scar tissue that is adherent to the pectoralis major muscle or with thin skin flap, fat grafting is performed prior to expander/implant reconstruction.

INTRODUCTION

Delayed breast reconstruction is reconstruction that is performed months to years after mastectomy. Despite the better aesthetic outcome, psychosocial advantage, and cost savings associated with immediate reconstruction,[1] 30% of breast reconstructions performed in the United States are delayed reconstructions,[2] for not all patients who undergo mastectomy are candidates for immediate reconstruction. The timing of reconstruction (ie, immediate or delayed) is dependent on a number of factors, including disease characteristics; patient comorbidity, body habitus, and preference; and neoadjuvant/adjuvant therapy. As with the subpectoral approach, prepectoral implant-based breast reconstruction can be performed as a delayed procedure.

INDICATIONS FOR DELAYED PREPECTORAL RECONSTRUCTION

Patients who have inadequate mastectomy flap perfusion and comorbidities that compromise flap perfusion are generally candidates for delayed prepectoral reconstruction (**Table 17.1**).[3] In patients with comorbidities that need medical management, the decision to perform delayed prepectoral reconstruction is typically made prior to mastectomy. In patients who do not have overt contraindications for immediate reconstruction, the decision to delay reconstruction is made after mastectomy following an objective assessment of flap perfusion and viability utilizing a tissue perfusion assessment device. If a perfusion device is not available, then careful clinical assessment of the mastectomy flap is undertaken. Signs of malperfusion include an absence of visible bleeding from incision margins, lack of subcutaneous tissue under the flap, or an extensive area of visible dermis. Delaying reconstruction allows the malperfused flap to heal, recover, and revascularize. As the expander/implant is placed subcutaneously in the prepectoral approach, a flap that is malperfused increases the risk of flap necrosis, infection, and expander/implant extrusion.

Comorbidities such as uncontrolled diabetes (HbA1c $> 7.5\%$) and active smoking can impair blood circulation and reduce tissue perfusion. Diabetic patients are advised to improve their HbA1c level to $\leq 7.5\%$ with medical treatment, and smokers are advised to cease smoking for at least 2 months before prepectoral breast reconstruction can be considered. HbA1c percentage depends on the blood glucose concentration and reflects the average glucose levels over the prior 6 to 8 weeks. While obesity per se is not a contraindication for immediate reconstruction, in those having morbid obesity (body mass index [BMI] >40 kg/m^2) and other comorbidities such as uncontrolled

TABLE 17.1 INDICATIONS FOR DELAYED RECONSTRUCTION

Reconstructive Considerations	Oncologic Considerations
Poorly vascularized/ ischemic flaps	Deep tumors
BMI >40 kg/m^2[a]	Chest wall involvement
Immunocompromised	High risk of recurrence (based on multidisciplinary approach)
HbA1c >7.5%	
Active smokers	

[a]With other associated comorbidities (eg, diabetes mellitus, hypertension); body mass index (BMI) alone is not a contraindication.

Adapted with permission from Sigalove S, Maxwell GP, Sigalove NM, et al. Prepectoral implant-based breast reconstruction: rationale, indications, and preliminary results. *Plast Reconstr Surg*. 2017;139:287-294.

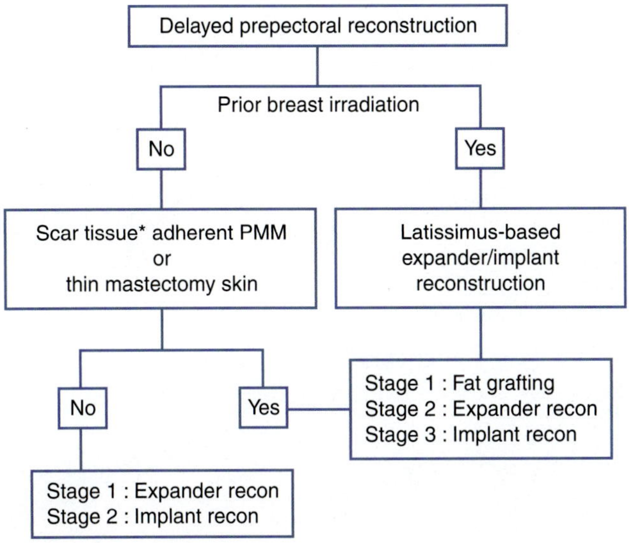

Figure 17.1 **Delayed reconstructive approach.**

diabetes or smoking, reconstruction is typically delayed, reducing the risk of reconstructive failure.

Prepectoral breast reconstruction can also be delayed in patients who have had prior breast irradiation and do not desire to have a concurrent autologous flap with an expander. Radiation has deleterious effects on the skin, affecting blood circulation and inducing fibrosis, which increase the risk of skin breakdown and capsular contracture (of the reconstructed breast), respectively. Traditionally, autologous reconstruction is the preferred reconstructive option for these patients; although delayed latissimus-based prepectoral reconstruction is an alternative option. Postmastectomy radiation is not an indication for delaying prepectoral reconstruction; refer to Chapter 18 for additional discussion on this topic.

Patients' disease characteristics may also influence the decision to delay prepectoral reconstruction (**Table 17.1**).[3] Posterior tumors lying near the pectoralis major muscle, chest wall involvement, and a high risk of recurrence should all prompt the decision to delay reconstruction, because the oncologic safety of prepectoral placement in these situations is unknown.

Lastly, patient preference for a delayed approach should be respected.

SURGICAL TECHNIQUE

Delayed prepectoral reconstruction is typically performed as an expander/implant procedure in the absence of prior breast irradiation or as a latissimus-based expander/implant procedure when the breast has been previously irradiated (**Figure 17.1**). In both cases, the use of expanders is critical. Generally, in patients without prior irradiation, the breast skin envelope has some degree of laxity, and the expander stage allows the skin to conform to the shape of the expander. In patients with prior breast irradiation, the expander stage provides an opportunity to improve the pliability of radiation damaged skin and tissues to better accommodate the definitive implant. This step involves the utilization of latissimus flap with a skin paddle. The size of the skin paddle depends on the extent of additional tissue needed to accommodate the missing skin envelope.

Preoperative Considerations

Preoperatively, to help guide expander placement, the position of the medial and lateral borders and inframammary fold is marked on the breast, creating a footprint of the future breast (**Figure 17.2A**). The mastectomy incision area is evaluated to determine whether there is adherence of scar tissue to the underlying pectoralis major muscle. As the muscle lacks a fascia after mastectomy, any scar adherence is directly to the muscle. To determine whether there is adherence, the skin over the scar tissue is pinched and moved over the scar area to feel for adherence (**Figure 17.2B**). Adequate nonadherent skin is needed for prepectoral reconstruction to minimize button holing through the existing central or vertical mastectomy scar because an inframammary incision is utilized for reconstruction. In the event of adherence to the pectoralis major muscle or inadequate skin thickness, fat grafting is performed as a first stage to augment subcutaneous tissue (**Figure 17.1**). Fat is grafted to the lower pole area and under the central incision area. Elevating the central scar minimizes complications of prepectoral reconstruction (**Figure 17.3**). Scar tissue is usually tenuous, and fat grafting helps strengthen the scar and reduce the risk of dehiscence during the expansion phase. Expander reconstruction is performed 3 months after first-stage fat grafting.

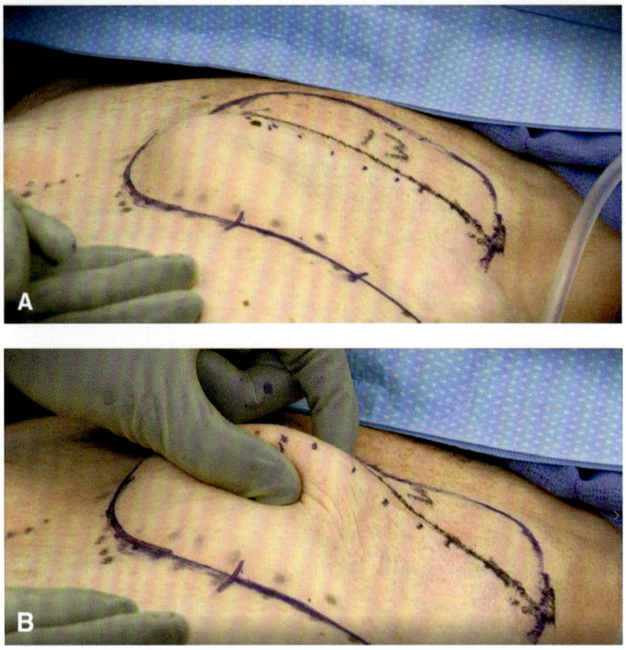

Figure 17.2 **Preoperative evaluation.** A, Footprint of breast marked on breast; B, Skin pinch test.

Expander Reconstruction

Reconstruction is performed via an inframammary incision in all cases, except in previously irradiated cases where a latissimus flap is being utilized at the same time. In the latter case, the central or breast splitting incision will be reopened as this is where the skin paddle will be placed. In nonirradiated cases, utilizing the previous central or vertical mastectomy incision is avoided. Reopening and closing the central incision contributes to flattening of the central projection of the reconstructed breast over time. An inframammary incision, in contrast, helps maintain the central breast projection. After making the incision, a snug prepectoral pocket, adequate to house the selected expander, is created by detaching and lifting the overlying subcutaneous tissue from the pectoralis major muscle (**Figure 17.4A**). A snug pocket (**Figure 17.4B**) is important to prevent seroma formation and ensure adequate contact between the acellular matrix and the skin flap, which is critical for matrix revascularization and recellularization and its incorporation into host tissue.

At times, when the skin and subcutaneous tissue are detached and lifted from the pectoralis major muscle for pocket creation, seroma pockets can be encountered. Seroma pockets can present in a variety of sizes and locations within the pocket and are addressed with capsulectomies. In rare cases, the seroma pocket fills the entire prepectoral pocket. In such an event, a capsulectomy is performed, drains are placed, and reconstruction is abandoned. Reconstructive surgery is revisited 3 months later after the pocket has healed.

In the event of a need to lower the inframammary fold or in the presence of thick lower pole tissue, radial scoring is performed at the transition zone between the subcutaneous tissue and the mastectomy flap at the lower pole. Radial scoring increases the surface area and allows for ease of subsequent lower pole expansion.

Prior to introduction of the expander, the pocket is irrigated with a triple antibiotic rinse (1 g cefazolin, 80 mg gentamicin, 50 000 IU bacitracin in 500 cc of normal saline) and 100% betadine. One 10″ French drain is placed in the lateral fold (**Figure 17.4C**).

Expander selection is guided by the patient's breast dimensions. For a patient with a generous skin envelope, an extra-full projection expander is utilized to allow greater projection to the lower pole over time. For a patient with a short breast height, a moderate-height variable expander is utilized, whereas for a patient with a tall breast height, a

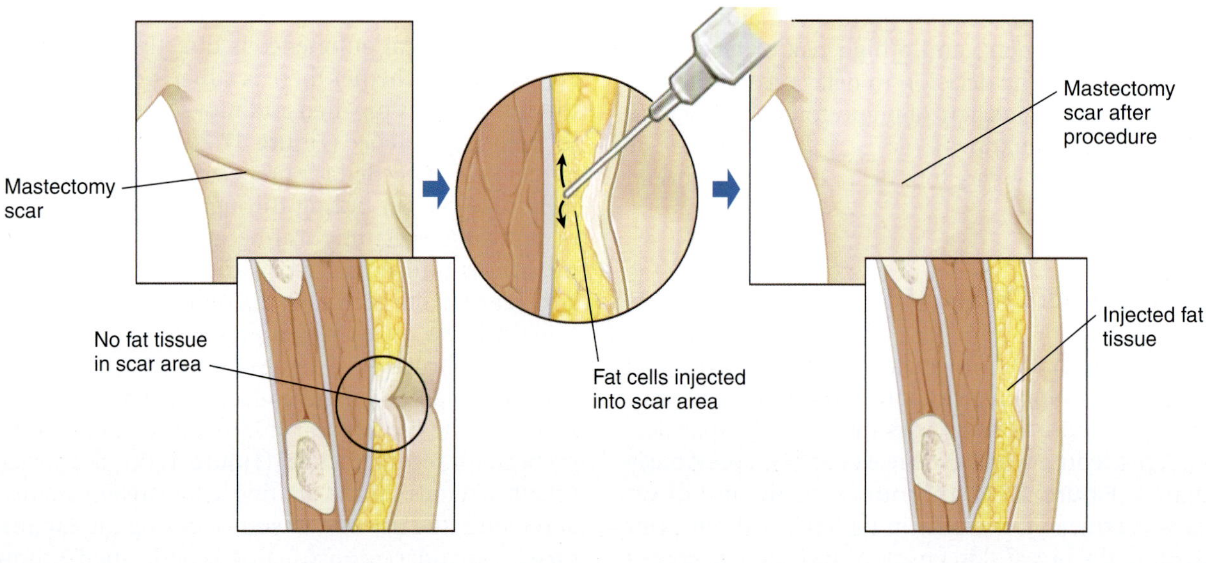

Figure 17.3 First stage of delayed reconstruction is fat grafting so the central breast-splitting scar can be elevated off the pectoralis major. This will make sure there is some subcutaneous tissue present when the expander is placed in the prepectoral plane through an IMF incision.

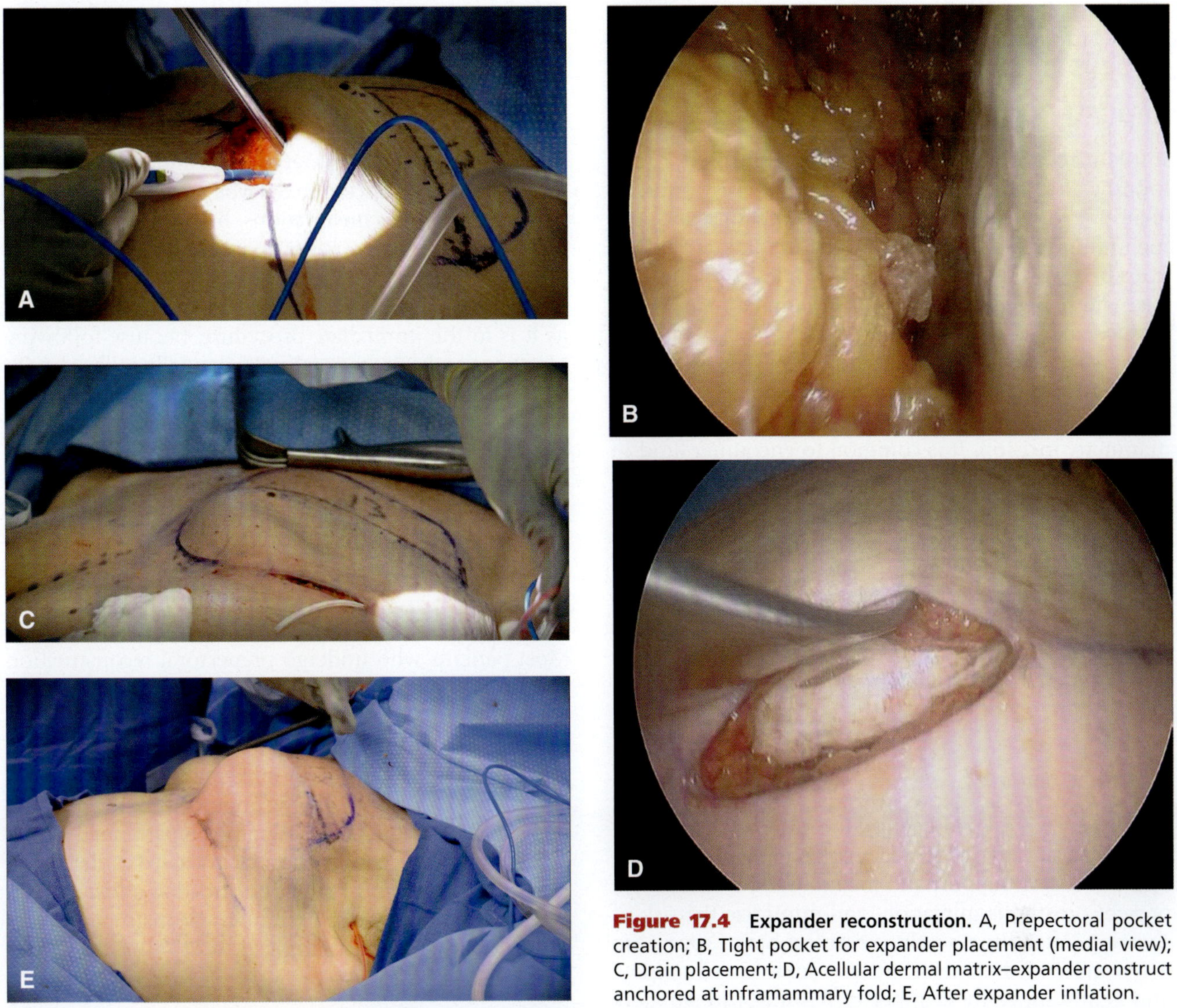

Figure 17.4 **Expander reconstruction.** A, Prepectoral pocket creation; B, Tight pocket for expander placement (medial view); C, Drain placement; D, Acellular dermal matrix–expander construct anchored at inframammary fold; E, After expander inflation.

full-height variable expander is utilized. Irrespective of the type of expander selected, the base width of the expander should be narrower (by 0.5-2.0 cm) than the base width of the final implant to ensure a snug fit of the final implant.

The expander is selected preoperatively and wrapped with a single 16 × 20 cm sheet of perforated acellular dermal matrix (ADM) that has been prepared according to the manufacturer's instructions. The thickness of the matrix utilized is guided by clinical assessment of flap thickness. For a flap of greater than 2 cm pinch thickness, a thin- to medium-thickness ADM is utilized, whereas for a flap of less than 2 cm thickness, a thick matrix is utilized. The anterior surface of the expander is completely covered by the matrix, whereas the posterior surface is covered to varying extents, depending on the size of the expander and the matrix. Wrapped constructs simplify reconstruction and allow for more efficient use of operating room time but are considered OFF-LABEL by the United States Food and Drug Administration.

ADM is a critical component of prepectoral reconstruction whether performed in the immediate or in a delayed setting. The matrix serves to define and stabilize the inframammary fold as well as to stabilize the expander preventing unwarranted displacements, bottoming out, and extrusion. It helps mask rippling/wrinkling and device visibility. Importantly, the matrix reduces chronic inflammatory response and the development of capsular contracture. Directly placing the expander or implant subcutaneously without an acellular matrix is associated with a significant increase in the rate of capsular contracture, an outcome that served as one of the reasons for abandoning the subcutaneous approach in the 1960s/1970s.

The wrapped construct is anchored at the inframammary fold by suturing the matrix to the pectoralis major muscle and chest wall tissues using barbed or 0-PDO sutures (**Figure 17.4D**). The expander may also be anchored via the suture tabs, but, in a snug pocket, there is no necessity to further anchor the construct. The expander is maximally or near maximally inflated with saline (**Figure 17.4E**). Air is generally not used in delayed reconstruction because there are no concerns with compromising mastectomy flap perfusion. The skin is allowed to reshape over breast the next several weeks before a further inflation, if needed.

The drain is removed when the output is less than 30 cc over a 24-hour period, which can take up to 1 to 2 weeks.

Implant Reconstruction

Implant reconstruction is typically performed 2 to 3 months after expander placement. Generally round or anatomic form-stable, highly cohesive gel implants and high-fill implants are utilized in prepectoral reconstructions because they are associated with less rippling. The base width, height, and shape of the implant are guided by the expander that is in place. Typically, an implant with a slightly wider (0.5-2.0 cm wider) base is selected to ensure a snug fit within the pocket.

Reconstruction is performed via the previous inframammary incision. It is common to encounter fluid in the prepectoral pocket, which is a normal finding and not a cause for concern because the fluid is sterile. After expander removal, the prepectoral space is observed to be completely lined by the incorporated ADM (**Figure 17.5**). The incorporated matrix provides stability to the prepectoral space and the future implant and eliminates the need for drains. The prepectoral space is rinsed with triple antibiotic solution before introducing the implant via a Keller funnel.

Postoperative Care

Patients are typically discharged the same day postoperatively. They are advised to wear a soft compression bra for 4 to 6 weeks to support and maintain the breast shape, prevent prosthesis migration, and minimize the risk of sheering. After 4 to 6 weeks, a comfort bra or sports bra is recommended. Patients are also advised to ambulate and gently move their upper extremities immediately after surgery but are kept on weight restrictions for 4 to 6 weeks. Patients are followed at regular intervals to assess for postoperative complications.

Hematoma, infection, and wound dehiscence are potential short-term complications in delayed prepectoral reconstructions. Infection may manifest as overt infection or as red breast (redness, erythema, and warmth). Skin necrosis is not a concern in delayed reconstructions, as it is in immediate reconstructions, because perfusion and viability of skin flaps are not an issue, except in the event of accidental skin damage from electrocautery. Likewise, seroma is usually not a concern in the delayed procedure, as it is in the immediate procedure, because following mastectomy, the prepectoral space naturally collapses with time. But, seroma can be a potential complication in the long term if contamination occurred during surgery or nonadherence of the acellular matrix was not addressed at the expander-to-implant exchange stage. Capsular contracture is rare in the author's early follow-up series with prepectoral reconstructions.[3]

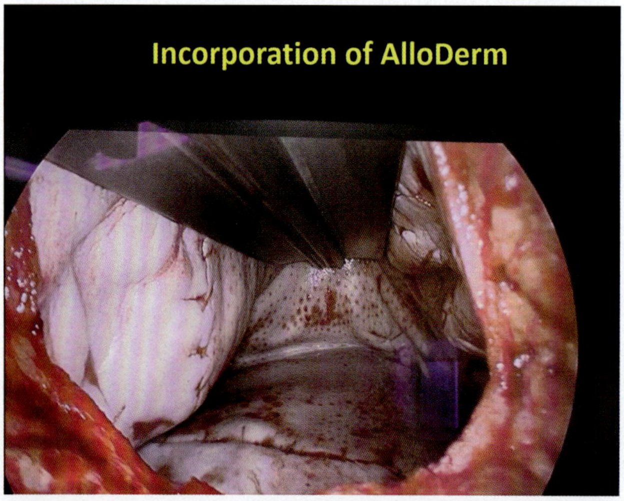

Figure 17.5 Fully incorporated acellular dermis. Prepectoral space lined with incorporated matrix after expander removal for implant reconstruction.

Additional Procedures

Most patients who undergo prepectoral reconstruction would require fat grafting to enhance breast thickness, contour, and/or shape as well as to mask implant visibility, rippling, and wrinkling at the upper pole. Fat grafting to the upper pole may also be needed to improve step-off for a smoother transition from the upper pole to the implant. In delayed reconstructions, fat grafting is performed mostly before expander reconstruction, as discussed earlier. In the event that fat grafting is not performed as a first stage, it is typically performed after implant reconstruction, after the reconstruction has stabilized.

Latissimus-Based Prepectoral Reconstruction

Autologous-based procedures are beyond the scope of this chapter. Nevertheless, a few points are worth mentioning. Recruitment of the latissimus muscle for prepectoral reconstruction negates the need for acellular matrix use for the muscle essentially replaces the matrix. If extensive fold lowering is required and there is concern for bottoming out, a sheet of thin acellular matrix can be added to the lower pole. There is no necessity for complete coverage of the expander with the matrix. Reconstruction is performed via an inframammary incision at the second stage so as not to disrupt the central pole and the latissimus muscle. If a portion of the skin paddle needs to be removed or thinned out for contralateral matching purposes, it is done without disrupting the latissimus muscle. Fat grafting is at times needed in the latissimus-based procedure to improve the upper pole transition. Duration of hospital stay is one day with the latissimus-based procedure, as would be expected given its more invasive nature. Latissimus flap necrosis is a potential short-term complication with this procedure.

CASE EXAMPLES

CASE 1 (FIGURE 17.6 A-D)

Forty-seven-year-old, morbidly obese female (BMI, 41 kg/m^2) diagnosed with left breast cancer. She was treated with neoadjuvant chemotherapy followed by bilateral mastectomy. Reconstruction was delayed because of her lack of desire for breast reconstruction. Her HbA1c was 6%.

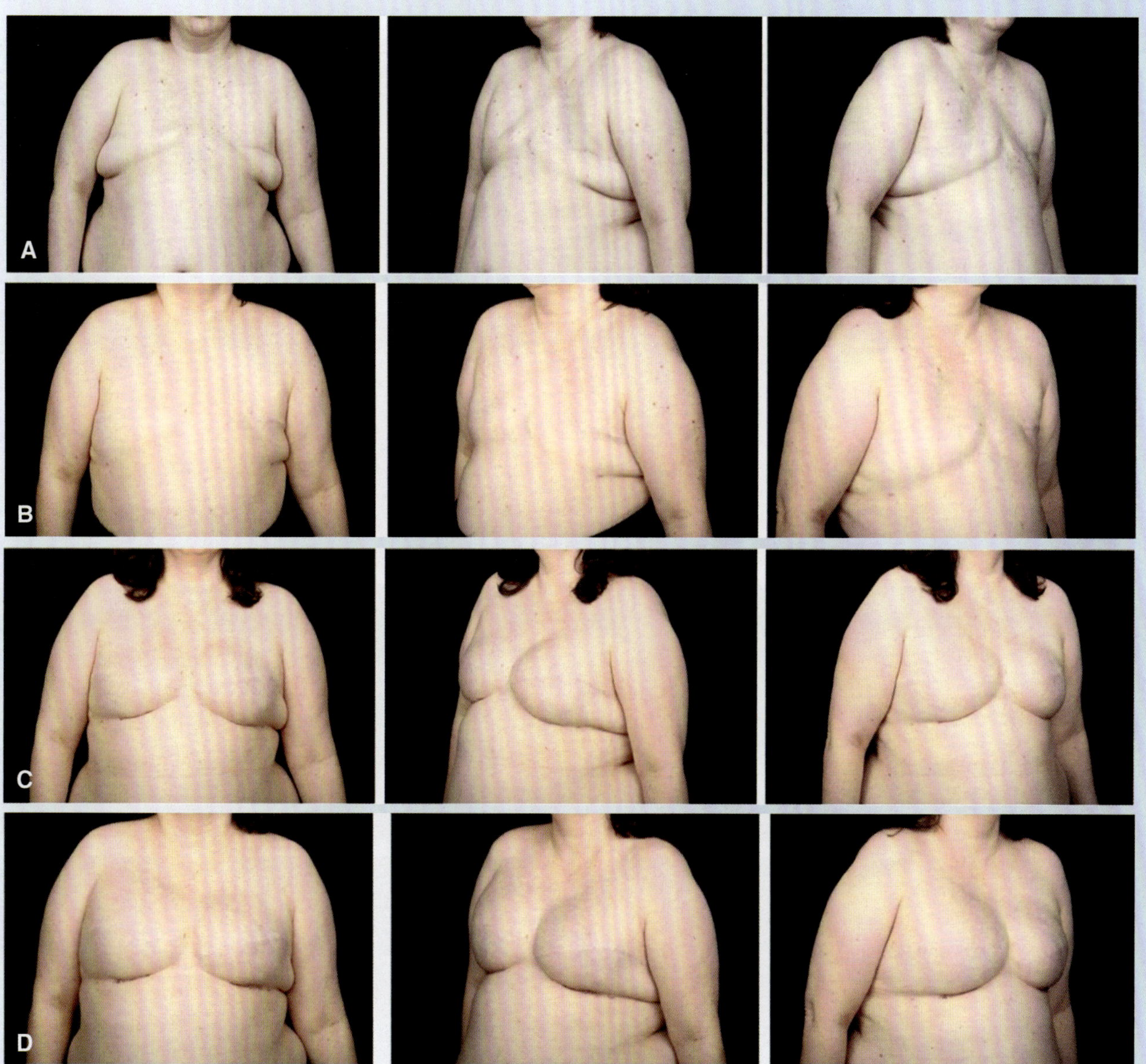

Figure 17.6 A, **Preoperative view.** B, **First-stage fat grafting.** Two months after liposuction of lateral chest and fat grafting to the central scar and lower pole flap. C, **Second-stage prepectoral expander reconstruction.** Five months after fat grafting, patient underwent bilateral breast reconstruction with 133 FV 500 cc (13 cm width) expanders and wrapped with upper pole AlloDerm and lower pole Artia. Expanders were fully inflated intraoperatively with saline to 420 cc. Patient is shown at 3 months after reconstruction. D, **Third-stage prepectoral implant reconstruction.** Four months after expander placement, patient underwent implant exchange with SRX 800 cc (width 15.5) silicone implants. Patient is shown at 6 months after implant exchange.

CASE 2 (FIGURE 17.7 A-D)

Fifty-year-old female (BMI, 21 kg/m^2) with right breast right breast cancer, treated with lumpectomy, radiotherapy, and chemotherapy. Her cancer recurred 2 years later following the end of her treatments. She underwent bilateral mastectomy followed by adjuvant chemotherapy. After her recurrence, patient was not sure if she wanted to have breast reconstruction and therefore her reconstruction was delayed until the completion of her chemotherapy so that she could think about her options.

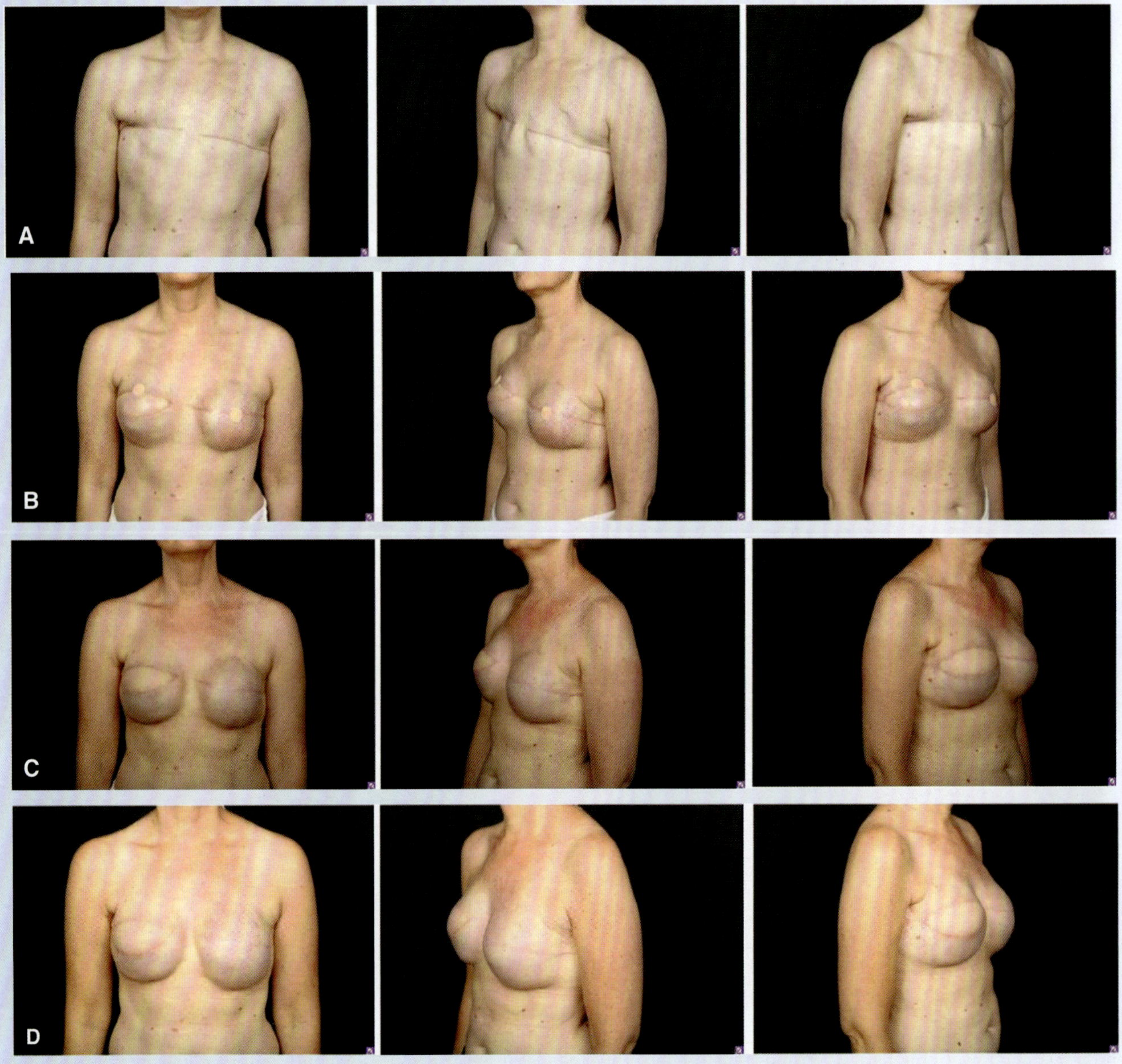

Figure 17.7 A, **Preoperative view.** B, **First-stage prepectoral expander reconstruction.** Right breast reconstructed with latissimus myocutaneous flap and left breast with prepectoral AlloDerm (upper pole) and Artia (lower pole). 133MX 400 cc (12 cm width) expanders were used. Patient is at 7 weeks after reconstruction. C, **Second-stage prepectoral implant reconstruction.** Fifteen weeks after expander reconstruction, patient underwent bilateral implant reconstruction with SCX 495 cc (12.5 cm width) silicone implants. Patient is shown at 7 weeks after her second stage. D, **Third-stage fat grafting.** Three months after second stage, 130 cc of processed fat was grafted to patient's left breast and 70 cc to her right breast. Patient is shown at 9 months after fat grafting and 12 months since her second stage.

SUMMARY

Delayed prepectoral breast reconstruction is a simple procedure that can be safely performed in all patients who are not candidates for immediate prepectoral reconstruction. Medical conditions should be managed prior to the reconstruction. When in doubt about the condition of the mastectomy flap, fat grafting should be done as the first stage of the reconstruction, followed by expander stage 3 months later.

KEY REFERENCES

1. Filip CI, Jecan CR, Raducu L, Neagu TP, Florescu IP. Immediate versus delayed breast reconstruction for postmastectomy patients. controversies and solutions. *Chirurgia (Bucur)*. 2017;112:378-386.
2. American Society of Plastic Surgeons. Plastic surgery statistics report 2016. https://www.plasticsurgery.org/documents/News/Statistics/2016/plastic-surgery-statistics-full-report-2016.pdf
3. Sigalove S, Maxwell GP, Sigalove NM, et al. Prepectoral implant-based breast reconstruction: rationale, indications, and preliminary results. *Plast Reconstr Surg*. 2017;139:287-294.

CHAPTER **18**

PREPECTORAL RECONSTRUCTION AND RADIATION THERAPY PLASTIC SURGEON'S PERSPECTIVE

Allen Gabriel, Steven R. Sigalove, Maurice Y. Nahabedian, and G. Patrick Maxwell

KEY POINTS

- Pectoralis major fibrosis is a major issue in patients undergoing radiation, and this muscle should not be included in the reconstructive process.
- Premastectomy radiated skin should be treated with caution, and, ideally, an autologous tissue should be included with or without a device in a prepectoral space depending on the extent of damage.
- If postmastectomy radiation therapy is planned, then every effort is made to place the device in a prepectoral space.

INTRODUCTION

Prosthetic breast reconstruction continues to be the most common form of reconstruction for women who undergo mastectomy and immediate reconstruction. In 2017, more than 80% of breast reconstructions were prosthetic reconstructions. Despite the success of prosthetic reconstruction, challenges remain with this mode of reconstruction, particularly with respect to reconstruction in the setting of radiotherapy. Radiation has a significant adverse impact on prosthetic reconstruction; notably, a reconstructive failure (implant or expander removal) rate of 20% to 50%,[1,2] a major corrective surgery rate of 40%,[3] and a capsular contracture rate of 17% to 60%.[1,2] Patient satisfaction and aesthetic outcomes are also diminished in the setting of radiotherapy.[4]

Prosthetic breast reconstruction has until recently been exclusively performed by placing the prosthesis in a subpectoral space. The placement of the prosthesis in a prepectoral space is currently emerging as a simpler, alternative approach to prosthetic reconstruction. Several studies have demonstrated the feasibility and safety of this approach.[5-7] Compared with subpectoral breast reconstruction, the current standard, prepectoral reconstruction is anatomically less invasive (pectoralis muscle sparing), technically less challenging, less time consuming, and associated with less pain; further, it reduces the requirement for intravenous pain management, eliminates animation deformity, and results in a more natural breast shape.[6,7]

Plastic surgeons typically encounter patients who have been exposed to radiotherapy at different stages of their cancer treatment journey. These patients can be categorized into four groups: patients who have failed breast conservation therapy (BCT; lumpectomy and radiotherapy) and present with recurrence or with pain and deformity necessitating a completion mastectomy; patients who have had expander reconstruction and are scheduled for planned postmastectomy radiotherapy (PMRT); patients who have had mastectomy and chest wall radiotherapy desiring delayed reconstruction; and, lastly, a unique group that has had dual-plane reconstruction followed by PMRT that requires revision to prepectoral. Each of these groups deserves a separate discussion because of differing reconstructive considerations.

Failed BCT With Patient Desiring Immediate Reconstruction

This group of patients can be challenging to treat, especially if aesthetic principles were violated during the original lumpectomy. Patients can present with a quadrant of the breast missing without any tissue rearrangement offered to avoid severe deformities and scarring (Figure 18.1).

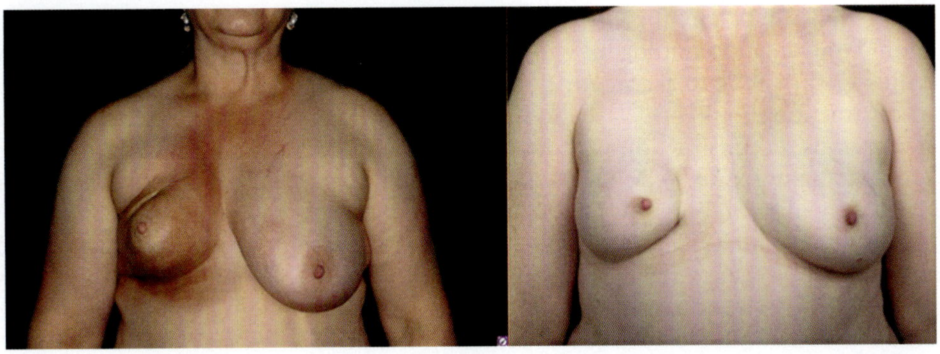

Figure 18.1 Patients post level 2 lumpectomy who were not offered reconstructive surgery (tissue rearrangement) before radiation therapy.

When evaluating a patient with prior lumpectomy for mastectomy, the lumpectomy scar location is identified, and the soft-tissue envelope mobility, deficit, and thickness are evaluated. If the scar is fixed and stiff, and if there is an obvious tissue deficit whether in the upper or lower pole, some form of autologous flap reconstruction with or without expander in the prepectoral space is needed to address the presenting issues. The size of the skin paddle for the autologous tissue is guided by the extent of scarring and the size of deformity that is present, such that a better match can be made to the contralateral side (**Figure 18.2**).

If the breast tissue is thick but mobile with minimal soft-tissue deficit, then the location of the lumpectomy scar becomes critical. If the scar is located at the lower pole where the radiation boost took place, the reconstructive approach is the same as when there is soft-tissue deficit. An autologous tissue with a skin paddle and an expander is utilized for prepectoral reconstruction. An autologous-based approach will allow for ease of lower pole expansion and will protect against lumpectomy scar dehiscence because there will be a layer of nonradiated vascularized tissue between the expander/implant and the soft-tissue envelope.

If the lumpectomy scar is in the upper pole, prepectoral placement of an expander without a latissimus flap can be considered only if the skin is supple and not fibrotic. In addition, the soft-tissue envelope asymmetry should be assessed with the contralateral breast because this can be a bigger concern following mastectomy considering the irradiated skin may retract and the asymmetry will be difficult to address. If there is any doubt of a lack of soft-tissue envelope, a latissimus flap with a skin paddle should be utilized and placed in the breast quadrant lacking the soft tissue. If reconstruction is attempted without a latissimus flap, the patient should be aware and advised that with any failure of the skin flap or concerns with the reconstruction, the patient would have to be mentally prepared to undergo salvage with latissimus flap reconstruction. If the patient is not willing to undergo a

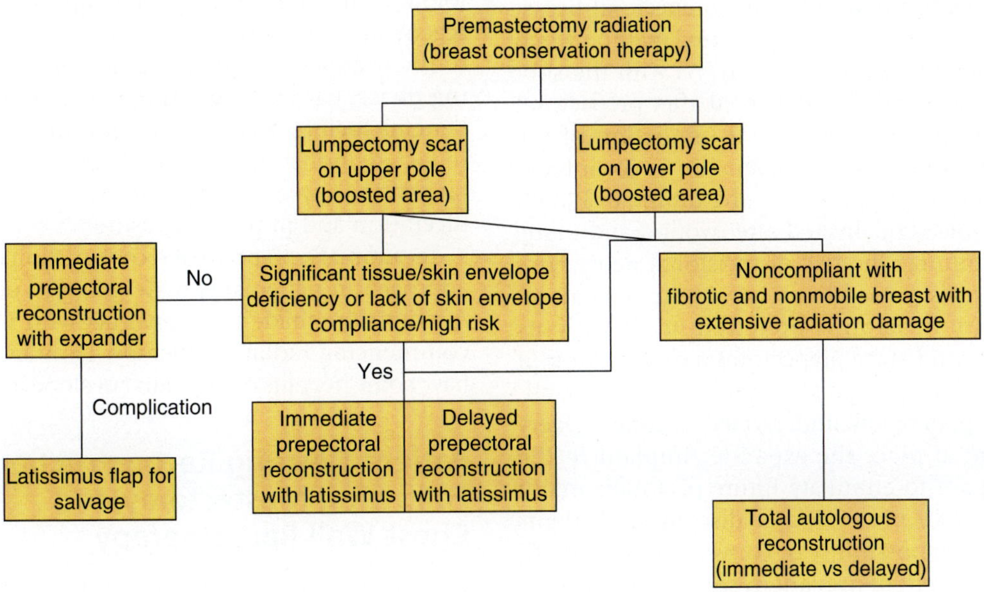

Figure 18.2 Reconstructive management of patients with premastectomy radiation therapy.

salvage latissimus flap, the initial reconstructive option should only include autologous with an expander. If the patient is unwilling to accept any donor site scars, then reconstruction should be delayed so she can think about her options. Reconstruction without latissimus should only be attempted in well-informed and mentally prepared patients with boosted scar in the upper pole. The authors' discussion for informed consent in these patients includes a 50% chance that they will undergo a latissimus flap if expander reconstruction is attempted without an autologous tissue. If the boosted scar is in the lower pole, then this option is never given to the patients because all of them require a latissimus flap.

In summary, in the latissimus-based approach, the latissimus muscle replaces the acellular dermal matrix for expander/implant coverage and support on the irradiated side. Soft tissue is introduced with the flap in areas where it is lacking; otherwise the procedure is performed with muscle flap only. Reconstruction is typically performed in two stages. The expander stage is critical to allow for skin and subcutaneous expansion. The lower pole is the most critical area for tissue expansion, and if the scar lies on the lower pole, then expansion will not be successful. Dual-plane reconstruction has no role in this case, because the pectoralis major muscle has also undergone radiation and has lost its expandability, and the patient will be better served with prepectoral reconstruction with latissimus flap to cover the lower pole. The authors always prefer to reconstruct a premastectomy radiated patient with autologous and expander versus autologous only if the skin and entire breast are fibrotic.

Patient Desiring Immediate Reconstruction With Planned PMRT

PMRT is not a contraindication for prepectoral breast reconstruction; it is the authors' preferred method when radiation is planned postoperatively. As with the subpectoral approach, PMRT is delivered after prepectoral expander or implant placement. If irradiation of the expander is planned, tissue expansion is completed before irradiation. Irrespective of the timing of PMRT, radiation is typically delivered after wound and tissue healing to minimize the risk of incisional dehiscence and skin necrosis caused by ischemia. In general, an inframammary incision is preferred in all patients undergoing second-stage prepectoral reconstruction, if possible. If PMRT is planned or there is a high likelihood that the patient will undergo the treatment, every effort is made to place the expander/implant in the prepectoral space to eliminate future pectoralis major fibrosis, distortion, and associated discomfort. Patients are advised of the possibility of conversion to a latissimus flap in the event of implant or soft-tissue concerns following completion of radiation therapy. This again depends on the field and the amount and duration of radiation that is administered, because it is unknown at what dose the severe irreversible changes occur. All published literature on breast reconstruction in combination with radiation does not include the duration, the extent of the field, and the amount of radiation that was applied. In addition, no information on boosting the incisions is provided because some centers continue to utilize this concept even though there is no evidence that there are recurrence benefits in patients undergoing mastectomy. Therefore, every patient is informed of the possibility of conversion to an autologous tissue if the damage of radiation on the skin envelope is severe. Even if there is conversion to full or partial autologous, the expander in the prepectoral space makes for a simpler conversion because there is no need to manipulate the muscle. If the patient presents with a failed dual-plane reconstruction that has been irradiated, a site change to the prepectoral space is performed with the addition of a partial or a full autologous flap. If a prepectoral, postirradiated expander or implant is to be converted to an autologous reconstruction, whether full autologous or with expander/implant, reconstruction would still be performed prepectorally to eliminate the deleterious effects of irradiation on the pectoralis major muscle.

Fat grafting following PMRT is typically delayed, allowing for tissue healing. Although it is current practice to perform fat grafting 3 to 6 months after PMRT, earlier fat grafting may be more appropriate and should be considered. An animal study that assessed radiation-induced skin changes over 6 weeks demonstrated the progressive nature of radiation-induced cutaneous thickening with decreased perfusion and elasticity.[8] Earlier fat grafting, before tissue perfusion, is severely compromised and before severe dermal thickening and fibrosis occurs, may present a more conducive milieu for fat graft retention and regeneration. In addition, the regenerative potential of fat cells may also be beneficial to the irradiated recipient tissue during the early healing phase. Earlier fat grafting may also lead to clinical benefits such as decreased complication rates. This was, in fact, demonstrated in a study by Ribuffo et al, where fat grafting 6 weeks after expander irradiation prevented ulceration and implant exposure.[9,10]

In summary, prepectoral reconstruction is the preferred approach in patients who are going to undergo PMRT. Attempts are made to reconstruct with implant before commencing radiation therapy. Early fat grafting may have some benefits on the skin envelope in the long term.

Patient Desiring Reconstruction Following Mastectomy and Chest Wall Radiotherapy

This group of patients who present for delayed reconstruction following mastectomy and radiation therapy can be challenging because of the severity of radiation and, at times, the lack of "workable" skin envelope. There is no doubt that these patients will have a prepectoral reconstruction, whether autologous, device based, or a combination of both, for the reasons stated previously because it relates to the pectoralis major. As discussed in the chapter titled *Delayed Prepectoral Breast Reconstruction* (Chapter 17), the consideration of fat grafting is made in the first stage of reconstruction to ensure central scar release from the pectoralis major and prepare the skin envelope, especially the lower pole, for a device-based reconstruction. If this is a unilateral case with severe dermal fibrosis and nonpliability, then the consideration for autologous reconstruction is made early, and there is no need for early fat grafting. If the consideration is made to move forward with device-based reconstruction, on the basis of appropriate patient selection, reconstruction on the radiated side is generally device-based autologous or device only. This is because of a lack of skin-envelope expansibility leading to complications during the early course of postsurgical recovery. The authors' preferred approach is to add a latissimus flap to an expander in delayed radiated reconstructions with varying sizes of skin paddles depending on the skin. Exceptions to this are patients with severe dermal fibrosis and inability to elevate and pinch the skin of the chest wall. These patients are better served with full autologous reconstruction, which is also always performed in a prepectoral space.

In summary, in patients presenting for delayed reconstruction after mastectomy and chest wall irradiation, the reconstructive option is autologous reconstruction with or without expanders, depending on the tissue quality.

Patient With Prior Implant-Based Dual-Plane Reconstruction and Either Premastectomy or PMRT

This group includes patients who have undergone a one-stage or two-stage device-based reconstruction and who have had either premastectomy or PMRT. These patients present with severe scarring and cephalad pull of the implant and desire correction of pain. This is another group that is difficult to treat, because the principles of premastectomy criteria can be utilized in these cases (**Figure 18.3**). The key here is that the muscle must be eliminated from the reconstruction because it is a major source of the issues, as previously stated. Now the plan is to convert this to prepectoral space but with a mastectomy flap that has been radiated and is scarred. Once again, some form of autologous tissue is going to be needed here to resurface the mastectomy flap with or without skin paddle, depending on the deficit of the skin envelope. When in doubt, a skin paddle can be included, and this can always be removed at the second stage when the implant is placed. These revisions are generally performed in two stages, with an expander first to minimize the stress on the damaged mastectomy flap and allow for ease of expansion over time. This is also where more projecting expanders are utilized. The authors also at times perform a preemptive fat grafting to better prepare the skin for the site change. This allows for a better dissection plane when the pectoralis major and lower pole acellular dermal matrix, if present, is being removed. These are very rewarding procedures for patients because there is an immediate sense of comfort once the radiated pectoralis major is excluded from the reconstruction, and this allows for more caudal movement of the skin envelope and breast mound.

In summary, when revising patients to prepectoral space from the previously radiated dual plane, an autologous tissue is advised with an expander; and this is performed in two stages. At times, the first stage includes fat grafting, depending on the quality and thickness of the starting mastectomy flap. Refer to Chapter 17 for similar principles that are utilized.

Surgical Technique

Prepectoral reconstruction has been described in detail in other chapters. Here, some considerations when working with radiated tissue are highlighted. In general, in prepectoral reconstruction, an expander with greater projection is chosen to better expand the lower pole, and this is also valid for patients who are radiated. The most important surgical pearl in irradiated cases is to avoid the original mastectomy scar during the second stage. Ideally, an inframammary fold (IMF) incision is utilized for the second stage; and if an IMF incision already exists, a more caudal and lateral IMF incision is chosen, so the same scar is not reutilized. During the mastectomy, if the suspicion of PMRT is high (because of node positivity) or radiation is planned, every effort is made to avoid an IMF incision unless it is a nipple-sparing mastectomy. If it is a skin-sparing mastectomy, the central scar is closed, and if it is a skin-reducing mastectomy, a vertical-only incision is made, and the horizontal component is avoided if possible. In this way, a new scar is utilized for the second stage. If there is a possibility of performing the second stage before radiation therapy, generally an IMF scar is utilized, and it is performed at 5 to 6 weeks following the mastectomy.

In patients who are scheduled to undergo radiotherapy after expander placement, tissue expansion is typically completed before delivery of radiotherapy. In patients who had air-filled expanders, the air is replaced with saline before radiotherapy. In patients who require additional soft-tissue coverage, autologous fat grafting is performed at the second stage unless a capsulotomy is performed or

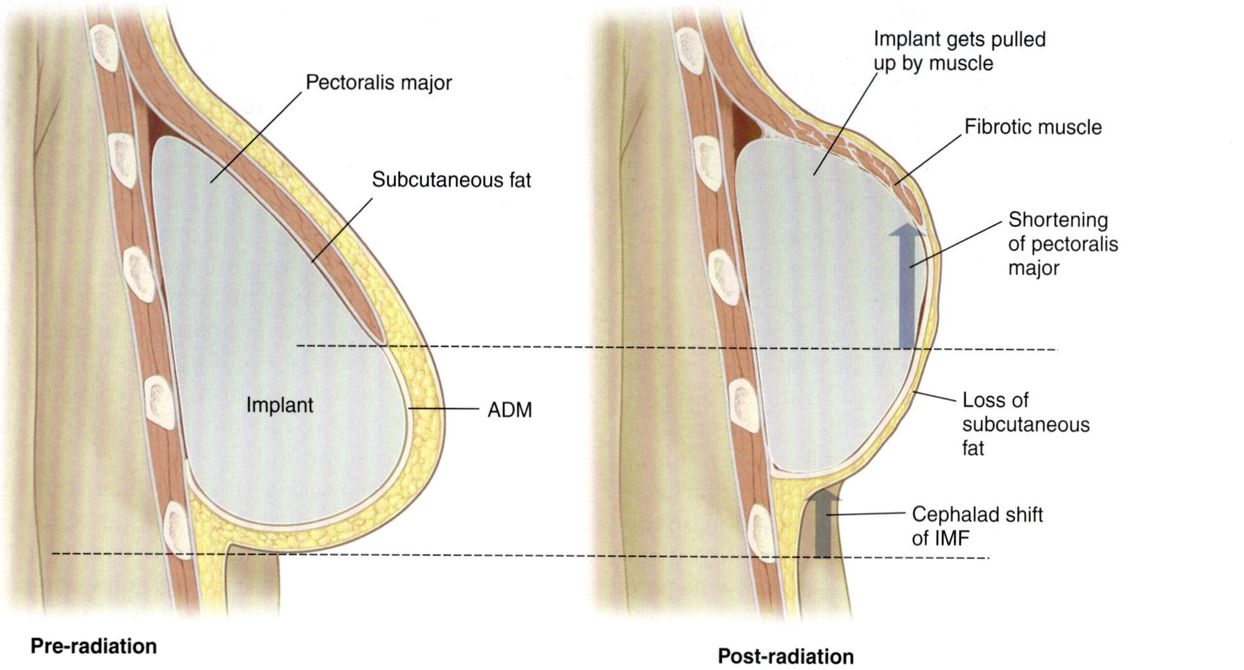

Figure 18.3 Effect of radiation on the pectoralis major. Severe shortening and fibrosis of the muscle is noted, and cephalad pull of the entire reconstructive breast is noted.

the patient is going to have radiotherapy after implant placement.

Fat grafting is usually necessary in irradiated breasts to improve overall aesthetics and is performed after tissue healing, typically 3 to 6 months after PMRT, although the authors are considering earlier fat grafting at 6 weeks following completion of PMRT. As irradiation progressively compromises tissue perfusion, early fat grafting allows the capitalization of perfused tissue for graft retention and regeneration. The regenerative environment created by the incorporated fat cells may also benefit the host tissue during the early healing phase post irradiation.

DISCUSSION

Radiation is the most significant risk factor for major complications in prosthetic reconstruction.[11] Radiation-induced injury is noticeable within days to weeks on breast skin and tissue as edema, inflammation, and desquamation. These acute effects may lead to complications such as incisional dehiscence, infection, delayed healing, seroma, and hematoma after breast reconstruction. Over months to years, radiation causes progressive deposition of fibrosis tissue in the skin and underlying breast muscles, resulting in dermal thickening and muscle fibrosis and atrophy. These delayed effects of radiation may lead to complications such as capsular contracture and implant malposition after reconstructive surgery.

The impact of premastectomy and PMRT on subpectoral implant-based reconstruction has been extensively studied and documented.[4,12] Given that prepectoral breast reconstruction is a relatively new technique, there is a paucity of data in the setting of radiotherapy. Nonetheless, a recent study by Sigalove et al showed that the timing of PMRT in prepectoral reconstructions appears to have little influence on postoperative outcomes.[13] In contrast, in subpectoral reconstructions, expander irradiation is generally associated with a higher risk of reconstructive failure and capsular contracture compared with implant irradiation.[2] However, the recent Mastectomy Reconstruction Outcomes Consortium Study reported no significant difference in complication rates between expander and implant irradiation in subpectoral reconstructions. This study concluded that the timing of PMRT is not a significant predictor of any complication, a major complication, or reconstructive failure,[8] corroborating Sigalove et al's findings in prepectorally reconstructed patients.[13]

The Sigalove et al study also reported a low rate of complications in irradiated breasts that included one incidence of seroma and one incidence of wound dehiscence followed by expander removal. There was no incidence of capsular contracture.[13] In speculating over reason(s) for the observed favorable outcomes after PMRT, particularly the absence of capsular contracture, one is reminded of a study by Cheng et al.[14] In this study, the authors described a novel technique to treat and prevent recurrent capsular contracture, which entailed using acellular dermal matrix to completely cover the implant anteriorly. Of 16 breasts treated, none developed recurrent capsular contracture over an average follow-up of 9.2 months (range, 2.4-18.8 months). Clinically, it is now well recognized that acellular dermal matrix mitigates capsular contracture, even if it partially covers the implant.[15,16] Histopathologic studies suggest that acellular dermal matrix diminishes the inflammatory and profibrotic signaling characteristics of breast capsule development, leading to capsules that are thinner than native breast capsules.[17] But in the setting of PMRT, the benefit of acellular dermal matrix appears to be diminished as reported by Spear et al.[18] This leads to the speculation that perhaps complete prosthesis coverage with acellular dermal matrix and sparing the pectoralis major may provide greater protection against the adverse effects of radiotherapy than partial coverage. Sparing the pectoralis major minimizes and eliminates the cephalad pull of the muscle, permitting the implant to remain in its preradiation location. Even if the pectoralis major is used, one must keep in mind that this is devoid of fascia and its function and scarring are changed given the lack of a protective and gliding surface. The skin reaction to radiation, however, is not eliminated in the prepectoral approach, which leads to dermal fibrosis and thickening of the skin envelope. This is where the addition of fat may play an important role in improving the overall skin envelope over time.

Patients with premastectomy radiation can also present challenges, and careful patient selection and understanding of the need for autologous muscle only versus with skin paddle tissue is made to ensure a successful outcome in these patients. The location of lumpectomy scar and lack of soft tissue and its expandability should be considered when evaluating the need for autologous tissue in these cases. The concern with this patient population is that premastectomy radiation may have caused changes to the skin envelope, as discussed earlier in this chapter. Following mastectomy, the radiation-damaged skin does not have the same recovery potential as a nonradiated skin, and even slight skin damage or contamination can lead to failure in this group.

A question that surgeons often ask is whether premastectomy radiation is a contraindication to prepectoral reconstruction. The short answer is no; it depends on the quality of tissue, and an addition of combined autologous flap should be considered in this patient population. Because the best outcome in this group is a prepectoral reconstruction no matter what the modality of reconstruction is, the next question that surgeons ask is whether the breast should be reconstructed with an expander/implant only, an expander/implant in conjunction with a latissimus flap, or a total autologous approach. The type of reconstruction depends on the quality of tissue that the patient is presenting with. If the lumpectomy scar is in the upper pole and the skin is supple, then a consideration for expander only can be made if the patient understands that she may need a latissimus flap for salvage if any complications occur. Otherwise, these patients undergo immediate latissimus/expander reconstruction. If the skin is damaged and adhered to the chest wall and there is damage to the surrounding skin, then a consideration for autologous only can be considered. This discussion then leads to delayed reconstruction of a previously radiated chest wall following mastectomy. These patients are reconstructed in the prepectoral space, but either with latissimus and expander or total autologous.

SUMMARY

In patients who have been radiated or scheduled for radiation, every effort is made to perform an implant-based prepectoral breast reconstruction with or without autologous tissue. In radiated premastectomy patients, the use of autologous tissue depends on the quality of the breast soft tissue and the location of the lumpectomy scar; whereas in the setting of PMRT, autologous tissue is utilized only if there is severe soft-tissue damage from radiotherapy or in salvage situations. In delayed postradiotherapy cases, the majority would require autologous or autologous and expander for a successful reconstruction. Prepectoral reconstruction in the setting of radiation therapy minimizes the adverse muscle contractions and pain associated with long-term fibrosis and the cephalad pull of the muscle.

CASE EXAMPLES

CASE 1 (FIGURE 18.4)

Sixty-eight-year-old female (body mass index, 24 kg/m^2) with a new diagnosis of stage III invasive ductal carcinoma (IDC) of the right breast who underwent neoadjuvant chemotherapy. She has had no prior submuscular augmentations through the nipple-areolar complex.

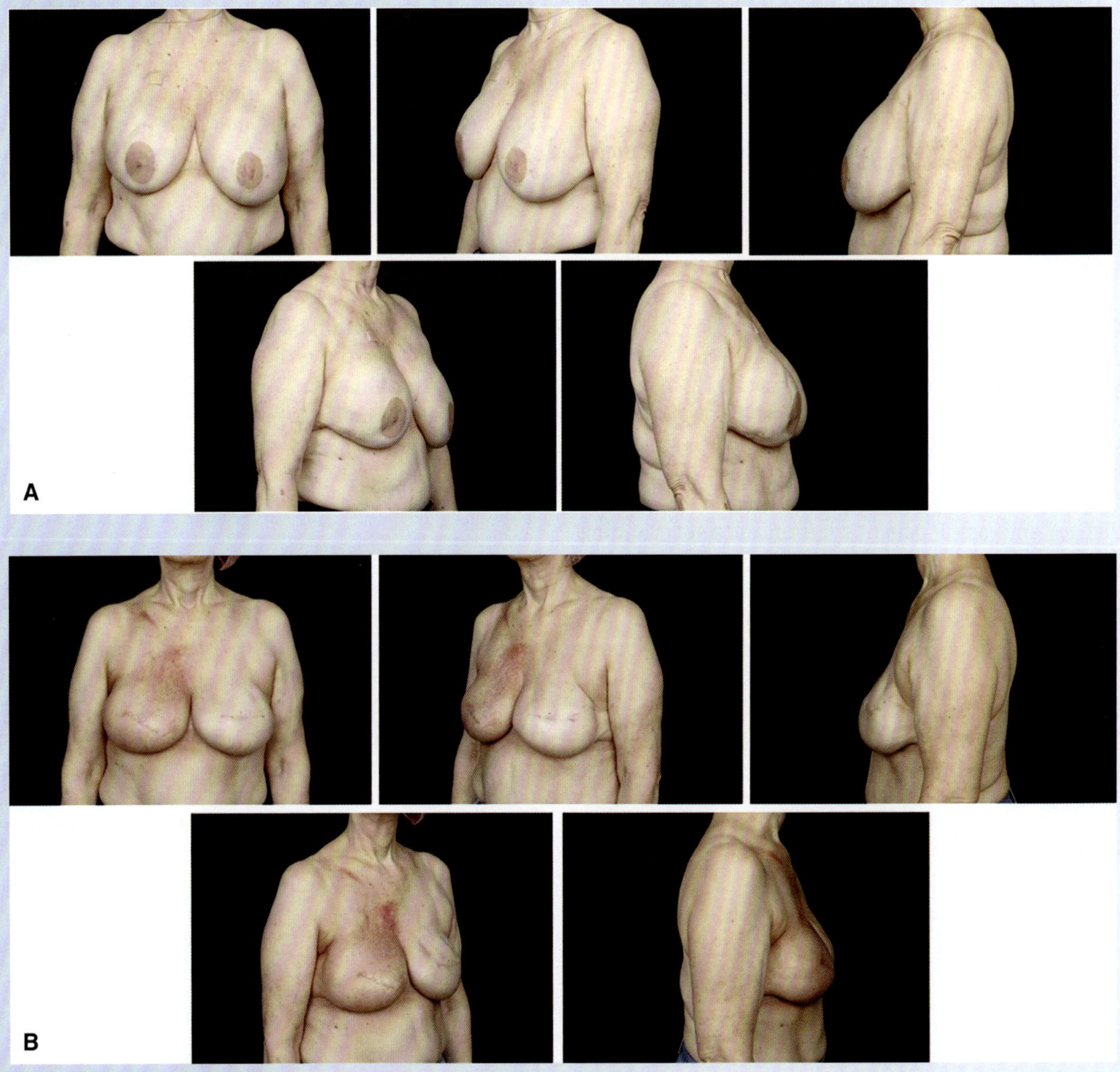

Figure 18.4 A, Preoperative views. B, Patient underwent bilateral skin-sparing mastectomy and prepectoral reconstruction with 133FV 550-mL expanders and upper pole AlloDerm and lower pole Artia followed by right breast irradiation. At 1 week following completion of her radiation therapy.

CASE 1 (FIGURE 18.4)

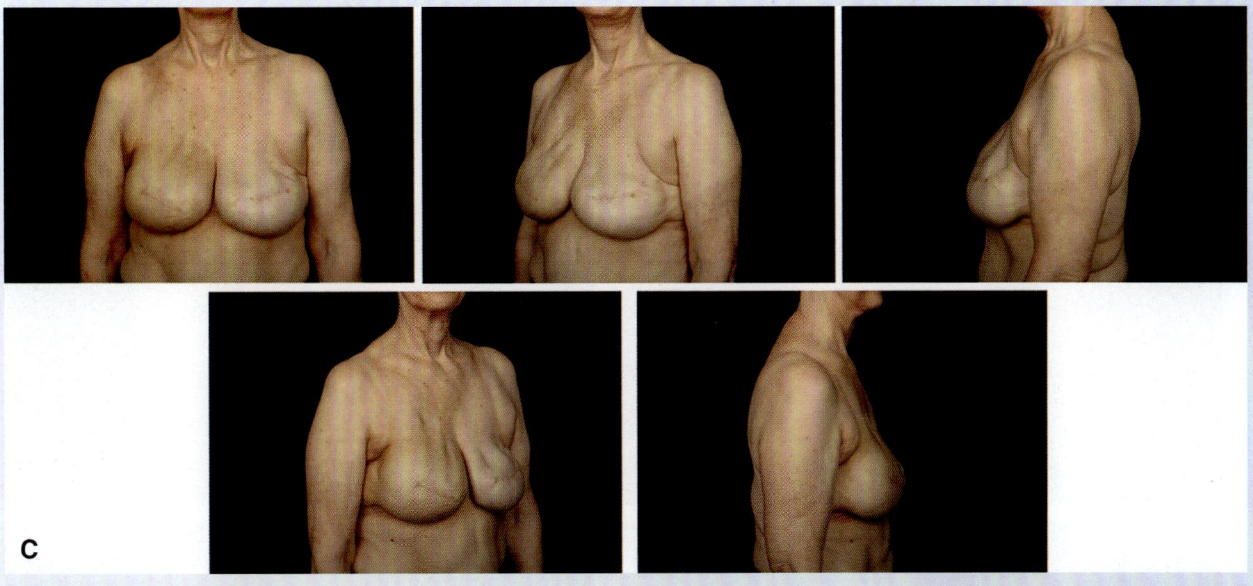

C

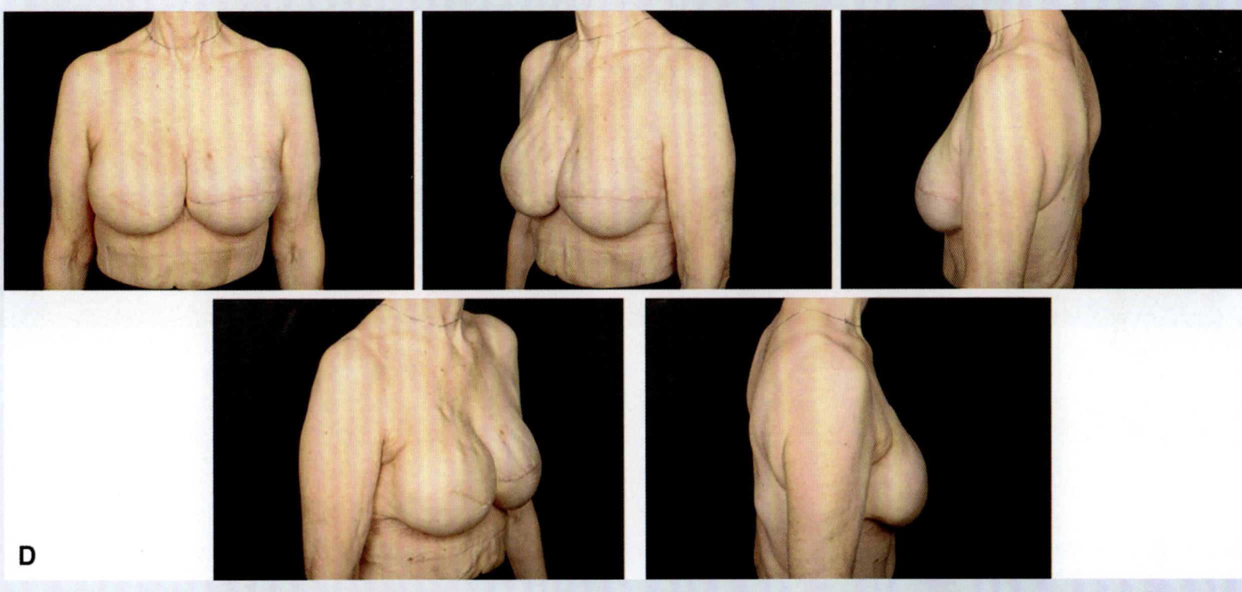

D

Figure 18.4 (*continued*) C, At 6 months following completion of radiation therapy. D, At 9 months following second-stage reconstruction with SRF 605-mL implant through an inframammary fold incision. Left breast skin envelope was addressed at time of exchange, but the implant pocket was not accessed through the central incision. The AlloDerm was imbricated to further tighten the pocket for an improved match.

CASE 2 (FIGURE 18.5)

Fifty-two-year-old female with a history of left lumpectomy and radiation therapy 4 years before her completion mastectomy with subpectoral two-stage, expander/implant reconstruction (**Figure 18.5**).

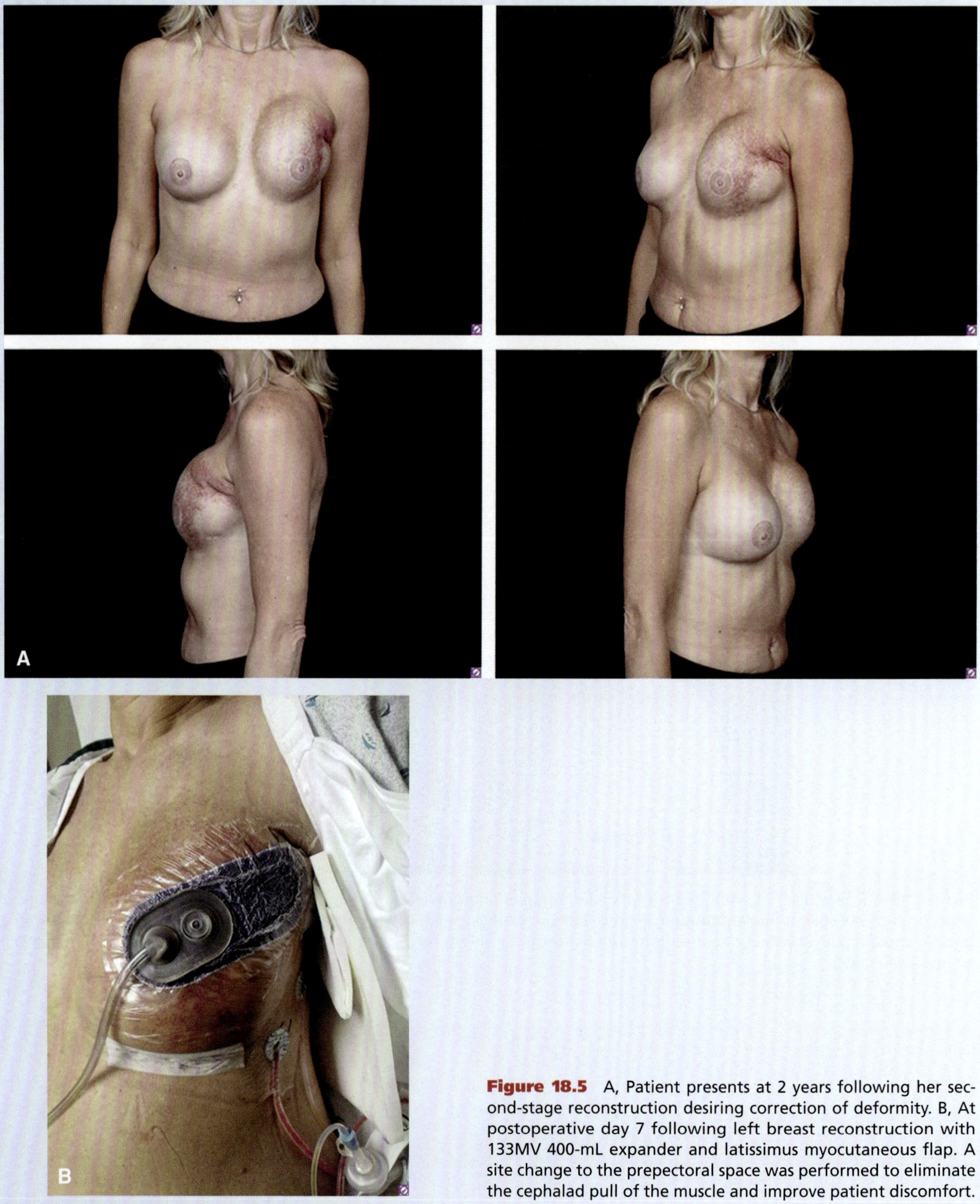

Figure 18.5 A, Patient presents at 2 years following her second-stage reconstruction desiring correction of deformity. B, At postoperative day 7 following left breast reconstruction with 133MV 400-mL expander and latissimus myocutaneous flap. A site change to the prepectoral space was performed to eliminate the cephalad pull of the muscle and improve patient discomfort.

CASE 1 (FIGURE 18.5)

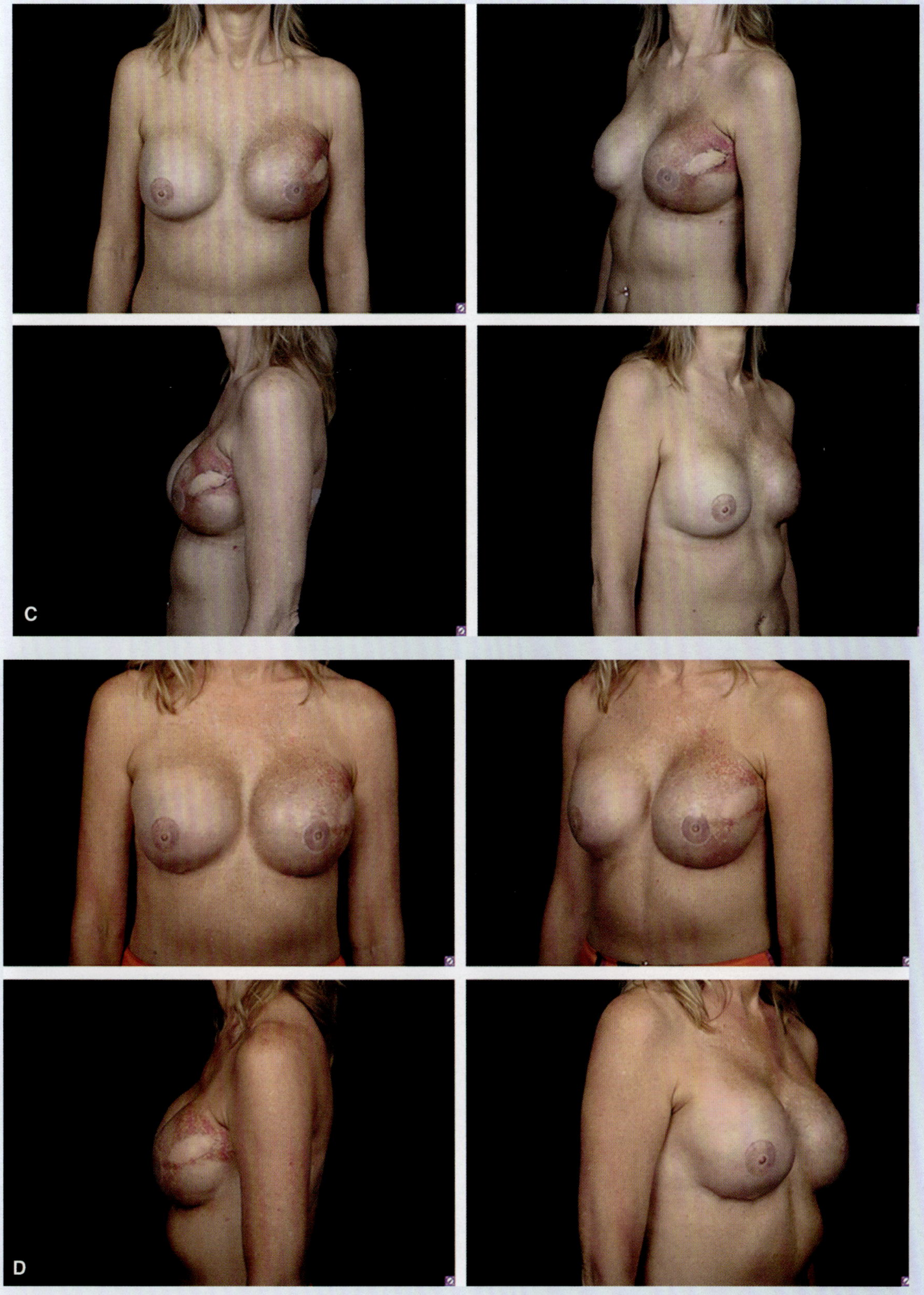

Figure 18.5 (*continued*) C, At postoperative day 21 following site change and reconstruction. D, At 3 months following the first stage, patient underwent bilateral second-stage reconstruction with SCX 560-mL implant on the left and SCX 580-mL implant on the right. Patient is shown at 9 months postoperatively.

CASE 3 (FIGURE 18.5)

Fifty-one-year-old female with a history of right lumpectomy and radiation therapy for right clinically stage IIA **IDC** presenting 2 years after completion of external radiation therapy. Patient has been undergoing numerous biopsies and imaging for surveillance every 6 months.

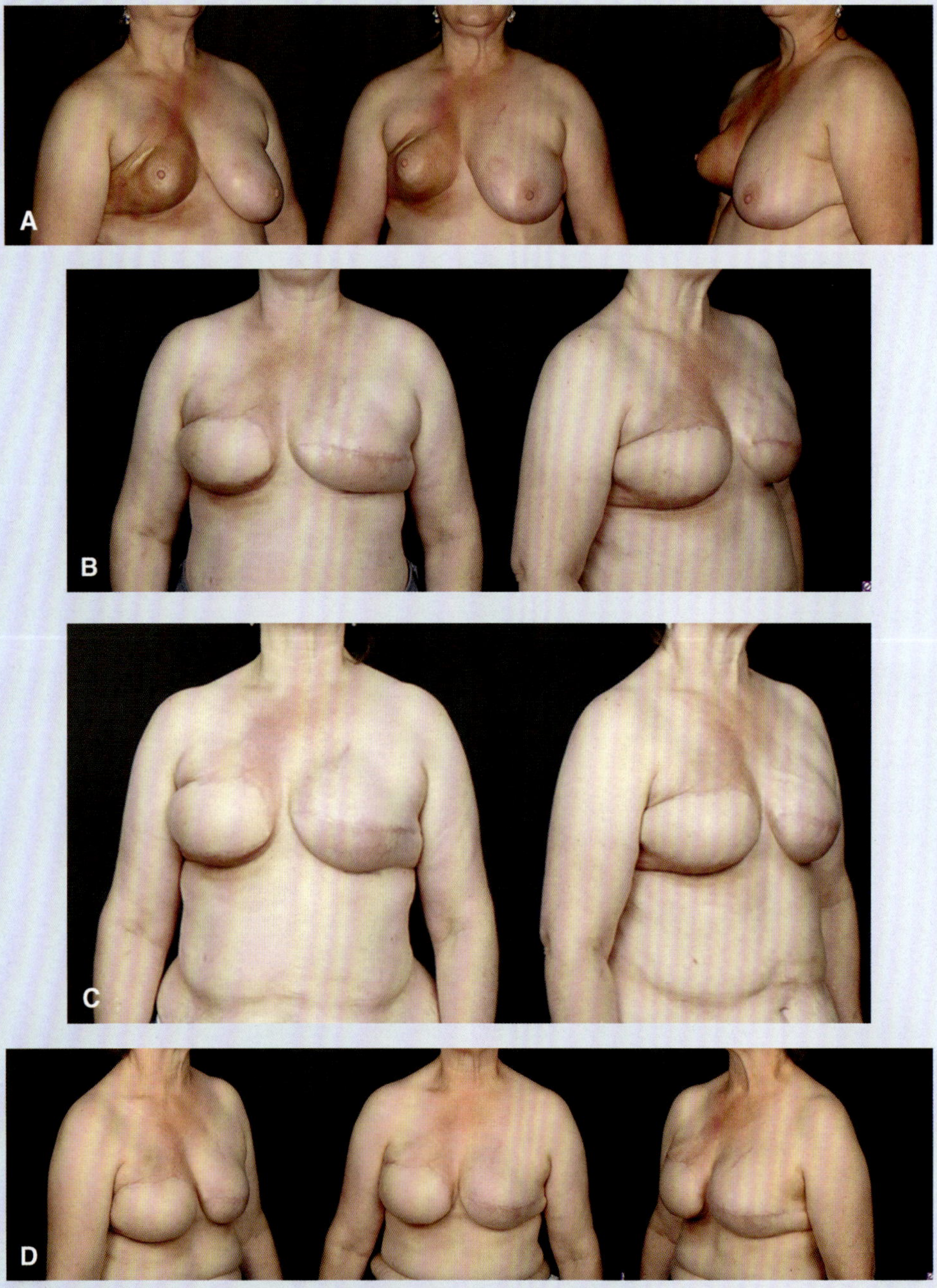

Figure 18.6 A, Patient presents at 2 years following her lumpectomy concerned about the imaging and biopsies issues and pain. B, At postoperative day 60 following bilateral mastectomy with immediate right latissimus flap reconstruction and left breast reconstruction 133FV 500-mL expander and acellular dermal matrix. C, At postoperative day 50 following right breast fat grafting and left breast reconstruction with SCF 560 mL. D, At 10 months following bilateral breast fat grafting.

KEY REFERENCES

1. Cordeiro PG, Albornoz CR, McCormick B, et al. What is the optimum timing of postmastectomy radiotherapy in two-stage prosthetic reconstruction: radiation to the tissue expander or permanent implant? *Plast Reconstr Surg*. 2015;135(6):1509-1517.
2. Nava MB, Pennati AE, Lozza L, Spano A, Zambetti M, Catanuto G. Outcome of different timings of radiotherapy in implant-based breast reconstructions. *Plast Reconstr Surg*. 2011;128(2):353-359.
3. Wong JS, Ho AY, Kaelin CM, et al. Incidence of major corrective surgery after post-mastectomy breast reconstruction and radiation therapy. *Breast J*. 2008;14(1):49-54.
4. Magill LJ, Robertson FP, Jell G, Mosahebi A, Keshtgar M. Determining the outcomes of post-mastectomy radiation therapy delivered to the definitive implant in patients undergoing one- and two-stage implant-based breast reconstruction: a systematic review and meta-analysis. *J Plast Reconstr Aesthet Surg*. 2017;70(10):1329-1335.
5. Nahabedian MY, Cocilovo C. Two-stage prosthetic breast reconstruction: a comparison between prepectoral and partial subpectoral techniques. *Plast Reconstr Surg*. 2017;140(6S Prepectoral Breast Reconstruction):22S-30S.
6. Sbitany H, Piper M, Lentz R. Prepectoral breast reconstruction: a safe alternative to submuscular prosthetic reconstruction following nipple-sparing mastectomy. *Plast Reconstr Surg*. 2017;140(3):432-443.
7. Sigalove S, Maxwell GP, Sigalove NM, et al. Prepectoral implant-based breast reconstruction: rationale, indications, and preliminary results. *Plast Reconstr Surg*. 2017;139(2):287-294.
8. Santosa KB, Chen X, Qi J, et al. Postmastectomy radiation therapy and two-stage implant-based breast reconstruction: is there a better time to irradiate? *Plast Reconstr Surg*. 2016;138(4):761-769.
9. Ribuffo D, Atzeni M. Protective lipofilling allows immediate expander-implant breast [corrected] reconstruction in the setting of postoperative radiotherapy. *Plast Reconstr Surg*. 2013;131(5):848e-849e.
10. Ribuffo D, Atzeni M, Guerra M, et al. Treatment of irradiated expanders: protective lipofilling allows immediate prosthetic breast reconstruction in the setting of postoperative radiotherapy. *Aesthetic Plast Surg*. 2013;37(6):1146-1152.
11. Berry T, Brooks S, Sydow N, et al. Complication rates of radiation on tissue expander and autologous tissue breast reconstruction. *Ann Surg Oncol*. 2010;17(suppl 3):202-210.
12. Clemens MW, Kronowitz SJ. Current perspectives on radiation therapy in autologous and prosthetic breast reconstruction. *Gland Surg*. 2015;4(3):222-231.
13. Sigalove S, Maxwell GP, Sigalove NM, et al. Prepectoral implant-based breast reconstruction and postmastectomy radiotherapy: short-term outcomes. *Plast Reconstr Surg Glob Open*. 2017;5(12):e1631.
14. Cheng A, Lakhiani C, Saint-Cyr M. Treatment of capsular contracture using complete implant coverage by acellular dermal matrix: a novel technique. *Plast Reconstr Surg*. 2013;132(3):519-529.
15. Salzberg CA, Ashikari AY, Berry C, Hunsicker LM. Acellular dermal matrix-assisted direct-to-implant breast reconstruction and capsular contracture: a 13-year experience. *Plast Reconstr Surg*. 2016;138(2):329-337.
16. Vardanian AJ, Clayton JL, Roostaeian J, et al. Comparison of implant-based immediate breast reconstruction with and without acellular dermal matrix. *Plast Reconstr Surg*. 2011;128(5):403e-410e.
17. Leong M, Basu CB, Hicks MJ. Further evidence that human acellular dermal matrix decreases inflammatory markers of capsule formation in implant-based breast reconstruction. *Aesthet Surg J*. 2015;35(1):40-47.
18. Spear SL, Seruya M, Rao SS, et al. Two-stage prosthetic breast reconstruction using AlloDerm including outcomes of different timings of radiotherapy. *Plast Reconstr Surg*. 2012;130(1):1-9.

CHAPTER 19

CANCER SURVEILLANCE FOLLOWING PREPECTORAL RECONSTRUCTION

Noemi M. Sigalove and Toni Storm-Dickerson

KEY POINTS

- Prepectoral reconstruction is a safe approach in carefully selected patients.
- Until FAST MRI is available, full breast MRI is offered to patients every 3 to 5 years.
- Self-breast examinations remain critical for patients.

INTRODUCTION

Early adoption of the prepectoral approach by breast and reconstructive surgeons has been driven by perceived and observed patient benefits. The elimination of animation deformity and the comfort derived from leaving the pectoralis muscle undisturbed have piqued the interest of patients in pursuing prepectoral reconstruction over other reconstructive options. Leaving the muscle in its native position allows for a procedure that is less invasive and better tolerated by patients than its subpectoral counterpart.[1,2] Postoperative complications with the prepectoral approach have been shown to be comparable in type and incidence to those reported with partial muscle coverage.[3-5] A less traumatic procedure leads to minimal pain with decreased need for narcotics, faster recovery, elimination of animation deformity, improved long-term comfort, as well as a more natural appearing breast.[1-2,6]

Although the prepectoral approach has been embraced by patients and surgeons alike, concern exists regarding adequate surveillance for recurrence once the prepectoral reconstructive device has been placed. For those patients who are at higher oncologic likelihood of recurrence, the inability to palpate a posterior recurrence may cause a delay in diagnosis and treatment. Critics of the approach have cited this difficulty in monitoring for recurrence as the main reason for their hesitance in becoming early adopters. Furthermore, the lack of published data on recurrence post prepectoral reconstruction, both local and distant, hold back some oncologic surgeons from recommending prepectoral reconstruction to their patients.

It is important to note that the prepectoral procedure is not suitable for all patients. Selection criteria for prepectoral reconstruction combine variables that are unique to each individual with parameters that are felt to be oncologically safe. Understanding and embracing these principles are at the core of delivering safe oncologic care. General exclusion criteria include ischemic, poorly vascularized skin flaps after mastectomy; patients with a history of preoperative breast irradiation or uncontrolled diabetes ($HbA_{1c} > 7.5\%$); patients who are active smokers, immunocompromised, or morbidly obese (body mass index > 40); and patients who lack fat donor sites (**Table 19.1**). As the technique gains wider acceptance and surgeons build increased experience, some of the original parameters are likely to be challenged and exclusion criteria narrowed. This is similar to the evolution of surgical technique and experience with nipple-sparing mastectomies.

We have also identified a number of oncologic contraindications for the prepectoral reconstructive approach (**Table 19.2**). Oncologic surgeons who feel ambivalent regarding the use of prepectoral reconstruction may start by choosing patients who are at low likelihood for tumor recurrence. Use of genomic testing, when available, may be of value in determining risk of recurrence. Patients with late-stage breast cancer, posterior tumors near to or involving the pectoralis major muscle, and patients at high risk for recurrence are felt to be poor candidates for prepectoral placement. As with subpectoral reconstruction, extreme caution should be exercised for large tumors and for clinically positive lymph nodes.[7]

TABLE 19.1 SUMMARY OF RECONSTRUCTIVE CONTRAINDICATIONS

Absolute reconstructive contraindications for **immediate** prepectoral reconstruction

- Poorly vascularized/ischemic flaps
- $HbA_{1c} > 7.5\%$
- Active smokers

Questionable reconstructive contraindications for immediate prepectoral reconstruction

- Body mass index > 35 kg/m^2
  - With associated comorbidities
- H/O premastectomy XRT
  - Unless latissimus is utilized

Abbreviations: H/O, history of; XRT, external radiation therapy.

For late-stage tumors, an attempt can be made to downstage the tumor using neoadjuvant chemotherapy. This is similar in concept to downstaging tumors to allow for breast conservation.[8,9] If a favorable clinical and radiographic response is achieved, prepectoral reconstruction becomes a possibility. We recommend obtaining a post neoadjuvant magnetic resonance imaging (MRI) before proceeding with surgery. Even though MRI is not absolute in its predictive value for pathologic response, it does allow for a more objective assessment of degree of response than physical examination alone.[10] It has been observed that the accuracy of MRI in estimating postchemotherapy tumor size varies with tumor subtype: highest in ER−/HER2+ (estrogen receptor negative/human epidermal growth factor receptor 2 positive) and lowest in luminal tumors.[11]

If MRI is not desired, and the tumor was originally visible on ultrasound, response can alternatively be evaluated using ultrasound.[12] Imaging should be assessed by the entire oncologic team, and recommendations should be made regarding optimal surgical and reconstructive options as well as the need for postoperative radiation therapy. If breast conservation becomes a possibility as a result of neoadjuvant chemotherapy, then breast conservation should also be discussed with the patient as a viable surgical alternative.

Although a history of radiation therapy negatively impacts prepectoral reconstruction, the converse is not the case. Radiation therapy can, and should, be used for prepectoral reconstruction patients who have oncologic indication for postmastectomy radiation. In our experience, to date, complications associated with adjuvant radiation are not significantly different from those seen with dual-plane reconstruction. Although complications of skin necrosis can occur, the more common complications tend to be skin tightening and stiffness with associated reduction in size. Therefore, if pathology or tumor biology warrants radiation therapy, radiation should be delivered on the basis of oncologic criteria and not on the type of reconstruction used.

Patient selection for prepectoral reconstruction should be approached from a multidisciplinary standpoint and should involve the entire care team. Reconstructive and oncologic surgeons, medical oncologists, and radiation oncologists should understand and be comfortable with the implementation of the prepectoral technique. Provided that oncologic safety criteria are upheld, prepectoral implant–based reconstruction can be used for both skin- and nipple-sparing mastectomies.

Placing implants in the prepectoral space can be likened to the positioning of tissue flaps in autologous breast reconstruction. Surveillance for cancer recurrence is thus recommended using a protocol similar to the one undertaken in autologous reconstruction. Autologous flaps are regularly monitored for cancer recurrence by clinical examinations, and at times by radiologic screening.[13,14]

TABLE 19.2 SUMMARY OF ONCOLOGIC CONTRAINDICATIONS

Absolute oncologic contraindications for **immediate** prepectoral reconstruction

- Inability to obtain clear margins
- Extensive skin involvement
- Chest wall involvement
- Inflammatory breast cancer

Questionable oncologic contraindications for immediate prepectoral reconstruction

- Palpable or matted axillary nodes
- Stages III and IV
- High risk of recurrence (based on multidisciplinary approach)

Because the majority of postmastectomy recurrence occurs in the subcutaneous breast tissue,[15-18] biannual clinical and monthly breast self-examinations are recommended. Mammography is of limited benefit in detecting local recurrence for myocutaneous flap–based reconstruction,[13] and routine use of mammography for prepectoral reconstruction is equally not advised. Diagnostic ultrasound and ultrasound-guided biopsy have been shown to be useful in assessing palpable subcutaneous nodules post reconstruction[14] and should also be utilized for assessing nodules with prepectoral implant–based reconstruction.

The major hesitance in the use of prepectoral reconstruction for the oncologic surgeon stems from the possibility of unrecognized chest wall recurrence resulting from implant position. Overall local recurrence of breast cancer after mastectomy with immediate reconstruction is noted to be 2.3%.[14] Of all recurrences, 28% recur at the chest wall.[15] Recurrence at the chest wall is detected later than recurrence in the subcutaneous tissues.[15] Chest wall recurrence is also more likely to be associated with concurrent distant metastatic disease,[15] and higher tumor stage is associated with increased incidence of recurrence.[18] When mastectomy is performed post neoadjuvant chemotherapy, the presence of lymphovascular invasion and lack of downstaging after neoadjuvant chemotherapy are strong predictors of adverse outcome in young women with locally advanced breast cancer.[19]

When proceeding with prepectoral reconstruction, it is important to minimize the likelihood of chest wall recurrence. In addition to appropriate oncologic patient selection, adequate mastectomy technique becomes imperative in decreasing the incidence of posterior recurrence. Glandular breast tissue and pectoralis major fascia must be removed anterior to the pectoralis muscle (**Figure 19.1**). For tumors close to the pectoralis muscle, knowledge of exact tumor location can be beneficial in guiding the extent of dissection. Mastectomy localization techniques may be utilized for cancers situated high in the upper inner and upper outer quadrants, especially when an inframammary incision is used. Having concrete knowledge of tumor position allows for more precise surgical tumor clearance at the location of the cancer. Using proper technique, the incidence and ability to detect recurrence is not anticipated to be any different than what we currently see in postmastectomy patients undergoing autologous reconstruction. The oncologic surgeon should be familiar with the expected area of reconstruction, acknowledging that maximum expander base width spans 15.5 cm. Residual breast tissue beyond the confines of implant base width can be monitored by palpation similarly to dual-plane reconstruction. There are areas that the oncologic surgeon should pay close attention to, so the areas are not devascularized or overdissected (**Figure 19.2**). It is also important to be aware of the sentinel injection sites, depending on the type of mastectomy that is planned (**Figure 19.3**).

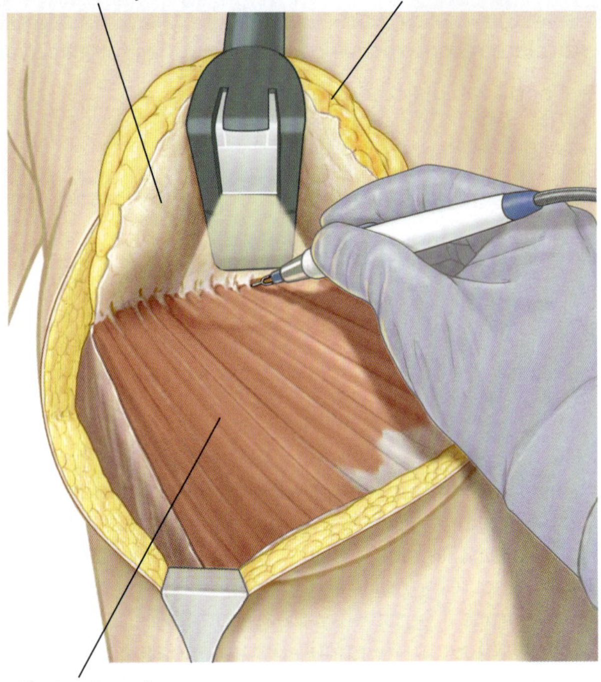

Figure 19.1 Removal of glandular breast tissue and pectoralis major fascia anterior to the pectoralis muscle.

Recognizing the controversies that exist regarding MRI in the care of the breast cancer patient, we were ambivalent about routinely using MRI for assessing local recurrence post prepectoral reconstruction. At our breast programs, we instituted imaging protocols for implant-based prepectoral reconstruction that coincide with the U.S. Food and Drug Administration (FDA)'s recommendation for implant surveillance with MRI at postoperative year 3, and every 2 years thereafter. Adding intravenous contrast to the MRI, we are able to monitor not only implant integrity but also potential mastectomy flap and chest wall recurrence. This is especially important for patients at higher risk for recurrence, such as young patients, patients with unfavorable receptor status, and those who

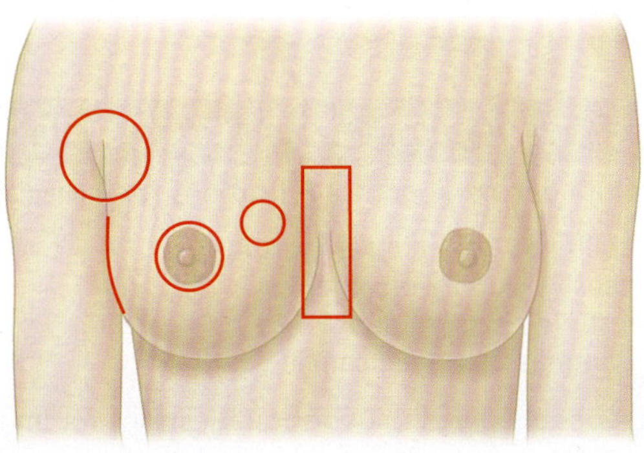

Figure 19.2 Areas that the oncologic surgeon should pay close attention to in order to minimize devascularization and overdissection.

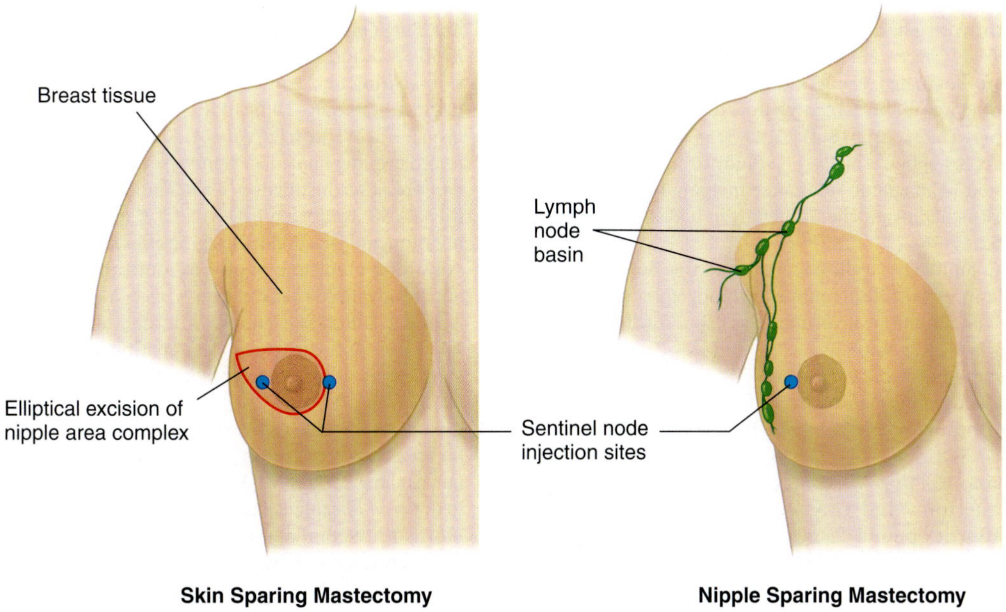

Figure 19.3 Sentinel injection sites depending on type of mastectomy.

have had mastectomies post neoadjuvant chemotherapy.[20] We intend to compile data on these patients, expecting to demonstrate that recurrence rates are similar in this population of patients to the rates of those who undergo autologous tissue reconstruction.

Because full breast MRI is not recognized as a cost-effective modality for breast cancer screening,[21] we are investigating alternate, less expensive ways to monitor for implant integrity and tumor recurrence. The rise of FAST MRI gives promise of the ability to lower cost and decrease the length of time spent in the machine. [21-23] Recall rates and false-positive rates of FAST MRI as compared to its full counterpart are not statistically significantly different,[22] making this imaging modality a viable option for screening high-risk patients for postmastectomy recurrence.

Until FAST MRI is available at our institutions, we continue to offer full breast MRI to our patients using the protocol described. To date, our patients have been receptive to obtaining MRI, because they recognize that surveillance for implant integrity is recommended by the FDA regardless of the type of implant-based reconstruction used.

SUMMARY

Overall, in our experience, the use of prepectoral reconstruction has been of great benefit to both patient and surgeon. Although there is a lack of published data regarding rates of cancer recurrence post prepectoral reconstruction, we feel that the technique is safe as long as appropriate oncologic criteria are applied in patient selection and vigilant surveillance is maintained for recurrence in high-risk patients.

KEY REFERENCES

1. Gabriel A, Sigalove S, Sigalove NM, et al. Can surgical technique impact length of stay and post-operative outcomes in breast reconstruction? Abstract: The American Society of Breast Surgeons 17th Annual Meeting; 2017; Las Vegas, NV.
2. Gabriel A, Sigalove S, Sigalove NM, et al. Does surgical technique impact post-operative outcomes of breast reconstruction? Abstract: International Society for Pharmacoeconomics and Outcomes Research 22nd Annual International Meeting; 2017; Boston, MA.
3. Cordeiro PG, McCarthy CM. A single surgeon's 12-year experience with tissue expander/implant breast reconstruction: part I. A prospective analysis of early complications. *Plast Reconstr Surg*. 2006;118:825-831.
4. Kim JY, Davila AA, Persing S, et al. A meta-analysis of human acellular dermis and submuscular tissue expander breast reconstruction. *Plast Reconstr Surg*. 2012;129:28-41.
5. Hunsicker LM, Ashikari AY, Berry C, Koch RM, Salzberg CA. Short-term complications associated with acellular dermal matrix-assisted direct-to-implant breast reconstruction. *Ann Plast Surg*. 2017;78(1):35-40.
6. Sigalove S, Maxwell PG, Sigalove NM, et al. Prepectoral implant-based breast reconstruction: rationale, indications, and preliminary results. *Plast Reconstr Surg*. 2017;139(2):287-294.
7. Maxwell GP, Storm-Dickerson T, Whitworth P, Rubano C, Gabriel A. Advances in nipple-sparing mastectomy: oncological safety and incision selection. *Aesthet Surg J*. 2011;31:310-319.
8. Manguso N, Gangi A, Giuliano AE. Neoadjuvant chemotherapy and surgical management of the axilla in breast cancer: a review of current data. *Oncology (Williston Park)*. 201529(10):733-738.
9. Read RL, Flitcroft K, Snook KL, Boyle FM, Spillane AJ. Utility of neoadjuvant chemotherapy in the treatment of operable breast cancer. *ANZ J Surg*. 2015;85(5):315-320.

10. Marinovich ML, Macaskill P, Irwig L, et al. Agreement between MRI and pathologic breast tumor size after neoadjuvant chemotherapy, and comparison with alternative tests: individual patient data meta-analysis. *BMC Cancer*. 2015;15:662.
11. McGuire KP, Toro-Burguete J, Dang H, et al. MRI staging after neoadjuvant chemotherapy for breast cancer: does tumor biology affect accuracy? *Ann Surg Oncol*. 2011;18(11):3149-3154.
12. Vriens BE, de Vries B, Lobbes, et al; INTENS Study Group. Ultrasound is at least as good as magnetic resonance imaging in predicting tumour size post-neoadjuvant chemotherapy in breast cancer. *Eur J Cancer*. 2016;52:67-76.
13. Lee JM, Georgian-Smith D, Gazelle GS, et al. Detecting nonpalpable recurrent breast cancer: the role of routine mammographic screening of transverse rectus abdominis myocutaneous flap reconstructions. *Radiology*. 2008;248(2):398-405.
14. Edeiken BS, Fornage BD, Bedi DG, Sneige N, Parulekar SG, Pleasure J. Recurrence in autogenous myocutaneous flap reconstruction after mastectomy for primary breast cancer: US diagnosis. *Radiology*. 2003;227(2):542-548.
15. Howard MA, Polo K, Pusic AL, et al. Breast cancer local recurrence after mastectomy and TRAM flap reconstruction: incidence and treatment options. *Plast Reconstr Surg*. 2006;117(5): 1381-1386.
16. Carlos GW, Styblo TM, Lyles RH, et al. Local recurrence after skin-sparing mastectomy: tumor biology or surgical conservatism? *Ann Surg Oncol*. 2003;10(2):108-112.
17. Kroll SS, Khoo A, Singletary SE, et al. Local recurrence risk after skin-sparing and conventional mastectomy: a 6 year follow-up. *Plast Reconstr Surg*. 1999;104(2):421-425.
18. Lee TJ, Hur WJ, Kim EK, Ahn SH. Outcome of management of local recurrence after immediate transverse rectus abdominis myocutaneous flap breast reconstruction. *Arch Plast Surg*. 2012; 39(4):376-383.
19. Khwaja SS, Ivanovich J, DeWees TA, et al. Lymphovascular space invasion and lack of downstaging after neoadjuvant chemotherapy are strong predictors of adverse outcome in young women with locally advanced breast cancer. *Cancer Med*. 2016;5(2):230-238.
20. Agresti R, Sandri M, Gennaro M, et al. Evaluation of local oncologic safety in nipple-areola complex-sparing mastectomy after primary chemotherapy: a propensity score-matched study. *Clin Breast Cancer*. 2017 ;17(3):219-231.
21. Chhor CM, Mercado CL. Abbreviated MRI protocols: wave of the future for breast cancer screening. *AJR Am J Roentgenol*. 2017;208(2):284-289.
22. Jain M, Jain A, Hyzy MF, Werth G. FAST MRI breast screening revisited. *J Med Imaging Radiat Oncol*. 2017;61(1):24-28.
23. Morris EA. Rethinking breast cancer screening: ultra FAST breast magnetic resonance imaging. *J Clin Onol*. 2014;32(22):2281-2283.

CHAPTER 20

COMPLICATIONS ASSOCIATED WITH PREPECTORAL RECONSTRUCTION

Maurice Y. Nahabedian, Allen Gabriel, and Steven R. Sigalove

KEY POINTS

- Postmastectomy tissue perfusion assessment is critical for prepectoral reconstruction to reduce the incidence of delayed healing.
- Capsular contracture is more common following prepectoral reconstruction without ADM compared to prepectoral reconstruction with ADM.
- Seroma formation can be minimized using perforated ADM and the use of one or two drains.
- Superior displacement of prosthetic devices following radiation therapy is more common following subpectoral reconstruction compared to prepectoral reconstruction.
- Rippling and wrinkling is more common following prepectoral reconstruction and can be minimized using highly cohesive implants and fat grafting.

INTRODUCTION

The goals of prosthetic breast reconstruction are to provide excellent surgical and aesthetic outcomes and to minimize the incidence of adverse events. Achieving ideal outcomes are dependent on proper patient selection, good surgical technique, and appropriate perioperative care. Adverse events can be attributed to patient-related factors such as poorly controlled diabetes mellitus, tobacco use, and obesity as well as poor or improper surgical technique.[1,2] As surgeons, we strive to control as many variables as we can; however, the reality is that some are within our control and others are not. In either event, the plastic surgeon must be able to safely and effectively manage adverse events to achieve a desirable outcome.

This chapter focuses on adverse events associated with prosthetic breast reconstruction in general and more specifically on prepectoral breast reconstruction. As mastectomy and reconstruction techniques have evolved over the years, the incidence of complications has changed. Fortunately, our ability to prevent or minimize some of these complications has improved because we have identified many of the factors that precipitate adverse events.

SUBCUTANEOUS PROSTHETIC BREAST RECONSTRUCTION: 1970S TO 1980S

Prosthetic breast reconstruction has evolved over the years and essentially come full circle. During the 1970s, radical mastectomies were common and breast reconstruction was rarely offered to women. Although breast implants had been available since the 1960s, their use following mastectomy was infrequent; thus, implant-based reconstruction was only offered to select patients. Because many women had the pectoralis major muscle removed with the mastectomy, subcutaneous placement of implants was the only option.

Schlenker et al (1978) reviewed their experience with 89 prosthetic reconstructions performed in the prepectoral position.[3] The reconstruction was performed immediately following mastectomy in 50 patients and on a delayed basis in 39. In all cases, a prefilled device was used. The primary reason for delayed reconstruction was thin mastectomy skin flaps with questionable viability. Patient follow-up ranged from 2 to 12 months. Complications were high and included infection (13.5%), skin necrosis (13.5%), implant extrusion (6.7%), capsular contracture (56%), and explantation (28%). It can be extrapolated that complication rates were high due to poorly perfused mastectomy skin flaps, aggressive mastectomies, and increased pressure and tension due to prefilled implants.

Radovan (1985) was the first to report the use of tissue expanders.[4] The initial application of the Radovan expander was in the subcutaneous space for the same reasons. Given that prefilled implants were fraught with high complication rates, the thought was that by inserting a minimally filled tissue expander and gradually filling it over months, skin necrosis and delayed healing could be minimized. In addition, these tissue expanders were placed 1 to 2 years following the mastectomy. Between 1976 and 1984, 68 patients had delayed breast reconstruction with the Radovan tissue expander. The intraoperative expander volume ranged from 100 to 150 mL and upon completion of expansion several months later ranged from 550 to 650 mL. Follow-up ranged from 1 to 2 years. Complications included hematoma in three patients (4.4%), infection in five patients (7.4%), skin necrosis in two patients (2.9%), and expander deflation due to pinhole rupture in one patient (1.5%). Capsular contracture was graded on the basis of the Baker classification and included grade 1 in 48%, grade 2 in 40%, and grade 3 in 12%. No patient developed a grade 4 capsule. Although the complication rates were much lower compared to the Schlenker study, initial enthusiasm for tissue expanders was low.

SUBPECTORAL PROSTHETIC BREAST RECONSTRUCTION: 1980S TO THE PRESENT

With the advent of the modified radical mastectomy in which the pectoralis major muscle was spared, the ability to place devices in the subpectoral space became the preferred method of prosthetic breast reconstruction. Total muscle coverage (TMC) and partial muscle coverage (PMC) techniques evolved and became the gold standard.[5] There was an increasing body of evidence that devices placed under muscle had less capsular contracture. In 2005, the use of acellular dermal matrices (ADMs) started to increase as a means of compartmentalizing implants that were placed partially under the pectoralis major muscle.[6,7] The use of ADMs was also postulated to reduce the incidence of capsular contracture by reducing the inflammatory reaction associated with the use of a breast implant.[8-11] In addition, ADMs provided additional tissue support along the lower pole of the breast to minimize the incidence of rippling and wrinkling as well as better define the inframammary and lateral mammary folds to minimize the risk of malposition.[7,12] With the introduction of autologous fat grafting, it became evident that contour abnormalities associated with prosthetic breast reconstruction could be readily corrected and that skin and subcutaneous fat quality could be improved.[13] This was especially true in the setting of radiation therapy.

In an outcome analysis comparing TMC to PMC with ADM, Antony demonstrated acceptable risk of morbidity with both.[14] Three cohorts that include 1170 patients in a TMC non-ADM group from 2002 to 2003, 2910 patients in a TMC non-ADM group from 2004 to 2008, and 153 patients in a PMC with ADM group from 2004 to 2008 were analyzed. The results are tabulated in **Table 20.1**. Seroma ranged from 1.6% to 7.2% and was more frequent using ADM. Cellulitis ranged from 1.4% to 3.9%. Mastectomy skin flap necrosis ranged from 4.6% to 8.7%. In another outcome analysis, Nahabedian compared two-stage prosthetic breast reconstruction following mastectomy with and without ADM.[15] Three cohorts were analyzed and included patients who received no radiation, premastectomy radiation/failed breast conservation therapy (BCT), or postmastectomy radiation. Findings included higher complications associated with prosthetic reconstruction

TABLE 20.1 COMPLICATIONS FOLLOWING PROSTHETIC RECONSTRUCTION IN THE SETTING OF TOTAL AND PARTIAL MUSCLE COVERAGE WITH AND WITHOUT ADM

	ADM 2004-2008	No ADM 2004-2008	No ADM 2002-2003
Patients	153	2910	1170
Seroma	7.20%	1.60%	3.20%
Cellulitis	3.90%	1.40%	3.40%
Reconstructive failure	5.90%	1.90%	2.20%
Infection	3.30%	1.30%	1.50%
Hematoma	2.00%	0.90%	3.20%
Mastectomy flap necrosis	4.60%	6.50%	8.70%
Device malfunction	0	0.10%	<1%
Total complication	23.60%	12.40%	17.60%

Abbreviation: ADM, acellular dermal matrix.

Antony AK, McCarthy CM, Cordeiro PG et al. Acellular human dermis implantation in 153 immediate two-stage tissue expander breast reconstructions: determining the incidence and significant predictors of complications. *Plast Reconstr Surg.* 2010;125(6):1606-1614.

TABLE 20.2 COMPLICATIONS FOLLOWING PROSTHETIC RECONSTRUCTION IN THE SETTING OF PARTIAL MUSCLE COVERAGE WITH AND WITHOUT ACELLULAR DERMAL MATRIX OR RADIATION THERAPY

Factor	Breasts (#)	Infection # (%)	Seroma # (%)	Dehiscence # (%)	Total Complications (%)
No radiation	77	3 (3.9)	2 (2.6)	1 (1.3)	11.70
Premastectomy radiation	9	1 (11)	1 (11)	2 (22)	44
Postmastectomy radiation	13	1 (7.7)	2 (15)	0	23
Pre- and postmastectomy radiation	1	0	0	1 (100)	

Nahabedian MY. AlloDerm performance in the setting of breast implants, infection, and radiation. *Plast Reconstr Surg*. 2009;124:1735-1740.

following mastectomy and failed BCT (44%) compared to postmastectomy radiation (23%) and no radiation (11.7%) (**Table 20.2**). In a systematic review of nine studies comparing TMC without ADM to PMC with ADM, Sbitany demonstrated that the only complication that was statically significant was seroma following PMC with ADM (8.4% vs. 4.3%, $P = 0.03$).[16] There was no difference between infection, hematoma, mastectomy skin flap necrosis, or explantation.

Another complication associated with subpectoral placement of breast implants following mastectomy was superior displacement and elevation of the inframammary fold. This was especially true following radiation and was presumed to be due to capsular contracture. Correction of this deformity was surgically challenging because of the soft-tissue radiation changes, inability to achieve tissue elasticity, and the propensity for incisional dehiscence.[15] In many cases, the best option for surgical correction was explantation and replacement with an autologous flap.

Given the relative failure and lack of acceptance of subcutaneous breast reconstruction and the relative success and acceptance of muscle coverage techniques, there was little impetus for change. The standard of care essentially evolved toward PMC or TMC of prosthetic devices for breast reconstruction. However, limitations of these muscle coverage techniques became increasingly appreciated and included animation deformity with pectoral muscle contraction, muscle spasm, contour abnormalities that included a wider than normal central cleavage space, and device malposition. Reoperation rates with subpectoral breast reconstruction were high depending on the results of the 6-, 8-, and 10-year core studies from Mentor, Sientra, and Allergan and are tabulated in **Tables 20.3 to 20.5**.[17-20]

PREPECTORAL PROSTHETIC BREAST RECONSTRUCTION: 2010 TO THE PRESENT

Prepectoral reconstruction reemerged as a viable option based on our ability to control certain variables such as mastectomy flap thickness and viability, minimizing the inflammatory response associated with implants, and using implants that were optimally filled with cohesive silicone gel. Prepectoral reconstruction could be performed with or without the use of ADM; however, many surgeons prefer to use ADM because it provides more control of the

TABLE 20.3 COMPLICATIONS FOLLOWING PROSTHETIC RECONSTRUCTION USING ALLERGAN DEVICES

Factor	Shaped Implant		Round Implant
	Reconstruction	Revision	Reconstruction
Number	225	68	98
Reoperation	54.60%	48.50%	71.50%
CC (grade 3, 4)	14.50%	26.80%	24.6
Malposition	5.70%	8%	2.30%
Infection	6.10%	8.50%	NR
Seroma	2.80%	6.20%	2.30%

Abbreviations: CC, capsular contracture; NR, not reported.

Spear SL, Murphy DK; Allergan Silicone Breast Implant U.S. Core Clinical Study Group. Natrelle round silicone breast implants: Core Study results at 10 years. *Plast Reconstr Surg*. 2014;133:1354; Maxwell GP, Van Natta BW, Bengston BP, Murphy DK. Ten-year results from the Natrelle 410 anatomical form-stable silicone breast implant core study. *Aesth Surg J*. 2015;35(2):145-155.

TABLE 20.4 COMPLICATIONS FOLLOWING PROSTHETIC RECONSTRUCTION USING MENTOR DEVICES

	Anatomic		Round (6 and 3 y)	
Factor	**Reconstruction**	**Revision**	**Reconstruction**	**Revision**
Number	191	68	251	60
Reoperation	44.50%	45.40%	33.90%	36.20%
CC (grade 3, 4)	10.10%	16.40%	13.70%	25.20%
Malposition	5.10%	6.50%	1.70%	8.50%
Infection	1.60%	3.00%	6.10%	0
Seroma	3.40%	4.60%	4.90%	1.70%

Abbreviation: CC, capsular contracture.

Hammond DC, Migliori MM, Caplin DA, Garcia ME, Phillips CA. Mentor contour profile gel implants: clinical outcomes at 6 years. *Plast Reconstr Surg*. 2012;129:1381.

periprosthetic space, decreases the inflammatory response associated with subcutaneous devices, and provides additional tissue support.[21-24]

Studies evaluating prepectoral reconstruction without ADM have demonstrated mixed results. In a retrospective review of 155 patients and 250 breasts with a mean follow-up of 55.5 months, Salibian et al demonstrated good to excellent results in 85.2% of patients and grade 3 to 4 capsular contracture in 7.6%.[25] Hammond performed prepectoral conversion in 19 patients without using an ADM and demonstrated patient satisfaction in 84.2% and grade 3 to 4 capsular contracture in 21.1% at a mean follow-up of 13.8 months.[26] Salibian performed a systematic review of prepectoral breast reconstruction with ADM and demonstrated implant palpability in 8.5%, rippling in 4.7%, infection in 1.2%, seroma in 2.9%, and grade 3 to 4 capsular contracture in 1.2%.[27] Sbitany reviewed his experience with prosthetic reconstruction by comparing the subpectoral and prepectoral approaches.[28] The adverse events are tabulated in **Table 20.6**.

Reducing the incidence of mastectomy skin flap necrosis with prepectoral reconstruction requires adequate perfusion and thickness of the flaps. Optimal thickness is difficult to quantitate; however, perfusion can be readily quantitated. The vascularity of mastectomy skin flaps can be assessed by arterial and venous bleeding from the incised skin edges, capillary refill, skin color, and perfusion angiography. Thicker flaps are associated with improved vascularity and enhanced tissue support; whereas, thin flaps are at increased risk for delayed healing and mastectomy skin flap necrosis. **Figures 20.1 to 20.3** illustrate partial necrosis along the incision (Figure 20.1), partial necrosis of the nipple-areolar complex (Figure 20.2), and total necrosis of the nipple-areolar complex (Figure 20.3).

Another concern with prepectoral reconstruction, especially in the setting of ADM, is the increased risk of seroma formation (**Figure 20.4**). There are various strategies to reduce seroma formation, which include the use of one to two drains.[7,23] Our standard protocol for drain use is to use one drain; however, in obese patients

TABLE 20.5 COMPLICATIONS FOLLOWING PROSTHETIC RECONSTRUCTION USING SIENTRA DEVICES

Factor	Primary Reconstruction	Revision Reconstruction
Patients/Implants	225/412	84/139
Round	87.60%	87.80%
Shaped	12.40%	12.20%
Reoperation (any)	46.30%	56.00%
Malposition	5.30%	8.60%
CC (grade 3, 4)	12.80%	14.60%
Infection	5.10%	1.20%
Seroma	2.40%	1.20%

Abbreviation: CC, .

Stevens WG, Harrington J, Alizadeh K, Broadway D, Zeidler K, Godinez TB. Eight-year follow-up data from the U.S. clinical trial for Sientra's FDA-approved round and shaped implants with high-strength cohesive silicone gel. *Aesthet Surg J*. 2015; 35(suppl 1):S3-S10.

TABLE 20.6 COMPLICATIONS FOLLOWING PROSTHETIC RECONSTRUCTION IN THE SETTING OF PREPECTORAL RECONSTRUCTION

Factor	Dual Plane	Prepectoral	P
Number of breasts	186	15 (17.9%	
Number (%) with complication	35 (18.8)	2 (2.4%)	0.49
Hematoma	2 (1.1%)	3 (3.6%)	0.59
Seroma	12 (6.5%)	3 (3.6%)	0.41
Partial nipple loss	3 (1.6%)	2 (2.4%)	0.65
Total nipple loss	3 (1.6%)	0	0.55
Cellulitis	17 (9.1%)	4 (4.8%)	0.33
Expander explantation	8 (4.3%)	1 (1.2%)	0.28

Sbitany H, Piper M, Pentz R. Prepectoral breast reconstruction: a safe alternative to submuscular prosthetic reconstruction following nipple-sparing mastectomy. *Plast. Reconstr Surg*. 2017;140:432.

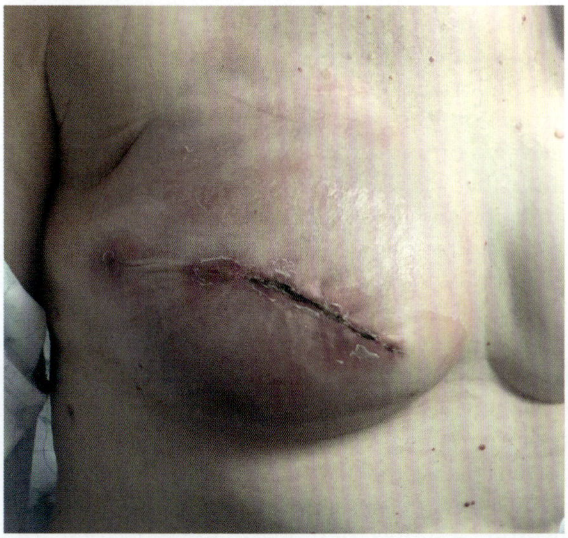

Figure 20.1 Skin edge necrosis and mastectomy skin flap ischemia are illustrated in this prepectoral reconstruction.

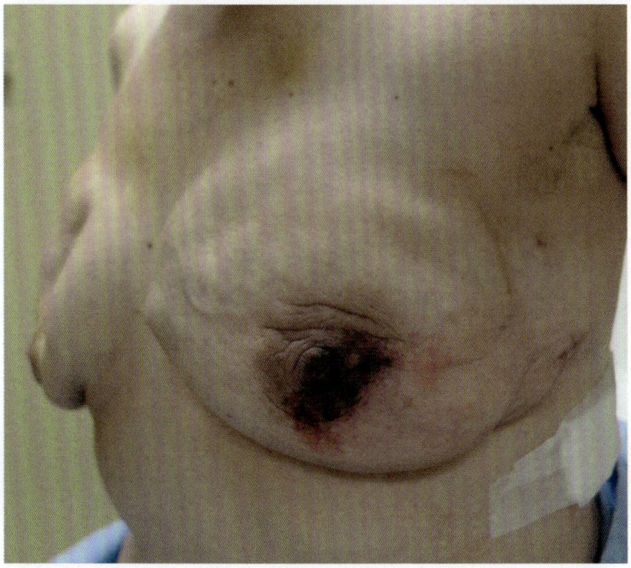

Figure 20.2 Superficial necrosis of the nipple-areolar complex is demonstrated. This went on to heal normally with local wound care.

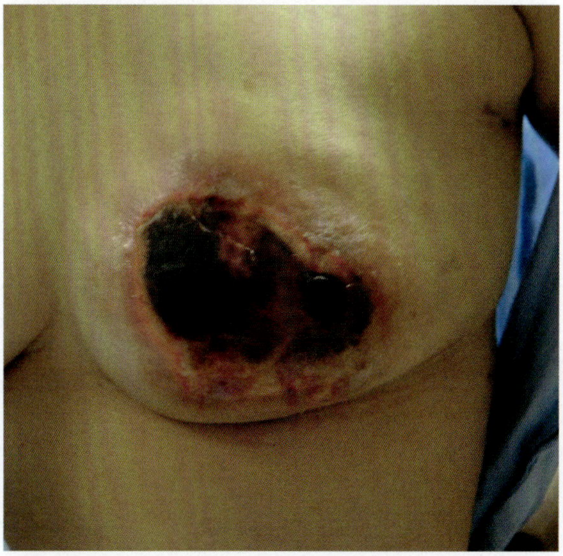

Figure 20.3 Full-thickness necrosis of the nipple-areolar complex. This was initiated by superficial necrosis that went on to become secondarily infected.

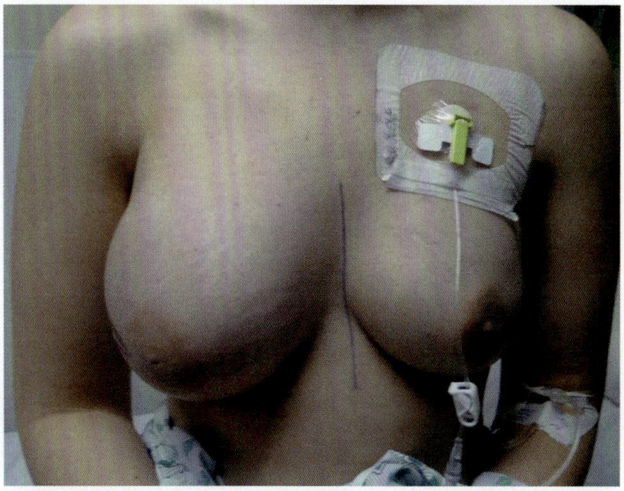

Figure 20.4 This patient developed a right breast seroma following bilateral prepectoral reconstruction. The seroma occurred following chemotherapy.

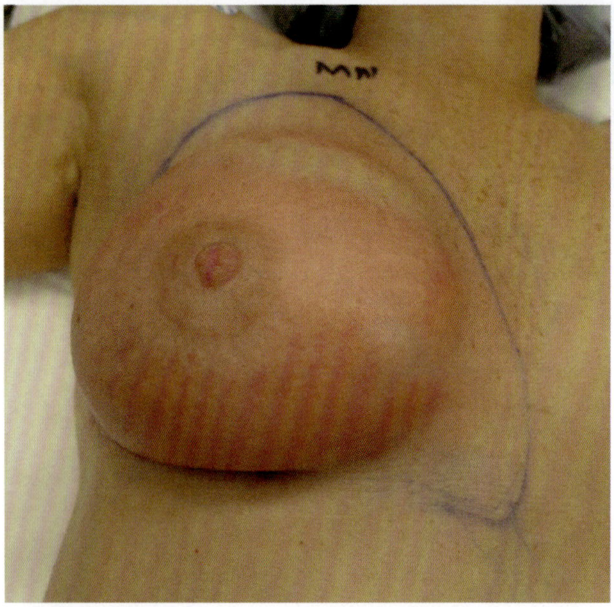

Figure 20.5 Cellulitis following prepectoral reconstruction is uncommon, but can result in reconstructive failure.

or those with more extensive axillary surgery, two drains are used. Drains are maintained for 1 to 2 weeks and removed sequentially when the drain output is less than 30 mL/24 hours. The use of perforated ADM can facilitate bidirectional flow of fluid between the mastectomy skin and the device and reduce the likelihood of sequestered fluid. In addition, the perforations or fenestrations can provide zones of adherence to the mastectomy skin flaps.

Infection associated with prepectoral reconstruction appears to be similar in incidence to that of dual-plane or subpectoral device placement.[15] Cellulitis is associated with an incidence of <5%.[28] (**Figure 20.5**). Our anti-infection protocol includes preoperative intravenous antibiotics, intraoperative antibiotic irrigation, and postoperative oral antibiotic therapy for 3 to 5 days. Antibiotic duration does not usually correlate with drain duration and is tailored to patient-related risk factors such as obesity or diabetes mellitus. The etiology of infection is multifactorial and may include native patient flora, operative contamination, delayed healing, mastectomy skin necrosis, and secondary seeding of the implant. It is important to appreciate that there is very little tolerance for delayed healing in the prepectoral setting because there is no muscle barrier between the device and the skin.

Rippling and wrinkling is another potential sequela of prepectoral breast reconstruction[21,28] (**Figures 20.6 and 20.7**). This is more common in patients with thin skin and in patients who have less cohesive silicone gel and saline implants. Another etiology for rippling is when the periprosthetic space or footprint of the breast is larger than the selected device. There should be a hand-in-glove fit between the implant and the pocket. The use of autologous fat grafting is frequently needed to add thickness to the mastectomy skin flaps and minimize the likelihood of rippling and wrinkling.

An important observation related to prepectoral reconstruction was the rarity of adverse events that were relatively common to subpectoral placement. These include the lack of animation deformity with pectoral contraction and the lack of superior displacement of the implant following radiation therapy.[21,28] It has become evident that the superior displacement associated with subpectoral device placement was due to the foreshortening of the pectoral muscle fibers that had the effect of pulling the implant in a cephalad direction. With prepectoral device placement, the pectoral fibers do not foreshorten and the patient does not have animation deformity. Animation deformity is a phenomenon related to subpectoral placement and is effectively managed by converting a subpectoral pocket to prepectoral. This is thoroughly reviewed in Chapter 16.

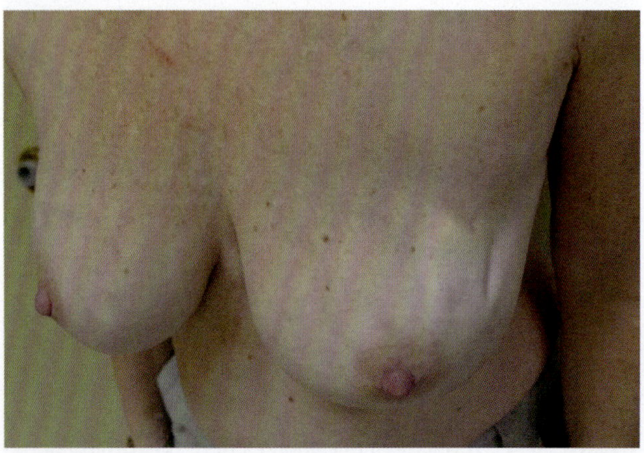

Figure 20.6 Mild lateral rippling following bilateral prepectoral reconstruction.

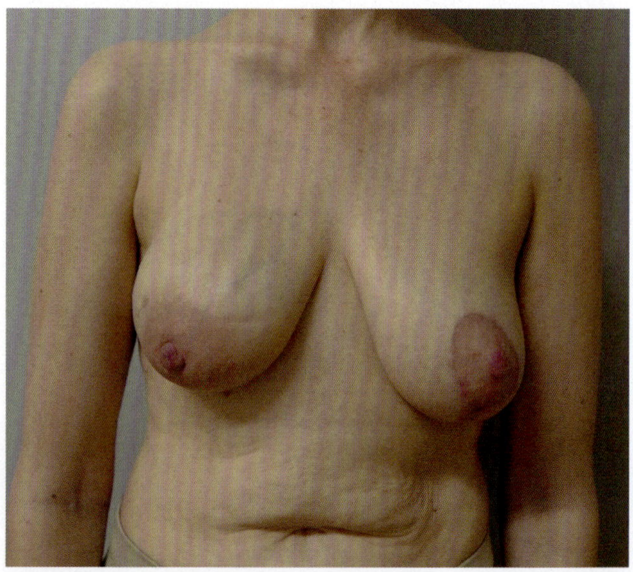

Figure 20.7 Mild upper pole rippling following unilateral prepectoral reconstruction.

SUMMARY

Complications following prosthetic breast reconstruction can occur and include seroma, infection, capsular contracture, mastectomy skin flap necrosis, hematoma, device malfunction, and reconstructive failure. Surgeons should be aware of these possibilities and make all efforts to prevent them. When they occur, strategies should be in place to minimize reconstructive failure. Prepectoral reconstruction has acceptable rates of adverse events that can be effectively managed utilizing the strategies mentioned.

KEY REFERENCES

1. McCarthy CM, Mehrara BJ, Riedel E, et al. Predicting complications following expander/implant breast reconstruction: an outcomes analysis based on preoperative clinical risk. *Plast Reconstr Surg.* 2008;121(6):1886-1892.
2. Nahabedian MY. Breast reconstruction: a review and rationale for patient selection. *Plast Reconstr Surg.* 2009;124:55-62.
3. Schlenker JD, Bueno RA, Ricketson G, Lynch JB. Loss of silicone implants after subcutaneous mastectomy and reconstruction. *Plast Reconstr Surg.* 1978;62(6):853-861.
4. Radovan C. Breast reconstruction after mastectomy using the temporary expander. *Plast Reconstr Surg.* 1982;69(2):195-206.
5. Cordeiro PG, Jazayeri L. Two-stage implant-based breast reconstruction: an evolution of the conceptual and technical approach over a two-decade period. *Plast Reconstr Surg.* 2016;138(1):1-11.
6. Salzberg CA. Nonexpansive immediate breast reconstruction using human acellular tissue matrix graft (AlloDerm). *Ann Plast Surg.* 2006;57:1-5.
7. Nahabedian MY, Mesbahi AN. Breast reconstruction with tissue expanders and implants. In: Nahabedian MY. *Cosmetic and Reconstructive Breast Surgery*. London, UK: Elsevier Publishers; 2009:1-20.
8. Prantl L, Schreml S, Fichtner-Feigl S. et al. Clinical and morphological conditions in capsular contracture formed around silicone breast implants. *Plast Reconstr Surg.* 2007;120:275.
9. Orenstein S, Qiao Y, Kaur M, Klueh U, Kreutzer D, Novitsky Y. In vitro activation of human peripheral blood mononuclear cells induced by human biologic meshes. *J Surg Res.* 2010;158(1):10-14.
10. Komorowska-Timek E, Oberg KC, Timek TA, Gridley DS, Miles DAG. The effect of alloderm envelopes on periprosthetic capsule formation with and without radiation. *Plast Reconstr Surg.* 2009;123:807.
11. Salzberg CA, Ashikari AY, Berry C, Hunsiker LM. Acellular dermal matrix-assisted direct-to-implant breast reconstruction and capsular contracture: a 13-year experience. Plast Reconstr Surg. 2016. 138(2):329-37.
12. Sbitany H, Sandeen SN, Amalfi AN, Davenport MS, Langstein HN. Acellular dermis–assisted prosthetic breast reconstruction versus complete submuscular coverage: a head-to-head comparison of outcomes. *Plast Reconstr Surg.* 2009;124:1735.
13. Rigotti G, Marchi A, Galie M, et al. Clinical treatment of radiotherapy tissue damage by lipoaspirate transplant: a healing process mediated by adipose-derived adult stem cells. *Plast Reconstr Surg.* 2007;;119(5):1409-1422.
14. Antony AK, McCarthy CM, Cordeiro PG et al. Acellular human dermis implantation in 153 immediate two-stage tissue expander breast reconstructions: determining the incidence and significant predictors of complications. *Plast Reconstr Surg.* 2010;125(6):1606-1614.
15. Nahabedian MY. AlloDerm performance in the setting of breast implants, infection, and radiation. *Plast Reconstr Surg.* 2009;124:1735-1740.
16. Sbitany H, Serletti JM. Acellular dermis–assisted prosthetic breast reconstruction: a systematic and critical review of efficacy and associated morbidity. *Plast Reconstr Surg.* 2011;128:1162.
17. Stevens WG, Harrington J, Alizadeh K, Broadway D, Zeidler K, Godinez TB. Eight-year follow-up data from the U.S. clinical trial for Sientra's FDA-approved round and shaped implants with high-strength cohesive silicone gel. *Aesthet Surg J.* 2015; 35(suppl 1):S3-S10.
18. Hammond DC, Migliori MM, Caplin DA, Garcia ME, Phillips CA. Mentor contour profile gel implants: clinical outcomes at 6 years. *Plast Reconstr Surg.* 2012;129:1381.
19. Spear SL, Murphy DK; Allergan Silicone Breast Implant U.S. Core Clinical Study Group. Natrelle round silicone breast implants: Core Study results at 10 years. *Plast Reconstr Surg.* 2014;133:1354.
20. Maxwell GP, Van Natta BW, Bengston BP, Murphy DK. Ten-year results from the Natrelle 410 anatomical form-stable silicone breast implant core study. *Aesth Surg J.* 2015;35(2):145-155.
21. Sigalove S, Maxwell GP, Sigalove NM, et al. Prepectoral implant-based breast reconstruction: rationale, indications, and results. *Plast Reconstr Surg.* 2017;139(2):287-294.
22. Woo A, Harless C, Jacobson SR. Revisiting an old place: single surgeon experience on post-mastectomy subcutaneous implant-based breast reconstruction. *Breast J.* 2017;23(5):545-553.
23. Nahabedian MY. Prosthetic breast reconstruction with acellular dermal matrices: achieving predictability and reproducibility. *Plast Reconstr Surg Global Open.* 2016;;4(5):e698.
24. Nahabedian MY. Acellular dermal matrices in primary breast reconstruction: principles, concepts, and indications. *Plast Reconstr Surg.* 2012;130(5)(suppl 2):44S-53S.
25. Salibian AH, Harness J, Mowlds DS. Staged suprapectoral expander/implant reconstruction without acellular dermal matrix following nipple-sparing mastectomy. *Plast Reconstr Surg.* 2017;139:30.
26. Hammond DS, Schmidt WP, O'Connor EA. Treatment of breast animation deformity in implant-based reconstruction with pocket change to the subcutaneous position. *Plast Reconstr Surg.* 2015;135:1540.
27. Salibian AA, Frey JD, Choi M, Karp NS. Subcutaneous implant-based breast reconstruction with acellular dermal matrix/mesh: a systematic review. *Plast Reconstr Surg Global Open.* 2016;4(11):e1139.
28. Sbitany H, Piper M, Pentz R. Prepectoral breast reconstruction: a safe alternative to submuscular prosthetic reconstruction following nipple-sparing mastectomy. *Plast. Reconstr Surg.* 2017;140:432.

CHAPTER **21**

POSTOPERATIVE CONSIDERATIONS FOLLOWING PREPECTORAL RECONSTRUCTION

John G. Apostolides

KEY POINTS

- One to two surgical drains are utilized depending on the size of the breast and the patient.
- Postoperative oral antibiotics are prescribed while surgical drains are in place.
- Closed incision negative pressure therapy and transparent film dressings are applied to immobilize and prevent shear forces.
- Second-stage implant exchange is performed after 3 months.
- In patients receiving chemotherapy, second-stage implant exchange is performed no earlier than 4 weeks after completion of therapy.
- In patients who will receive postoperative radiation therapy, second-stage implant exchange is performed at least 4 weeks before commencement of radiation.
- Fat grafting is performed separately from implant exchange surgery.

In the setting of thin mastectomy flaps, nipple reconstruction is not performed unless previous autologous fat grafting occurs to thicken the subcutaneous layer.

INTRODUCTION

Prepectoral breast reconstruction is a growing and popular reconstructive technique in prosthetic-based breast reconstruction. The clinical benefits of utilizing the prepectoral space, and avoiding the manipulation of pectoralis major muscle, are well described and documented.[1] In the setting of this minimally invasive technique, postoperative management must be tailored to the shorter hospital stay or outpatient setting. The surgical success of this procedure is based on well-perfused mastectomy skin flaps and incorporation of acellular dermal matrix (ADM). Taking into consideration these key factors, postoperative management must create the optimal environment for these to occur. Proper and strategic immediate postoperative management will complement the prepectoral surgical reconstruction. In the late-stage postoperative period, deliberate and thoughtful surgical timing for additional procedures is important to allow for maintained and improved results.

THE IMMEDIATE POSTOPERATIVE PERIOD

The immediate postoperative period consists of the time from the completion of surgery and the application of the dressings to the sixth postoperative week when patients no longer have physical restrictions to their postoperative activity. This is a crucial period that starts with optimizing the healing and recovery and continues with restrictions and management to limit complications.

The Surgical Dressing

In prepectoral reconstruction, the mastectomy skin flaps are self-reliant and isolated from the underlying pectoralis muscle and chest wall. It is this fact that makes tissue perfusion and skin flap viability essential to success. In the operating room, the surgical dressing has the vital function of maintaining and optimizing this vascular and viable environment. In addition, it is important to safely immobilize these skin flaps over the underlying ADM to allow for tissue ingrowth and incorporation. Closed incision negative pressure therapy and complete breast coverage with transparent film occlusive dressing allow for a vascular and safe environment while simultaneously immobilizing the mastectomy skin flaps and preventing shearing forces. This negative pressure therapy is applied to the incisions and nipple-areola complex. The benefit of this therapy includes protection from contamination, minimizing tissue edema, promoting vascular flow, and minimizing skin tension.[2] The result is an environment that is optimal for ADM incorporation, tissue ingrowth, and incisional healing. In complement with the negative pressure therapy is a drain site dressing utilizing chlorhexidine gluconate disks and occlusive dressings to create an aseptic environment at the skin drain site. Proper drain dressings are important, especially in the setting of prolonged drain placement. Drains are common in place for 2 to 3 weeks and minimizing infection potential is essential (see **Figure 21.1**).

After postoperative day 7, closed incision negative pressure therapy is commonly removed, at which point the occlusive transparent film dressing can be reapplied, or soft compressive bras can be worn to continue the "immobilizing" effect. The goal of these garments and dressings is to prevent shearing as the patient's activity begins to increase. This supportive garment or bra is encouraged for 4 to 6 weeks following surgery.

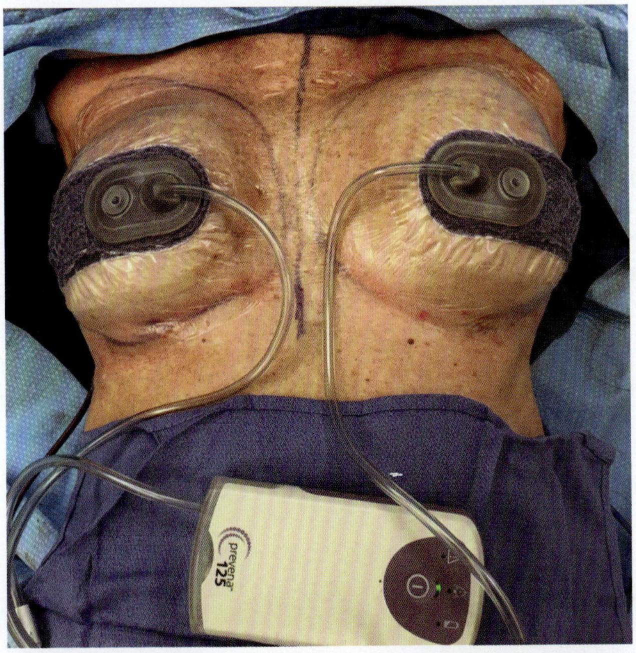

Figure 21.1 Image of the surgical dressing demonstrating the closed incision negative pressure dressing and transparent film dressing. This surgical dressing allows for complete coverage and immobilization of the breast without compromising tissue perfusion.

Drain Management

Closed suction drains are widely used in reconstructive breast surgery. Elimination of dead space, prevention of seroma, and optimizing apposition of mastectomy skin flaps to ADM is essential to prepectoral surgical success. Drain placement, as previously discussed, is a significant component of the postoperative management.[3] One or two closed suction drains are utilized between the mastectomy skin flaps and the ADM. Average drain duration is 2 to 3 weeks, based on drain output. When drain output levels reach 25 mL/24-hour period or less, they are removed. In cases where drain output is still high at 3 weeks, expansion is performed to further eliminate dead space and the drains are removed by the 4th week. Antibiotics are administered during the postoperative period until all drains have been removed. Postoperative practices vary among physicians, but showering is typically restricted until the closed incision negative pressure therapy is removed. At that point, after postoperative day 7, patients are permitted to shower. Soaking, bathing, and swimming are restricted for the first 6 weeks.

Expansion

The process of eliminating dead space within the breast pocket begins at the time of surgery with expansion of the tissue expander. Utilizing saline or air, the expander is filled to the point of ADM apposition to the overlying skin flaps and elimination of dead space. It is important to avoid overexpansion at the time of surgery to minimize risk of tissue necrosis. During the postoperative period, expansion resumes after the second week if needed. Additional air or saline can be injected to help decrease drain output, or to begin the shaping and expansion of the breast pocket. Underfilling of the tissue expander, in relation to final implant volume, is recommended to ensure a precise and snug fit of the final implant in the second stage of reconstruction. In patients who are going to fly, visit high-altitude destinations, and patients who are scheduled to receive postoperative radiation therapy, air-filled expanders must be converted to saline fills.

THE LATE POSTOPERATIVE PERIOD

Subsequent surgery in the prepectoral patient is similar to the traditional dual-plane or subpectoral approach in both order and timing. Among the various postoperative courses and treatments, there are several combinations and approaches to second- and third-stage reconstruction. With regard to the prepectoral patient, it is important to adjust the reconstructive algorithm to the individual patient. Various factors such as radiation therapy, chemotherapy, flap thickness, and nipple-sparing status can alter the order, timing, and/or feasibility of the remaining reconstructive procedures. Following the mastectomy and first-stage prepectoral expander surgery, patients must strategically receive (1) implant exchange, (2) autologous fat grafting, and (3) nipple reconstruction. We address the combinations of factors and subsequent order and timing of procedures to best navigate these issues (see **Figure 21.2**).

Thin Mastectomy Flap, No Radiation

Prepectoral reconstruction in the thin patient is performed in a manner similar to that of other patients. Second-stage implant exchange is typically performed as early as 3 months from the time of mastectomy. At this stage, pocket revision and sizing modifications can be performed and proper implant selection can occur without concern for tissue and skin viability. The postoperative period allows for ADM incorporation, skin and pocket maturity, and elimination of dead space from the previous mastectomy. These factors allow for a more precise and snug implant fit and positioning.

In the thin patient, lack of subcutaneous fat and thin mastectomy flaps play a role in the timing and feasibility of nipple reconstruction and autologous fat grafting. When nipple reconstruction is performed in thin skin flaps, the resulting reconstruction commonly loses projection and flattens. In addition, this nipple flap will commonly expose the underlying ADM, or even the implant when perforated ADM is used. It is for these reasons that autologous fat grafting is recommended as a third-stage procedure and separate procedure before nipple reconstruction. In many cases, nipple reconstruction is abandoned all together in favor of nipple-areola tattooing. The autologous fat stage is preferably performed on its own, at least 3 months from the time of implant exchange. This allows for pocket modification and implant exchange and allows tissues to heal and settle for more accurate fat transfer.

Thick Mastectomy Flap, No Radiation

In the patient with thick mastectomy flaps, prepectoral reconstruction is performed in a similar manner. Second-stage implant exchange is also performed as early as 3 months from the time of mastectomy. Similarly, pocket revision and sizing modifications can be performed and proper implant selection can occur. The postoperative period allows for ADM incorporation, skin and pocket maturity, and elimination of dead space from the previous mastectomy. In these patients, it is again preferred to perform implant exchange separate from any autologous fat transfer for the same reasons. In addition, these patients may find that they do not require autologous fat transfer based on the amount of subcutaneous tissue. If fat grafting is required, it can be combined with nipple reconstruction as a third stage or it can be during the second stage as long as no capsulotomies are performed.

Radiation, Rapid Implant Exchange

When postoperative radiation therapy is planned, it is important to have a well-planned and coordinated strategy

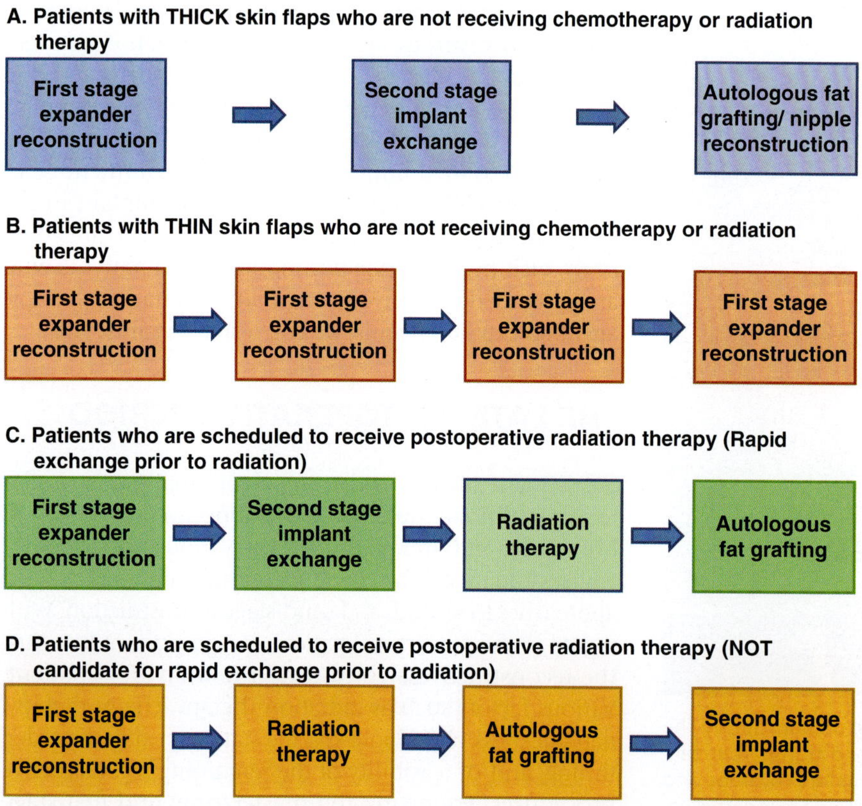

Figure 21.2 The surgical algorithm for subsequent reconstructive procedures specifying timing of implant exchange, fat grafting, and nipple reconstruction.

for timing of subsequent reconstructive procedures in relation to the radiation regimen. When patients have healthy viable mastectomy flaps, well-tolerated expansion, and the radiation oncologist concurs with the beginning of radiation therapy approximately 8 weeks post mastectomy, then rapid implant exchange surgery can be performed before radiation. In the traditional dual plane/subpectoral reconstruction, radiation-induced fibrosis leads to progressive pectoralis muscle fibrosis, tightening, and dermal thickening, which distorts the implant reconstruction.[4] In this traditional approach, it is preferred to radiate the fully filled expander before subsequent procedures. In the prepectoral setting, the absence of pectoralis major muscle over the implant appears to result in less contracture and deformity. This finding allows for implant exchange within approximately 4 weeks of mastectomy, with adequate time for wound healing before radiation therapy. It is essential that all members of the medical and surgical team are in agreement and coordinate the various treatment modalities and plans.

Upon completion of radiation therapy, current practice is to perform autologous fat grafting 3 to 6 months later. Recent studies, however, indicate a potential benefit to early autologous fat grafting in the acute post radiation therapy period.[5] In this setting, autologous fat transfer is performed throughout the subcutaneous plane of the breasts approximately 6 weeks after radiation therapy is completed. In these radiated cases, it is also preferable to avoid nipple reconstruction because of the inability to achieve adequate projection and potential risk and complications to the reconstruction. In the setting of radiation, nipple-areola tattooing (micropigmentation) is the preferable aesthetic procedure.

Radiation, No Rapid Implant Exchange

When postoperative radiation therapy is planned, there will be occasions where the patient or clinical scenario is not compatible with rapid implant exchange before radiation. In these scenarios, the prepectoral expander will be radiated before subsequent surgery. Following radiation therapy, implant exchange should no longer be the next reconstructive procedure. These cases benefit from autologous fat grafting either acutely, approximately 6 weeks post radiation, or 3 to 6 months after radiation. The autologous fat is beneficial to the radiated breast by creating a nonradiated layer of autologous cells within the subcutaneous plane, as well as decreasing potential complications of both the expander and future implant surgeries.[6] Once the autologous fat has had a 3- to 4-month period of recovery, final stage reconstruction is performed to place the permanent implants. As in the rapid exchange patients, it is preferable to avoid nipple reconstruction because of the inability to achieve adequate projection and potential risk and complications to the reconstruction. In the setting of radiation, nipple-areola tattooing (micropigmentation) is the preferable aesthetic procedure (see **Figure 21.3**).

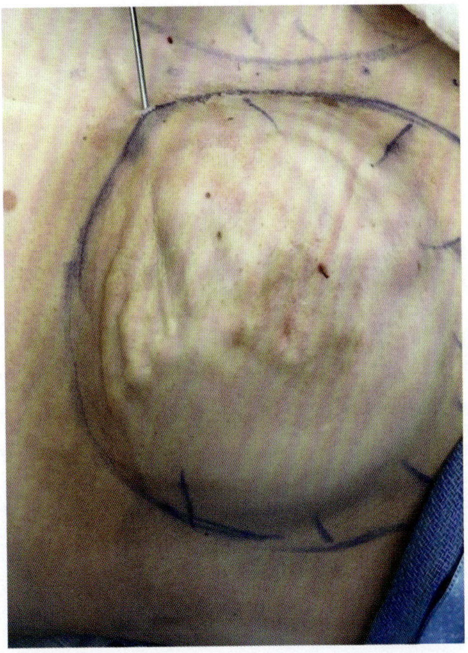

Figure 21.3 Intraoperative image of autologous fat transfer to the subcutaneous plane of the radiated breast with expander inflated and in place.

SUMMARY

Prepectoral breast reconstruction is an effective, aesthetic, and growing surgical technique. It is important to tailor the postoperative management of the surgical patient to the prepectoral approach. To complement the surgical procedure, it is important to utilize the latest advances in surgical dressings, proper drain management, and strategic surgical planning. The goal is to create the optimal environment for tissue health and surgical healing.

KEY REFERENCES

1. Sigalove S, Maxwell GP, Sigalove NM, et al. Prepectoral implant-based reconstruction: rationale, indications, and preliminary results. *Plast Reconstr Surg*. 2017;139:287-294.
2. Semsardzadeh NN, Tadisina KK, Maddox J, et al. Closed incision negative pressure therapy is associated with decreased surgical-site infections: a meta-analysis. *Plast Reconstr Surg*. 2015;136(3):592-602.
3. Unalp HR, Onal MA. Analysis of risk factors affecting the development of seromas following breast cancer surgeries. *Breast J*. 2007;13:588-592.
4. Thanik VD, Chang CC, Zoumalan RA, et al. A novel mouse model of cutaneous radiation injury. *Plast Reconstr Surg*. 2011;127:560-568.
5. Ribuffo D, Atzeni M, Guerra M, et al. Treatment of irradiated expanders: protective lipofilling allows immediate prosthetic breast reconstruction in the setting of postoperative radiotherapy. *Aesthetic Plast Surg*. 2013;37:1146-1152.
6. Salgarello M, Visconti G, Barone-Adesi L. Fat grafting and breast reconstruction with implant: another option for irradiated breast cancer patients. *Plast Reconstr Surg*. 2012;129(2):317-329

CHAPTER 22

BUILDING AN ECONOMIC MODEL FOR PREPECTORAL BREAST RECONSTRUCTION

Scot Bradley Glasberg

KEY POINTS

- Prepectoral reconstruction is promising on the basis of early data.
- Benefits are less associated pain and lower incidence of animation deformities.
- Economic benefits are due to early activity, less narcotic use, and earlier function of daily living.

Long-term stable results can lead to less future revisionary surgery.

INTRODUCTION

Implant-based breast reconstruction remains the number one surgical technique for breast reconstruction in the United States.[1,2] Improvements in mastectomy procedures, and specifically advanced incisions, have yielded improved aesthetics especially since the advent of the use of the nipple-areola sparing method.[3,4] The past several years, however, have seen the focus shift dramatically to discussions of which plane to place the tissue expander or implant in. Specifically, the prosthetic breast reconstruction world has seen practice turned on its head with a shift back to the subcutaneous space, turning back the clock completely. A reversion to placing tissue expanders and implants in a prepectoral space has yielded surprisingly superior and consistent results and benefits[5] considering the immense complications encountered the last time such efforts were undertaken in the 1960s and 1970s during the beginnings of prosthetic breast reconstruction.[6,7] This is most definitely not a simple return to a previous operation, but instead has been made possible only due to improvements in a variety of reconstructive techniques and technologies over the past two to three decades. Advances in fat grafting, acellular dermal matrices (ADMs), better methods for assessing breast flap viability, and improved implants and tissue expanders have all helped make prepectoral breast reconstruction feasible as well as enhance its results.[8-11] The main benefits of a switch to prepectoral breast reconstruction clinically appear to be less associated pain, lower incidence of animation deformities, and its associated symptoms as well as presumably better aesthetics.[12]

As in any developing technique, given the current health care environment, consideration must be given to the issues of cost and associated expense when considering the long-term implications of such a procedure. Although clinical results are early, economic considerations are even more premature, and the data is, therefore, limited. However, given the positive nature of the techniques and their outcomes, one can envision building an economic model that could show significant fiscal benefits for this evolving surgical procedure. Clearly, the major obstacle to a positive fiscal model in the setting of prepectoral breast reconstruction is the cost of the needed larger piece of ADM associated with the technique. Sizes of ADM used for this procedure tend to be three to four times the magnitude of those used for subpectoral breast reconstruction.[13] However, other clinical and economically enhancing variables that appear to not only offset those expenses but also, perhaps, suggest a model of economic benefit overall for this enhanced operation are clearly apparent. Finally, any economic model proposed should clearly consider who are the actual monetary and financial beneficiaries, specifically, the patient, the surgeon, the hospital, or the third-party payor.

PAIN

The most clearly evident and data-driven clinical benefit of prepectoral breast reconstruction to date appears to be the significantly lower associated pain.[14] Several early retrospective papers appear to show such an advantage. This relates directly to the lower level of dissection associated with this technique especially due to the lack of need for submuscular dissection and rearrangement of soft tissues. The patient is clearly the most direct beneficiary of less postoperative pain. However, this benefit often yields improved ratings and statistics for both surgeons and hospitals by their patient base, potentially yielding improved referrals as well as generally better reviews.

LESS NARCOTIC USE

Less postoperative pain most closely ties to the lower use of both intravenous and oral postoperative opioids and analgesics.[14] This variable is clearly of economic advantage because it tends to lead to many of the other associated cost variables and savings. In addition, given the current health care climate and noted state of federal emergency surrounding increased opioid abuse, the decreased use of these medications should be of benefit to not only patient safety but to the overall social environment as well. The potential benefits associated with a technique that could eventually be free of opioid use are immeasurable.

DECREASED LENGTH OF STAY/ INCREASED AMBULATORY SURGERY

Early studies surrounding prepectoral breast reconstruction appear to show a direct benefit of decreased length of hospital stay from approximately 2 to 3 days to 1 to 2 days on average.[12,14] Some authors have also suggested that this could yield a change in implant-based breast reconstruction being converted from an inpatient to an outpatient procedure. Early data is too minimal to yet show this change in a statistically significant light. In most health care–related economic models, decreased length of hospital stay usually translates to the single greatest factor of cost savings possible. Everyone benefits from the positive financial implications and scenarios of decreased length of stay including the patient, the hospital, and the third-party payor. In addition, surgeons can use this quality metric to report improved outcomes for enhanced reimbursement under the current quality payment programs being utilized.[15]

SHORTER OPERATIVE TIME/EASIER TECHNIQUE

When looking at the specific varied techniques of prepectoral breast reconstruction that have been outlined, specifically either wrapping the device or completely covering the prosthesis by suturing the ADM directly to the chest wall (see **Figures 22.1 and 22.2**), several authors have now shown a significant decrease in actual operative time.[14,16] This probably results from the ability to prepare the tissue expander or implant with the ADM in some instances on the back table while the mastectomy is still taking place. In addition, the time saved by not having to elevate the pectoralis muscle and prepare a subpectoral pocket is translated to this decreased surgical time. Given the ever-increasing costs of operative time, this could yield a significant benefit in any proposed prepectoral economic model. The most direct beneficiary of this enhancement is the hospital, which can both cut costs and more efficiently run the operating rooms. Indirectly, patients may benefit from a decreased operative time and anesthetic exposure.

LESS POSTOPERATIVE EXPANSIONS

Several authors have now shown both increased initial intraoperative fill volume of the tissue expander as a percentage of final desired fill capacity and further decreased numbers of expansions postoperatively in two-stage breast reconstruction.[17] Although the decreased number of required expansions yields both less procedural interventions and an associated lower incidence of postoperative complications, it can also translate to enhanced patient satisfaction. The patient benefits most directly from fewer interventions postoperatively and there are some associated cost savings for the surgeon in their offices because

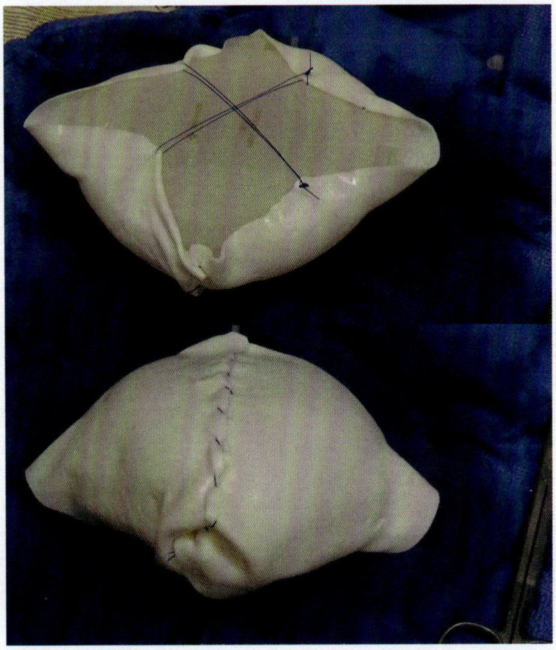

Figure 22.1 These photographs show a tissue expander wrapped on the back table during the mastectomy with acellular dermal matrix. Note the tabs are left free for suturing to the chest wall.

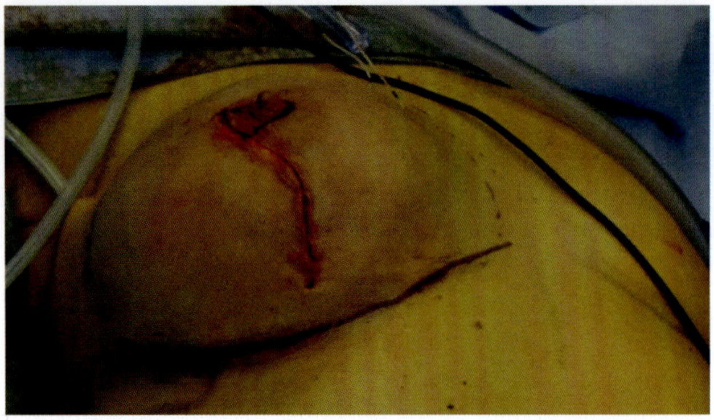

Figure 22.2 The tissue expander once placed intraoperatively into the prepectoral space.

of decreased use of equipment and potentially less time consumption.

QUICKER RETURN TO WORK

Given the associated decreased pain, lower use of analgesics, and decreased length of hospital stay, several early studies suggest that patients are returning to work earlier.[12,14,18] The direct beneficiary of this variable is the patient who is required to take less days off from work with its obvious financial advantages. That said, the entire public and health care environment also benefits in an indirect manner from these cost savings through greater numbers of work days. Multiple economic models have shown that earlier return to work translates to increased productivity in the community and the workforce.

IMPROVED AESTHETICS

Several authors have now suggested that because of the lack of the pectoralis muscle restricting breast contour and the easier ability to mold a breast mound in a more controlled environment with simply the ADM and the breast flaps providing support, the result will be improved patient outcomes and aesthetics.[19,20] Although the data is clearly not yet apparent or conclusive, improved early aesthetics should translate to less secondary procedures to improve all types of outcomes and results. Less operative interventions lend themselves to less complications overall. The patient benefits directly from less associated secondary operations and the insurers profit from the lower outlay of monies for these procedures.

EARLIER RANGE OF MOTION/ ENHANCED RANGE OF MOTION/LESS PHYSICAL THERAPY

With the lack of pectoral muscle dissection, early adopters of prepectoral breast reconstruction appear more willing to allow patients to start full range of motion earlier in the postoperative period.[5,12,14,16,18,19] This early use of the upper extremities translates to less patient discomfort, earlier mobility, and easier return to normal functionality. Authors have noted not only the lack of postoperative animation deformity but have also realized a better and more normal maintenance of shoulder girdle strength. In addition, many breast reconstruction patients are often referred to specialists for both physical and occupational therapy. This earlier range of motion and return to normal function should lower the number of patients who require this type of postoperative intervention. That said, this is clearly yet to be proved, but could yield further financial savings to both the patient and the third-party payor.

ENHANCED PATIENT SATISFACTION

Many of the postoperative benefits noted should yield enhanced patient satisfaction results as well as patient-reported outcomes. Early reports tend to confirm this patient approval.[5,12,14,16,18-21] As patient-reported outcomes become a key component of quality measurements moving forward, this improvement in care should translate to enhanced reimbursement for surgeons and hospitals because of the associated cost savings and its primary focus within quality payment programs.[22]

DECREASED INCIDENCE OF CAPSULAR CONTRACTURE

One of the greatest benefits of ADM-assisted subpectoral breast reconstruction appears to be the decreased incidence of capsular contracture both in the short and long term.[23-25] This has presumably yielded a significantly decreased number of secondary corrective procedures over time. Early data with prepectoral breast reconstruction seems to suggest an even lower incidence of capsular contracture in the postoperative period.[14,18,19] One theory is that this is because of the complete or near-complete wrapping or coverage of the tissue expander or implant with ADM when performing this technique. Although the data is not yet conclusive and further long-term data is clearly necessary, this would further yield those associated cost savings as noted in the earlier sections.

LESS REVISIONAL SURGERY

Overall, better aesthetic outcomes, lower capsular contracture rates, and improved patient satisfaction should all yield a lower incidence of secondary revisional surgery in this cohort of patients. Clearly more and longer term data needs to be analyzed to prove this conclusively. However, if current trends hold, this should be of significant economic and financial benefits to both patients and third-party payors.

SUMMARY

Early indications appear to show that this next phase and shift of prosthetic breast reconstruction from the subpectoral into the prepectoral space and realm appears to be yielding significant clinical benefits to patients. Clearly, more evidence-based data needs to be researched and analyzed to confirm these potential findings. However, early assessment seems to show that surgeons are adopting this operation at a much quicker pace than previously expected despite only early available clinical data. As of the writing of this chapter, the incidence of the use of this procedure appears to be in the 15% to 22% range for all prosthetic breast reconstructions. Although it is unclear what is prompting this dramatic swing, ease of technique coupled with initial reported improved outcomes appear to be key to this early enthusiasm. As was seen with the early and rapid adoption of subpectoral breast reconstruction with ADM, any improved techniques that can enhance outcomes and aesthetics are often adopted quickly by surgeons to meet the many challenges of prosthetic breast reconstruction. From an economic perspective, additional work needs to be done to both build an efficient economic model and continue to show financial benefits for patients, surgeons, hospitals, and third-party payors. If the early clinical signals are any clue, the future looks bright for attaining a truly beneficial economic outcome and model for prepectoral breast reconstruction. On a clinical basis, if the current trends continue, this could result in a generational and seismic shift in how prosthetic breast reconstruction is performed.

DISCLOSURES

Dr. Glasberg is a consultant for LifeCell Corp., an Allergan affiliate, and Allergan Corp. No compensation or support was received for this manuscript.

KEY REFERENCES

1. ASPS procedural statistics. www.plasticsurgery.org. Accessed May 2017.
2. Albornoz CR, Bach PB, Mehrara BJ, et al. A paradigm shift in U.S. breast reconstruction: increasing implant rates. *Plast Reconstr Surg.* 2013;131:15-23.
3. Mallon P, Feron JG, Couturaund B, et al. The role of nipple-sparing mastectomy in breast cancer: a comprehensive review of the literature. *Plast Reconstr Surg.* 2013;131:969.
4. Cemal Y, Albornoz CR, Disa JJ, et al. A paradigm shift in U.S. breast reconstruction: Part 2. The influence of changing mastectomy patterns on reconstructive rate and method. *Plast Reconstr Surg.* 2013;131:320e-326e.
5. Woo A, Harless C, Jacobson SR. Revisiting an old place: single surgeon experience on post-mastectomy subcutaneous implant-based breast reconstruction. *Breast J.* 2017;23(5):545-553..
6. Schlenker JD, Bueno RA, Ricketson G, Lynch JB. Loss of silicone implants after subcutaneous mastectomy and reconstruction. *Plast Reconstr Surg.* 1978;62(6):853-861.
7. Gruber RP, Kahn RA, Lash H, Maser MR, Apfelberg DB, Laub DR. Breast reconstruction following mastectomy: a comparison of submuscular and subcutaneous techniques. *Plast Reconstr Surg.* 1981;67:312-317.
8. Nahabedian, MY. Prosthetic breast reconstruction with acellular dermal matrices: achieving predictability and reproducibility. *Plast Reconstr Surg Glob Open.* 2016;4(5):e698.
9. Spear SL, Coles CN, Leung BK, et al. The safety, effectiveness, and efficiency of autologous fat grafting in breast surgery. *Plast Reconstr Surg Glob Open.* 2016;4(8):8.
10. Gabriel A, Maxwell GP. The evolution of breast implants. *Clin Plast Surg.* 2015; 42(4):399-404.
11. Phillips BT, Munabi NC, Roeder RA, et al. The role of intraoperative perfusion assessment: what is the current state and how can i use it in my practice? *Plast Reconstr Surg.* 2016; 137(2):731-741.
12. Salibian AA, Frey JD, Choi M, Karp NS. Subcutaneous implant-based breast reconstruction with acellular dermal matrix/mesh: a systematic review. *Plast Reconstr Surg Global Open.* 2016;4(11):1139.
13. Maxwell GP, Gabriel A. Bioengineered breast: concept, technique, and preliminary results. *Plast Reconstr Surg.* 2016;137(2):415-421.
14. Sigalove S, Maxwell GP, Sigalove NM, et al. Prepectoral implant-based breast reconstruction: rationale, indications, and results. *Plast Reconstr Surg.* 2017;139(2):287-294.
15. Squitieri, L, Chung, KC. Value-based payment reform and the Medicare Access and Children's Health Insurance Program Reauthorization Act of 2015: a primer for plastic surgeons. *Plast Reconstr Surg.* 2017; 140(1):205-214.
16. Vidya R, Iqbal FM. A guide to prepectoral breast reconstruction: a new dimension to implant-based breast reconstruction. *Clin Breast Cancer.* 2017;17(4):266-271.
17. Zhu L, Mohan AT, Abdelsattar JM, et al. Comparison of subcutaneous versus submuscular expander placement in the first stage of immediate breast reconstruction. *J Plast Reconstr Aesthet Surg.* 2016;69:e77-e86.
18. Sbitany H, Piper M, Lentz R. Prepectoral breast reconstruction: a safe alternative to submuscular prosthetic reconstruction following nipple sparing mastectomy. *Plast Reconstr Surg.* 2017;140(3):432-443.
19. Bernini M, Calabrese C, Cecconi L, et al. Subcutaneous direct-to-implant breast reconstruction: surgical, functional, and aesthetic results after long-term follow-up. *Plast Reconstr Surg Glob Open.* 2016;3:e574.
20. Chopra, K, Houssock, C, Cai, SS, et al. Submuscular versus prepectoral immediate implant based breast reconstruction. Abstract/Presentation at Northeastern Society of Plastic Surgeons; 2017 (in manuscript).
21. Kobraei EM, Cauley R, Gadd M, Austen WG Jr, Liao EC. Avoiding breast animation deformity with pectoralis-sparing subcutaneous direct-to-implant breast reconstruction. *Plast Reconstr Surg Glob Open.* 2016; 4(5):e708.
22. Squitieri, L, Chung, KC. Measuring provider performance for physicians participating in the merit-based incentive payment system. *Plast Reconstr Surg.* 2017; 140(1):217e-226e.
23. Glasberg, SB, Light, D. AlloDerm and strattice in breast reconstruction: a comparison and techniques for optimizing outcomes. *Plast Reconstr Surg.* 2012; 129(6):1223-1233.
24. Basu CB, Leong M, Hicks MJ. Acellular cadaveric dermis decreases the inflammatory response in capsule formation in reconstructive breast surgery. *Plast Reconstr Surg.* 2010; 126(6):1842-1847.
25. Salzberg CA. Nonexpansive immediate breast reconstruction using human acellular tissue matrix graft (AlloDerm). *Ann Plast Surg.* 2006;57:1-5.

INDEX

Note: Page numbers followed by "*f*" and "*t*" denote figures and tables respectively.